T0374698

How the Clinic Made Gender

How the Clinic
Made Gender

The Medical History of a
Transformative Idea

SANDRA EDER

The University of Chicago Press   Chicago and London

The University of Chicago Press, Chicago 60637
The University of Chicago Press, Ltd., London
© 2022 by The University of Chicago
All rights reserved. No part of this book may be used or reproduced
in any manner whatsoever without written permission, except in
the case of brief quotations in critical articles and reviews. For more
information, contact the University of Chicago Press, 1427 E. 60th St.,
Chicago, IL 60637.
Published 2022
Printed in the United States of America

31 30 29 28 27 26 25 24 23 22   1 2 3 4 5

ISBN-13: 978-0-226-57332-8 (cloth)
ISBN-13: 978-0-226-81993-8 (paper)
ISBN-13: 978-0-226-57346-5 (e-book)
DOI: https://doi.org/10.7208/chicago/9780226573465.001.0001

Library of Congress Cataloging-in-Publication Data

Names: Eder, Sandra, author.
Title: How the clinic made gender : the medical history of a transformative idea / Sandra Eder.
Description: Chicago : University of Chicago Press, 2022. |
    Includes bibliographical references and index.
Identifiers: LCCN 2021047903 | ISBN 9780226573328 (cloth) |
    ISBN 9780226819938 (paperback) | ISBN 9780226573465 (ebook)
Subjects: LCSH: Gender identity—United States. | Intersex people—United States. |
    Medicine—United States—History.
Classification: LCC HQ1075.5.U5 E33 2022 | DDC 305.30973—dc23
LC record available at https://lccn.loc.gov/2021047903

Contents

Introduction   1

1   Sex before Gender: From Determining
True Sex to Finding the Better Sex 18

Robert: Hope 45

2   Happy and Well Adjusted: The Psychologization
of Sex in the 1930s and 1940s 53

Karen: Coming of Age 76

3   Culture, Gender, and Personality 84

4   Making Boys and Girls: Gender at Johns Hopkins 110

5   Gender in the Clinic: The Process of Normalization 141

6   The Circulations of Gender, Cortisone,
and Intersex Case Management 166

Janet: Despair 187

7   The Life of Gender: Reformulations and Adaptations 195

Epilogue 225

Acknowledgments 231
List of Abbreviations 235
Notes 237
Bibliography 291
Index 317

Introduction

Charles was born in 1955. He was a sickly infant, a poor eater, and prone to vomiting, but by the age of fifteen months his health had improved. His doctor described him as a "very happy and healthy boy."[1] When he was two years old, his parents became increasingly concerned that his penis appeared too large for his age and that he had started growing pubic hair. They first saw "a local physician," who tested the child's androgen production, measured his bone age, and did a buccal smear test to determine his sex chromosomes. Charles, it turned out, had a female XX pattern. He was, the physician told his parents, actually a girl.

At the time, doctors referred to Charles as a female pseudohermaphrodite.[2] He had ovaries, an XX sex chromosome pattern, and male-appearing genitals. As physicians eventually explained to his parents, he had a condition called congenital adrenal hyperplasia (CAH). An inborn hyperplasia of the adrenal glands, CAH results in a lack of cortisol and an overproduction of androgen. In Charles it had caused his genitals to "virilize" in utero and appear male after birth. The diagnosis also explained why Charles had failed to thrive in infancy, since CAH can cause metabolic problems such as salt loss. Today, medicine refers to individuals like Charles as having intersex traits or disorders of sex development (DSD).[3] These terms indicate variations from what we commonly understand as male and female anatomy. Often, the sexual anatomy of children with DSD is only slightly different from what many perceive as standard or average male or female bodies, but sometimes their anatomies result in confusion and debates about whether they should be considered male or female.[4] Although Charles's anatomy had always been perceived as male, after diagnosing him as a female pseudohermaphrodite, the local physician recommended that he undergo plastic repair on his genitals and be raised as a female.

Charles's parents objected to this plan, which came two years after they had been raising him as a son. Their doctor referred them to the Johns Hopkins Hospital in Baltimore to get further evaluations, and three months later, in the spring of 1958, Charles was admitted there. At Hopkins, Lawson Wilkins, whose Pediatric Endocrinology Clinic was located at the adjacent Harriet Lane Home for Invalid Children, was one of the nation's leading experts on CAH. In 1950, he had introduced cortisone as treatment for CAH, and starting in 1951 his team consisting of the psychologist John Money and the psychiatrists Joan Hampson and John Hampson had studied the psychological health of children with CAH and developed recommendations for medically managing cases of DSD. Money had introduced the term *gender role* in 1954 based on a three-year longevity study of patients with intersex at Wilkins's clinic. The team claimed that gender role was determined by the sex in which the child had been raised rather than by sex chromosomes or other biological sex characteristics.

Money evaluated Charles and interviewed his mother and grandmother, then rendered the opinion that the child's gender role was male, even though a repeat buccal smear test again revealed an XX chromosome.[5] Charles had been assigned as a boy at birth, and thus his acquired gender role was male. In his psychological report, Money pointed out that Charles's "entire family [was] strongly oriented in the direction of masculine gender for this patient." He recommended that Charles remain a boy despite his chromosomal female sex. Charles's parents agreed, and Hopkins doctors removed his ovaries and uterus and prescribed cortisone. Had doctors decided to change his sex to female, his penis would have been declared a clitoris, and physicians would have recommended drastic genital surgery: the amputation of what they perceived as an unacceptably large clitoris and the construction of a vulva and vagina.

The team at Hopkins recommended such operations in early infancy to make children's genitals look more convincingly male or female. Their study had shown, they maintained, that children's gender role matched the sex in which they were raised regardless of biological factors. Masculinity and femininity were learned in the course of growing up. In order for children to learn their gender role and convincingly become a boy or a girl, their body had to be adjusted to the sex they were raised in. These procedures, the Hopkins team insisted, were therefore essential in helping children develop the gender role consistent with their assigned sex at birth. This recommendation quickly became the standard approach in the treatment and management of children with intersex traits, normalizing the surgical "correction" of their genitals and reproductive organs.

Charles's parents may have readily accepted the notion that their child's upbringing meant more than his chromosomal sex, but the word *gender* was completely unfamiliar to them in this context. Before the 1950s, *gender* had been mostly synonymous with *sex* or had referred to linguistic distinctions in languages that have them. If anything, anthropologists and sociologists would have used *sex roles* to discuss culturally specific male and female behavior. But based on Money's coinage of *gender role*, the word *gender* slowly but steadily won popular currency, signifying the separation between biological sex and a culturally and environmentally shaped gender that would become the orthodoxy of feminist theory and women's liberation in 1970s and 1980s America.

Today, the term *gender* is ubiquitous. A simple online search produces over 1.1 million results, ranging from *gender spectrum, gender unicorn,* and *transgender* to *the gender inequality index* and *gender discrimination.* Google's Ngram Viewer reveals a steady climb in the usage of *gender* since the 1960s—with a sharp increase from the mid-1980s onward. By the 1980s, the terms *gender role* and *gender identity* had become part of the vocabulary of scholars in the social sciences and the humanities. The WHO defines *gender* as "the socially constructed characteristics of women and men— such as norms, roles and relationships of and between groups of women and men."[6] Most commonly, we now use *gender identity* to refer to personal gender identity and *gender norms* to address the social norms of masculinity and femininity, while *gender roles* refers to the roles or behavior learned by a person as "appropriate" to his or her gender. For historians, since the 1980s gender has been a "useful category," one that for some in its rejection of essentialism surpassed the narrower confines of women's history.[7]

How the Clinic Made Gender historicizes the emergence of the sex/gender binary. It tells the story of how "gender" was invented within US medicine and how it transformed over the span of two decades: from a pragmatic tool in the sex assignment of children with intersex traits in the 1950s, to an essential category in newly established gender identity clinics for "transsexual" patients in the 1960s, to a focal point of new feminist debates about the sex/gender binary in the 1970s. The book's primary focus is the Johns Hopkins Hospital and the adjacent Harriet Lane Home for Invalid Children, where a new theory about gender and protocols for the medical management of children with intersex traits were first developed in the early 1950s. Previous literature on this subject focuses predominantly on the psychologist John Money and his work, without acknowledging either the important role of existing practices within clinical settings where these conceptualizations took place or several decades of debates about the role of culture in shaping human behavior.[8] *How the Clinic Made Gender* expands this scope by focusing on the practices of sex assignment based on behavior and personality that had existed before Money's influence and by assessing the role of pediatric endocrinology, psychology, psychiatry, and the social sciences in the transformation of sex. At the Hopkins clinic, Money was one of several figures coming from different specialties who converged on an understanding of gender in the context of a particular clinical problem. Lawson Wilkins, a pediatrician who established at the Johns Hopkins Hospital the first Pediatric Endocrinology Clinic; the psychiatrists Joan Hampson and her husband, John; and the surgeons Howard W. Jones and William W. Scott were the most prominent members of a group of clinicians who were trying to assess how to determine the sex of children with intersex traits. They did so through consultations, discussions, and deliberations with colleagues who were addressing similar questions at other clinics.

This is not a tidy story about the introduction of a liberating concept which professed that experiences rather than biology shape much of what we identify as masculine and feminine behavior.[9] Nor does this book simply focus on the development of a medical regime that subjected infants with intersex traits to irreversible operations on their genitals.[10] Rather, *How the Clinic Made Gender* shows the intrinsic links between these two stories by examining the shifting landscapes of discussion about sex, gender, and sexuality. The process by which ideas about gender became medicalized, enforced, and popularized was messy, contradictory, and inconsistent. How the concept of gender came to be understood and applied through clinical practices of treating patients with intersex traits at the Johns Hopkins Hospital and beyond was fraught and contested. This book is above all a story about how gender was "made"— the intricate way in which ideas were put into practice and practices informed ideas.

Making Gender

Nonetheless, I contend that "gender role" emerged as a new way to think about a person's sex in mid-twentieth-century US clinical practice.

Many concurrent and enduring debates about the true nature of sex; the role of culture, experience, and learning in shaping human behavior and personality; and a normative definition of health coalesced at Hopkins's Pediatric Endocrinology Clinic in the 1950s. To talk about the nature of sex was not a new discussion. The clinical formulation of a learned gender role emerged at the tail end of three decades in which social scientists and psychologists debated and accepted the idea that culture rather than biology shaped human behavior. Psychiatric and psychologic evaluation in the assessment of a person's sex further normalized the idea that a person's masculinity or femininity might not be purely biological. Many physicians, faced with contradictions between sex determiners and behavior in patients with intersex traits, had been operating with some kind of construct of "gender role" in their clinical practice well before the introduction of the term, although in theory they believed that biology determined sex. These convergent ideas were then utilized to solve a particular clinical problem of what sex to assign to children with intersex traits.

This is an uneasy origin story. The shift from sex to gender was not a paradigm shift or radical break but a gradual and uneven change that consolidated several currents in the social sciences, psychology, and psychiatry with medical practice and social norms and practices. This transition occurred slowly and did not have the same impact in all places. Indeed, this inconsistent history is with us to this day in recurring highly contested debates about the true nature of gender and sex. Whereas previous scientific and public discussions conflated the categories of sex, gender, and sexuality, Money's and the Hampsons' particular formulation of gender role aimed to disentangle these categories. Their work at the Johns Hopkins Hospital thus became one important station in the long emergence of gender and a hub where clinicians and psychologists applied diverging and at times contradictory approaches to promote a formulation of our modern sex/gender binary. This pragmatic concept, devised to solve a specific clinical problem, does not easily map onto our many modern concepts of gender. Clinical practices and clinical needs shaped the formulation of gender role at Johns Hopkins. There gender was never entirely social but part of a feedback loop between the biological and the social. Yet this work remains critical to a genealogy of the sex/gender binary from which many subsequent discussions of gender are drawn.

Gender was (and is) a dynamic category. Depending on the particular problem it was utilized to solve, it delineated various relationships between nature and nurture, biology and culture. As the concept of gender proliferated in the decades after it was first formulated, its meaning changed as it was absorbed into and adapted to different fields. For example, in the 1950s Money and his associates the Hampsons relied on social norms of masculinity and femininity to evaluate a person's gender role. The biological binary of sex might have fallen, but a social binary of sex was still important to maintain. Feminists, women's rights activists, and female academics have debated and contested the true nature of sex differences since the nineteenth century and argued, in the words of the French feminist Simone de Beauvoir, that "one is not born, but rather becomes a woman."[11] In the 1970s, some feminists took the Hopkins findings to argue that if gender roles were learned, then they could also be unlearned or reconfigured. Women and girls could be boisterous, independent, play with cars, fall in love with other women and girls and still be female. All these behaviors would have been deemed masculine in the Hopkins model and considered a failure of proper gender role adjustment.

Gender was also a particularly American reformulation of sex. For one, it emerged in a certain post–World War II moment when the debates around cultural relativism shifted from a discourse about how all cultures were equally valid to debates about how one could ensure and socially engineer the development of a particular kind of American personality. In its abandonment of biological determinism, the 1950s formulation of gender role was an endorsement of social engineering that demanded individual adjustment to a mainstream status quo of prescribed and binary sex roles and behavior. In the 1950s, discussions about socially engineering US citizens lay at the heart of the nation's Cold War concerns with social roles and emotions.[12] Scientists, politicians, and the public grew increasingly anxious about the proper upbringing of children within the nuclear family, especially by a loving mother who enforced appropriate gender roles.[13] The mother/child dyad, then, became the focus of calls for the proper rearing of emotionally well-adjusted children—always within the conviction that children's environment and upbringing shaped their personality. Yet ironically, these debates coexisted with seemingly contradictory theories that privileged hormones or instinct as primary factors in human behavior.[14]

Cold War social and environmental determinism proved just as restricting as biological determinism. The idea of social malleability led to the strong belief that Americans must perpetuate firm and binary gender roles and that social engineering could help establish normativity and implement required social values in a new American generation. In intersex case management, treatment recommendations often relied on a vague prognosis of future happiness. The American gender concept was specific in its emphasis on social roles and functionality and its insistence that the ultimate goal was to produce happy and well-adjusted citizens. Clinician-researchers, psychiatrists, psychologists, and parents alike emphasized the pursuit of happiness, a right as American as apple pie. Medicine had the tools to fit intersex children into this paradigm, be it the prescription of hormones, surgery to "fix" ambiguous genitals, psychological analysis, or the decision about what sex would be better for each child. At the center of these medical interventions lay a concept of health that did not halt at restoring biological normativity; it encompassed a notion of functionality and happiness that was historically specific to American Cold War culture.

Sexuality and sexual norms also changed tremendously in the twentieth century as American society slowly embraced a new understanding of sexuality as a deeply personal expression of individual freedom and personhood.[15] By the 1950s, the American public was widely discussing sex and sexuality in forums such as print media and television, university campuses, and newsletters and discussion groups of a newly emerged homophile movement.[16] The biologist Alfred C. Kinsey in his massive sex surveys, which both garnered praise and scandalized the American public, introduced a new quantitative approach to sexuality by documenting the erotic practices of American men (1948) and women (1953), which became known as the Kinsey Reports.[17] His data, gleaned from seventeen thousand face-to-face interviews with ordinary citizens, showed that many of these practices surpassed the narrow prescription of heterosexual intercourse in wedlock. Homosexual behavior, masturbation, petting, and premarital sex were fairly common and therefore, according to Kinsey's new quantitative understanding of sexuality, also normal sexual behavior. Based on these insights, he devised a heterosexual–homosexual rating scale that conceptualized sexuality as a spectrum rather than a binary. For the scale, Kinsey counted sexual acts to determine whether a person's sexuality was predominantly heterosexual, homosexual, or somewhere in between the 0–6 scale. Most important, this was a dynamic concept, since sexual practices could shift and change over a lifetime of experiences.[18]

At the same time, the widely publicized sex change of Christine Jorgensen from male to female in 1952 gripped the American public and alerted it to the plasticity and malleability of the human body and mind.[19] To be sure, these changes did not come out of nowhere. The question of sex had been on the minds of many scientists and physicians in the first half of the century, even though the historically specific categories of sex, gender, and sexuality were very much entangled in these debates.[20] In early twentieth-century Europe, the British sexologist Havelock Ellis had conceptualized homosexuality as sexual inversion, a form of cross-gender identification.[21] The German physician Magnus Hirschfeld had postulated a theory of sexual intermediaries, naturally occurring sexual variations such as hermaphroditism, homosexuality, and transvestitism. In the 1920s and 1930s, scientists had utilized the idea of so-called sex hormones to remap the human body, hoping the new wondrous substances would cure many ills, reverse aging, and cure sexual deviance. The emergence of a theory of universal hormonal bisexuality based on the detection of male and female sex hormones in both men and women postulated that sex was a matter of quantity rather than quality and could be easily altered through hormones.[22] US biological and social scientists also embraced this new universal biological bisexuality, which was paralleled by social and psychological understandings of masculinity and femininity as existing on a spectrum. Yet as we have seen, by the 1950s ideas of biological plasticity and social engineering had been paralleled by anxieties about proper roles, behavior, and personality.

Race plays a central role in the history of the sex/gender binary despite the relative absence of patients of color.[23] Most historians who analyzed the few published case studies of Black patients with intersex traits suggest that, in line with the history of racism in medicine, doctors rarely involved these patients or their family in treatment decisions and often cast them as problematic patients—unruly, unreliable, and sexually deviant.[24] At Hopkins, physicians and surgeons published the three major works on diagnosis, treatment, and surgical intervention in intersex cases between 1937 and 1958; each text references more than a hundred patients, only six of whom were Black.[25] Yet African Americans accounted for between 9.6 and 10.5% of the US population between the 1930s and the 1960s.[26] While this undercount could easily reflect bias on the part of the doctors, or omission of the race of patients either by these authors or by those of the published cases they cite, the more general absence of patients of color in the archive is puzzling. The low numbers of cases stand in stark contrast to a documented depiction of Black bodies in medical textbooks and publications that generally is disproportionally higher. Though intersex is a rare condition and the most inclusive estimation proposes that about 1.7% of all births have intersex traits, Hopkins was a center of research where physicians would encounter a disproportionally greater number of patients.[27] It was also, until desegregation, the only white hospital in Baltimore treating Black patients.[28] In 1900, around 20 percent of patients treated at Hopkins were listed as "colored"; by 1923 the number had risen to 24 percent.[29] The Harriet Lane Home for Invalid Children, which housed Lawson Wilkins's Pediatric Endocrinology Clinic, was integrated as early as 1928. Structural differences in health practices and access, mistrust of white medical authority, varying conceptions of what constituted a medical problem and appropriate solution, and different referral practices are among the reasons why we are left with an absence of accounts of how Black patients and other patients of color understood and experienced DSD.[30] As the historian Saidiya Hartman reminds us, "Every historian of the multitude, the dispossessed, the subaltern, and the enslaved is forced to grapple with the power and authority of the archive and the limits it sets on what can be known, whose perspective matters, and who is endowed with the gravity and authority of historical actor."[31] Might the absence in the medical archives suggest a history of intersex to be told outside the realms of medicalization and of people with intersex traits who do not become patients, a history which may be reconstructed by creating alternative archives that give a voice to these individuals?

Yet race matters no less for the production of whiteness. Significantly, our conception of the sex/gender binary is profoundly a story of white agency and personhood. At Hopkins, white and predominantly male doctors used norms to determine a patient's correct gender role that were based on their own culturally specific understandings of white masculinity and femininity.[32] The sociologist Zine Magubane, in her analysis of the "intersection of race and nation in the production and reproduction of intersex bodies," similarly argues that "from the sixteenth to nineteenth centuries the archetypal intersex person—whose case history, childhood, type of life, and morphology were featured in medical texts after undergoing examination and forcible sex reassignment—was a white adult."[33] Hermaphroditism and the doubting of sex had profound consequences for a person's economic, social, and political status. The right to vote or run for office, to inherit or own property, to pursue an education, career, or profession, to marry and divorce, were largely organized according to a person's sex. Until the late nineteenth century, only a white male person could inhabit the subject position at stake in the doubting of somebody's sex in the United States. By the 1950s, the medical focus had shifted from adults to infants and children, but the representative intersex patient who was subjected to the Hopkins model of intersex case management and gender role management was still quintessentially white. "The masculine and feminine states of being" to which John Money's concept of gender referred, Magubane argues, "were already and inherently coded as white and in opposition to blackness."[34]

At the Hopkins clinics and its peer institutions, the understanding of gender role and the correct assignment of sex was inseparable from white heteronormativity in Cold War America. The whiteness of sex/gender, a binary fashioned through medical encounters with intersex bodies, subsequently underwrote US feminist practices and theories and has proved insufficient for the experiences of Black women and women of color.[35]

A Medical History

In recent decades, historians of gender have explored the cultural intertwinement of medicine, sex, and sexuality in the history of intersex and transgender, and they have revealed the medical profession's role in defining and determining sex. Their work has exposed how social norms such as heterosexuality and marriage shaped medical decisions, how new medical technologies in endocrinology and plastic surgery enabled a particular deployment of gender as separated from sex, and how scientists and physicians have constructed the bodies of intersex individuals to fit a binary of male/female division that does not exist in nature.[36] The mid-twentieth century is considered a turning point in an already sexualized American society. Other scholars have focused on the impact, logics, and ethics of current intersex case management as well as patient resistance to the normalizing procedures inflicted on infants and children without their consent. They have critically evaluated both the heteronormativity that underwrites the insistence that a person be consistently sexed and gendered and the violence gender nonbinary individuals experience at the hands of medicine, psychology, and society.[37]

Not surprisingly, the emergence of gender in opposition to biological sex in midcentury medical discourse (and thus John Money) is central to the historiography of how sex was transformed in the twentieth-century United States, even though the differentiation of the sex of the mind, the sex of the body, and sex roles along with the myriad combinations of these factors in producing sex had been debated, weighed, and studied earlier. The historian Joanne Meyerowitz's groundbreaking social history of "transsexuality" in the United States, which chronicles the history of the medical ideas and transgender activism, ascribes central meaning to the emergence of Money's concept of gender in midcentury medical discourse.[38] While Money is an important figure in this book, his formulation of gender is discussed within a longer history of clinical practices pertaining to intersex and of theories in the social sciences that privileged learned behavior; the inconsistencies and tensions surrounding the emergence of gender are placed front and center. Similarly, in the scholarship on intersex medicine at times appears as a homogenously oppressive institution—a view that distorts the complex and at times inconsistent ways in which medicine was practiced. Furthermore, although heteronormativity is certainly one of the reasons doctors (and parents) insisted on clear-cut and binary sex divisions, it is the matrix within which these practices are embedded and through which doctors, patients, and their families made sense of the world, not the primary cause of those practices.

How the Clinic Made Gender is a medical history of gender. Historians of medicine have long stressed that "disease" is more than a "a biological event." It is, to quote the medical historian Charles Rosenberg, also "a generation-specific repertoire of verbal constructs reflecting medicine's intellectual and institutional history, an aspect of and potential legitimation for public policy, a potentially defining element of social role, a sanction for cultural norms, and a structuring element in doctor/patient interactions." "In some ways," he writes, "disease does not exist until we have agreed that it does—by perceiving, naming, and responding to it."[39] In that sense, we frame medical conditions and anatomical variations in the social and cultural context in which we historically experience them. In the study of sex differences, scientists do not discover the truth in nature; rather, as the feminist biologist Anne Fausto-Sterling points out, "scientists in analyzing male/female differences peer through the prism of everyday culture. More often than not their hidden agendas that are articulated bear strong resemblances to broader social agendas."[40] Scholars who have engaged with the history of how doctors have viewed individuals with intersex traits over time have stressed how medical practitioners made intersex into a medical problem. This engagement gathered steam in the 1990s, inspired by the emerging patients' rights movement and intersex activism. Scholarship since then has focused on the modern history of the medical engagement with intersex individuals and the ethical problems arising from current standards of intersex case management.

Historicizing medical practices and technologies that have fallen into disrepute allows us to explore the multiple factors that made sense of specific treatment protocols at a particular moment. It is tempting to assume that the acceptance of medical innovation is evidence of a given treatment's efficacy: procedures work and enter the medical record—or they don't work and fall into disuse. However, as the historian Jack Pressman emphasizes in his history of lobotomy, the question, Did it work?

distorts our historical vision.[41] The question of how medicine functions cannot be answered outside the prevailing culture within which the patient and the doctors are situated. As he writes, "Clinical assessment is a contingent historical product," and investigating contested treatments of the past shines a light on why one particular treatment appeared worthwhile to physicians at a specific time and place.[42] Medicine is a social practice that plays out within a complex web of ideas, practices, technologies, relationships, materiality, experiences, and emotions.

The contribution of *How the Clinic Made Gender* is to show how convergent and multidisciplinary ideas about masculinity and femininity coalesced in the practices of those working in the Pediatric Endocrinology Clinic at Hopkins. Focusing on this clinic allows us to explore how medical practices had developed before they were theorized, reconstructing the material conditions under which physicians approached the body and engaged with their patients.[43] In order to do so, I utilize unique and previously unavailable as well as overlooked primary sources, including a selection of patient records that allow an intimate glimpse into the clinical practices by which sex was transformed in addition to verbatim transcripts of discussion among the medical practitioners featured in this history. The patient records reveal the clinician-researchers' actual methods for determining a patient's sex, their observations, their techniques, and the concepts of health and medical logics they relied on. These practices often differ from medical accounts polished for publication. The records thus reveal how knowledge about particular bodies was produced amid the messiness of daily life in the clinic and how physicians' convictions of what constituted health and sex often differed from the beliefs of their patients and their patients' parents.

While other studies have focused on published medical cases or retrospective interviews with intersex patients, I use patient records from the Johns Hopkins University clinic to reconstruct clinical encounters at the time when gender was first being formulated. Focusing on these patient records has allowed me to write about patients and their experiences as much as the medical logics that led to the conceptualization of gender and the development of standardized intersex case management protocols. The patient records I use here are highly formalized yet strikingly intimate sources, providing patient histories, graphs, blood counts, and chemistry lab and X-ray reports as well as photographs of the child and letters from parents and social workers. They comprise a diary of the daily practices in the medical encounters among physicians, patients, and their families. Patient records allow us to explore the strategic relationships between patient and physician as well as "the relationship between the medical practices and medical ideas, between ideology and behavior."[44] They provide a rare glimpse into how this clinic ran each day, illustrating the specific medical logic that structured clinical encounters between doctors, parents, and patients. A careful reading of the clinical records shows how clinical practice structured enactments of sex and gender, and of health and disease. I have tried to avoid a narrative of perpetrators and victims and to avoid juxtaposing a medically defined objective sex to a subjective inner truth of sex.[45] My close reading of the patient records allows me to show normalization as a process in which treating somatic effects and assuring psychological health were deeply enmeshed in the conviction that only a clearly gendered and sexed person could have a "normal" and happy life.

I use patient records from the Pediatric Endocrinology Clinic to get to the nitty-gritty, disclosing the often messy ways in which doctors actually diagnosed sex, assessed gender, attributed treatment, evaluated health and medical success—in short, how gender was made and embodied in practices that were then written up, formalized, and published. Through these cases I explore how sex is enacted through clinical practices rather than simply conceived scientifically.[46] The materiality of the clinic and the medical technologies that shape the diagnosis and maintenance of sex and gender there emerge in these accounts. For example, while published case studies often simply state the diagnosis of sex and the method by which physicians achieved this diagnosis, patient records reveal how contentious and time-consuming the diagnosis of sex was in some of these cases. Charles's case was typical in that the Barr body test to determine sex chromosomes, which the Hopkins clinic began using as early as 1952, did not particularly simplify the diagnosis of his sex.

Patient records have their limitations, and these limitations shape the stories that can be gleaned from them. One problem is accessing the patients' perspectives through these highly mediated sources. Patient records privilege the physician's voice and, in pediatric records, to a certain extent the parents' narrative.[47] Scholars have long debated how the patient's perspective, once central to the practice of medicine, disappeared in modern biomedicine.[48] In the twentieth century, with the rise of the modern hospital and the dominance of the clinic in medical care, a new form of record taking took hold. Previously, doctors noted patients' information in individual casebooks. Often, each laboratory and clinic also kept their own leather-bound ledgers, noting several different patient histories on one page.[49] In the first third of the twentieth century, patient records expanded: hospitals began keeping a dedicated folder for each patient that remained at their facility. Increasingly, technical data and test results were collected in an unbound format that theoretically could extend indefinitely. This folder would be accessible to all medical and bureaucratic personnel. New medical specialties, a focus on technology and tests, separate billing procedures, and bureaucratic routines that came into being with the modern hospital amplified this shift from storing information by the treating doctor to storing it by the patient.[50] The change facilitated scientific research, as it provided standardized information both easily accessible and easily comparable. The records' standardized format and focus on tests and examination often negate or reinterpret the patients' perspective on health, disease, and their clinical encounters.

The life stories that I find in the patient records resist chronology; some stretch over many decades, and many patients had long breaks in between visits. Thus, these narratives interact with different aspects of the history that I reconstruct in this book. Yet the records contain glimpses of patients that allow access, however limited, to how they might have experienced their lives inside and outside the clinic. This book includes three stories that reconstruct the patients' lives and experiences. They are separated from the main part of the book, inserted between the chapters to provide a counterpoint or complicate the previous chapter, and they focus on the lives of children who grew up under the gaze of modern biomedicine. These stories concern how hope is medical currency, what it means to live a life mediated by medicine, how patients' relationships with the clinic changed over time, and how patients' illness experiences differed from medical disease categories. These stories reveal the disjunctions between what patients say and what is noted as fact in the record, and they raise the question of who can speak with authority about their conditions, their lives, and their gender.

Book Outline

By constructing a series of chronologically overlapping episodes, in *How the Clinic Made Gender* I historicize and situate the formulation of the sex/gender binary in the clinic and chart the genealogy of gender from the 1940s to the 1970s. Chapter 1, "Sex before Gender," examines the practices of sex assignment before and at the brink of the formulation of the concept of gender at Hopkins's Pediatric Endocrinology Clinic. In the 1940s, Lawson Wilkins was already making decisions on whether his patients with congenital adrenal hyperplasia (CAH) should be assigned as boys or girls based on a socially rather than a biologically determined idea of sex. His focus had shifted from determining a person's true sex to the practice of finding the "better" sex—the sex that patients could live in and whose role they could fulfill. Presuming that it might be difficult for male-appearing women with CAH to marry, he recommended assigning them as male under the "reasonable" assumption at the time that it would make it easier for them to support themselves. Wilkins operated within a notion of health that encompassed social aspects; his main treatment goal was to restore both biological and social functioning.

Chapter 2, "Happy and Well Adjusted," contextualizes Wilkins's clinical approach by investigating the psychologization of American society and the popular acceptance of the paradigm of adjustment and maladjustment that by the 1950s had long since become part of the medical evaluation of sex. Medical practitioners agreed on the importance of a new group of experts, psychiatrists and clinical psychologists. They acknowledged that psychological sex could differ from anatomical sex and shared the assumption that environment, social situation, upbringing, and cultural patterns could determine a person's psychological sex. They insisted on the malleability of the human body and its secondary sex characteristics, which could be adapted to the psychological sex. Chapter 3, "Culture, Gender, and Personality," shifts the focus to the social sciences and that discipline's ideas about the culture and environment shaping human behavior and personality. I use the eccentric yet familiar figure of John Money to show how these ideas were incorporated into clinical practices. Money's intellectual biography, accessible through his diary and vast correspondence, allows an exploration of a particular branch of behavioral sciences in the 1940s and 1950s, one in which social scientists had largely accepted the idea that culture and not biology shaped human behavior and explored how children developed their personalities in specific environments. The aspiring psychologist integrated this idea, the postwar focus on social engineering, and the contemporaneous belief in scientific authority into the way he conducted his first case studies for his doctoral research.

Chapter 4, "Making Boys and Girls," surveys the concept of a learned gender role formulated at Lawson Wilkins's clinic between 1951 and 1956 by focusing on shared practices and on debates among health experts, psychologists, psychiatrists, and sex researchers. Wilkins hired the team of Joan Hampson (later joined by her husband, John) and John Money to study the psychological health of his CAH patients, and by 1954 they had discussed their findings with clinicians who consulted with the Hopkins team at medical and scientific conferences and to solve individual cases. The chapter analyzes how Money and the Hampsons produced their recommendation about intersex case management, developed the concept of gender, and tested their concepts and recommendation in discussions with clinicians, endocrinologists, and sex researchers.

Chapter 5, "Gender in the Clinic," explores how "gender role" was folded into medical practices pertaining to the diagnosis, treatment, and management of CAH. Based on patient records from the clinic, it reveals the process of normalization in which social and biological norms were conflated to achieve health—that is, to enable patients to function in the world. This process consisted of three parts. Diagnosis included the determination of sex to design a gendered treatment approach specific to the desired social outcome. Treatment involved urgent intervention to prevent death through salt loss in children with CAH as much as chronic and sustained interventions specific to the assigned sex of the child. As social norms were integrated into the medical norms of health, correct "gender role" became part of the treatment process. Maintenance—the long-term care for a chronic condition such as CAH—included all aspects of the patient's life in the prescribed goal of "adjustment" and health. Gender role became one aspect of successful treatment and management.

Finally, chapters 6 and 7 address the afterlife of gender as a new concept of sex and as an essential component of intersex case management. Chapter 6, "The Circulations of Gender, Cortisone, and Intersex Case Management," shows how the new concept of gender traveled beyond the boundaries of the Hopkins clinic, how it was circulated in the United States and internationally, and how it was adapted to different locales and disciplines. This chapter follows "gender" and the Hopkins recommendations as they left the clinic, and it traces their translation into a clinical setting in Zurich, Switzerland, in the early 1950s. By the 1960s, major American medical and surgical textbooks had integrated and adapted the Hopkins recommendations. Chapter 7, "The Life of Gender," explores how the notion of psychological sex and the idea of a learned gender role were reformulated as gender identity in the field of psychology. It was this reformulated notion of gender that returned to Hopkins when Money opened the Hopkins Gender Identity Clinic in 1965—the first "sex-change" clinic at a US research hospital.

In the 1970s, feminists and queer communities adopted the term *gender* and used it in an uneven and unrestrained manner. Some feminists engaged critically with the medical and psychological literature from which gender emerged; others used these concepts side by side with earlier studies from the social sciences as evidence that masculinity and femininity were learned; and many activists and queer communities used gender indiscriminately to replace sex or to describe new practices such as gender-fuck (sending mixed messages about one's gender). In all these transitions, gender was a dynamic concept informed by social and cultural changes in the United States. Our current idea of gender might not map exactly onto these earlier formulations, but we still live with the legacy of this genealogy. There is no doubt that something new, transformative, and enduring about the concept of gender had developed through clinical practices at a pediatric endocrinology clinic in the mid-twentieth century. The history of gender laid out in this book shows that these ideas held no single, unified meaning within the clinic or outside it, and "gender" was shaped by the practices and needs of those who utilized and adapted it.

ONE

Sex before Gender: From Determining True Sex to Finding the Better Sex

Mary was born in December 1948. When she was only a few weeks old, she was referred to Johns Hopkins's Harriet Lane Home for Invalid Children (HLH) because of a genital anomaly and an inability to retain salt.[1] She failed to thrive on the formula she was fed. As chances of survival seemed slim, Dr. Lawson Wilkins, the treating pediatrician, decided to risk an adrenalectomy, the surgical removal of the adrenal glands, in the spring of 1949. After the adrenalectomy, at least "the danger of progressive virilization would be eliminated." One month after the operation to remove her second adrenal gland, the baby developed a high fever and died despite all efforts to save her life. In a letter to the referring physicians, Wilkins wrote, "We realize fully that the bilateral adrenalectomy in her case was a heroic measure, especially in view of the fact that the adrenal hormones for substitution therapy are not yet available in adequate amounts." The parents, however, were "far from resigned to the outcome."

Shirley was born the same year that Mary died, but unlike Mary, she did not come to the HLH until she was five years old.[2] Her mother had taken her to the local hospital when she was four because she "was worried about the hair in her pubic region." The mother was told that Mary's bone age was advanced, and Wilkins was called in for a consultation. A year later, in 1954, the five-year-old, of "feminine appearance," was admitted to the HLH. She was put on cortisone and became part of a study to set up the regulation of the hormone treatment. Before her discharge, Shirley was taken to see the psychologist John Money in his office, and she left Hopkins with regular returns already scheduled with her parents.

Mary and Shirley came to Hopkins because it housed Lawson Wilkins's Pediatric Endocrinology Clinic, the nation's first medical center devoted to hormonal problems in children. Moreover, the clinic had a special emphasis in congenital adrenal hyperplasia, or CAH; it saw more cases of this disease than any other clinic in the world. Both children were diagnosed as having CAH, an adrenal disorder that affects the body's metabolism and its ability to retain salt, as well as growth, sexual development, and general appearance. It affects the whole body, though its sexual effects, such as "virilization" and precocity, are most noticeable. Girls with CAH often looked "male" and were sometimes raised as boys. Boys with CAH showed symptoms of precocity such as advanced growth and early sexual development.[3]

The diagnosis and treatment of CAH changed in many ways during the short interval between the cases of Mary and Shirley. In 1949 at the Pediatric Endocrinology Clinic, with only limited substitution therapy available, the clinic's director, Lawson Wilkins (fig 1.), used a surgical approach to Mary's case that had been developed at Johns Hopkins by the renowned genitourinary surgeon Hugh Hampton Young;[4] by 1953, Wilkins had developed a profoundly different, nonsurgical approach that he used in Shirley's case. Wilkins was a pediatrician-turned-innovator in biomedicine: in 1950, he introduced a novel therapy centered on the steroid hormone cortisone as a treatment for CAH. Any doctor in the country who saw a young patient with these symptoms knew, with a phone call or two, to send the child to Hopkins. Mary's and Shirley's experiences, like those of the other CAH patients at the Pediatric Endocrinology Clinic, were profoundly shaped by the sweeping changes in both American culture and biomedicine taking place in the early post–World War II period. Moreover, their experiences were shaped by the presence of Wilkins and by the local peculiarities of the clinic, the Harriet Lane Home, and the Johns Hopkins Hospital.

Wilkins, the "father of pediatric endocrinology,"[5] sought to anchor the new field in science, add blood chemistry measurements to the pediatric routine, accurately diagnose endocrine disease and pathologies in children, and train a new generation of fellows to become experts in the field. For more than a decade, he studied CAH and framed it as an often life-threatening adrenal pathology. Yet in the course of treating an

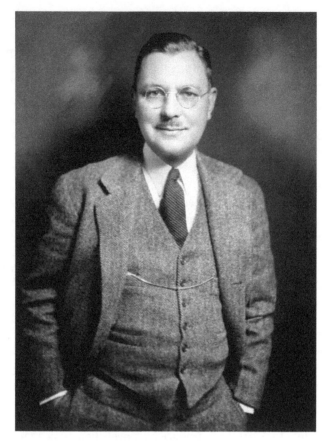

Figure 1   Lawson Wilkins, 1940

increasing number of infants and children with CAH in his clinic, he found himself confronted with questions concerning their lives outside the clinic. For one thing, how should girls with CAH live? They were chromosomally female and had internal reproductive organs such as ovaries and uteruses, but they had been born with male-appearing genitals and looked increasingly male as they grew up.

These concerns forced Wilkins to reconsider the meaning of sex through his clinical practice. This chapter shows how shifting meanings of health, worried parents, lacking or limited therapeutics, surgical techniques, disease-centered clinical practices, medical research on adrenal health and sex determination, and a wide range of symptoms—some of them related to sex and many not—shaped his construct of gender before the sex/gender binary was formulated in the Pediatric Endocrinology Clinic. As he experimented with different treatment strategies, he devised a strategy for determining the sex assignment that would be better for a child by focusing on social functionality rather than biological certainty. This strategy of a workable gender, shaped by medical pragmatism and a concept of health that encompassed biological and social norms, would profoundly inform the formulation of the sex/gender binary.

A New Medicine

The HLH (figs. 2–3), built with private funds in 1909 on the Johns Hopkins Hospital site and staffed with Hopkins's medical and nursing personnel after its opening in 1912, was the first children's hospital in the United States associated with a medical school.[6] From 1927 onward, the HLH's third director, Edward Park, head of the Department of Pediatrics at Johns Hopkins School of Medicine and pediatrician-in-chief at the Johns Hopkins Hospital until 1946, supported and encouraged the establishment of specialty clinics at the HLH.[7] Park introduced a new collaborative style and a disease-centered organization of the hospital, with particular focus on epilepsy, cardiac disease, and behavior/psychiatry. These specialty clinics were linked to the laboratory and allowed the study of particular patient groups over longer periods of time. Together with meticulous record keeping, this new practice established a continuity of data with one goal in mind: to produce a better understanding of long-term effects as children grew up to become adult patients.

In 1935, Park asked Lawson Wilkins to establish a Pediatric Endocrinology Clinic at the HLH.[8] The forty-one-year-old pediatrician felt himself to be an odd candidate to lead the new facility. Born in 1894, the son of a Baltimore physician who "had pulled himself up by his own bootstraps from the mire of the Dismal Swamp of Virginia," Wilkins also pursued a medical career, graduating from Johns Hopkins Medical School in 1918.[9] He received his degree while serving as an orderly in the Johns Hopkins Hospital Unit in France during World War I.[10] During his internship in internal medicine at the Yale New Haven (Connecticut) Hospital in 1919, he decided to go into pediatrics. Afterward, he returned to Baltimore and the Johns Hopkins Hospital as a pediatric resident at the HLH, where he claimed to have learned of the advantage of organization in clinical care, the value of good record keeping, and the importance of appropriate follow-up.[11]

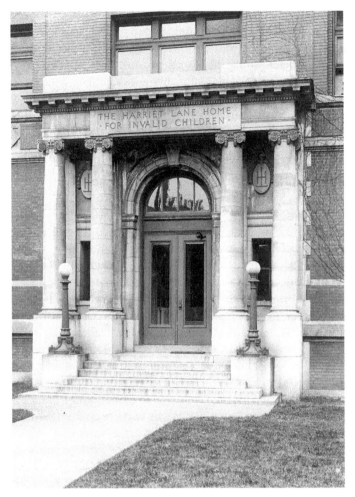

Figure 2 Exterior view of the entrance of the Harriet Lane Home, 1950–74

Wilkins's interest in scientifically grounded medicine was matched by his concern about patient care and his ambition to organize this care efficiently. As an intern at Hopkins, he initiated a clinic for congenital syphilis to improve the care of the children who came to the HLH by organizing medical and social care and follow-up. This effort eventually led to the first subspecialty clinic at Hopkins for children with congenital syphilis, which remained the only such clinic until Park became the director in the 1920s.[12] Faced with the decision between an academic career and private practice, Wilkins decided to follow in his father's footsteps and became a pediatrician in Baltimore for the next twenty-five years. In his private practice, he was described as empathetic and passionate with his patients while employing an organized approach to patient care. His practice, said to have been one of the largest in Baltimore, was described by Park as "eminently democratic," as it was open to and affordable by all social classes.[13] During this time, Wilkins continued visiting the hospital to get treatment advice and collaborate with clinicians there.[14]

Wilkins's emergence as America's first pediatric endocrinologist makes more sense contextualized within the history of medicine and the rise of scientific medicine, or biomedicine, in the United States in the early twentieth century. When Wilkins graduated from Johns Hopkins Medical School, it was at the forefront of scientific medicine, bringing a new European format to the practice of medicine in the United States. Hopkins was the first US research hospital to incorporate bedside teaching and laboratory research, combining a French pathological model of medicine with German lab sciences. The establishment of disease-centered specialty clinics was part of both the professionalization of medicine in this period and the attempt to build clinical knowledge from a systematized approach to medical practice. Specialization was seen as essential for the advancement of the medical sciences, and reformers

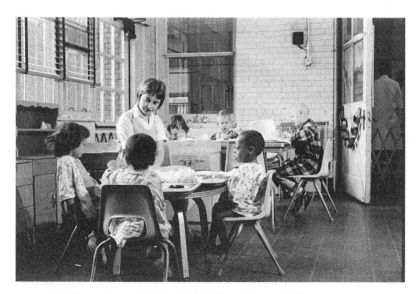

Figure 3   Children and nurse in the Harriet Lane Home playroom, 1959

argued optimistically that the observation of many cases of the same disease would produce new medical knowledge. Within a clinical setting, this new, systematically derived knowledge would in turn further the development of new understandings of disease and enable the systematic study of rare diseases.[15]

In pediatrics, endocrinology was still a new perspective in the 1930s. Since the nineteenth century, the study of glands and internal secretions, named hormones in 1905 by the British physiologist Ernest Starling, had been associated with sensational claims of bodily rejuvenation, exaggerated therapeutic hopes, and startling notions of the body's sexual malleability.[16] The 1920s and 1930s were the golden age of endocrinology, with many discoveries, including the purification of insulin in 1922 and the isolation and characterization of ovarian and testicular hormones between 1927 and 1934, which sparked a hormone fever that captured popular attention.[17] In the eyes of many medical researchers, however, the more sensationalized aspects of endocrinology tainted the clinical application of hormones.[18] Despite the impact that the introduction of insulin in the 1920s had on the lives of diabetic children, investigative pediatrics focused mostly on infectious disease, nutritional disorders, and disease prevention in the first half of the twentieth century. With the scientific advances in biochemical and metabolic clinical investigation between the two world wars, the role of hormones in children and adolescents became increasingly accessible to pediatricians.[19]

When Park invited Wilkins to establish the Pediatric Endocrinology Clinic, the subspecialty may not have existed yet, but it was clearly on the horizon as a new perspective in pediatrics. Within a few years, in 1942, the pediatrician Nathan B. Talbot established a second clinic, at Massachusetts General Hospital in Boston. During the 1950s and 1960s, both clinics and their fellowship and training programs produced the second generation of pediatric endocrinologists in the new field, along with national and international networks of collaborators.[20] Wilkins's consolidation of knowledge in the field's first textbook in 1950, followed by Talbot's in 1952, was essential in shaping the gradual birth of pediatric endocrinology as a new subspecialty, making Wilkins the unofficial "father" of the field.[21]

Sexing the Adrenal

First described anatomically in the sixteenth century by Eustachius, the adrenal, or suprarenal, glands sit atop the kidneys, as the name suggests.[22]

Physiological experimentation during the nineteenth century showed that the adrenal glands were vital for survival.[23] Physicians pursued physiological experimentation on animals to determine the glands' function in the healthy body, usually through the classic physiological ablation experiment in which the glands were removed, the effects of the removal on the animal were studied, and those effects were then countered by feeding chopped-up glands to the animal.[24] Research on the adrenals was part of a general development in medicine in which researchers started to imagine internal secretions as part of a complex bodily system.[25] Since the 1890s, physicians had suggested that these "internal secretions" were fundamentally important for understanding physiological processes. From the beginning, three sites were crucial for the development of the study of these secretions and the glands that produced them: the clinic, the pharmaceutical industry, and the laboratory. Although these sites were often in conflict, their relationship was close and structured by the role of research material—at first animal glands, then isolated and purified hormonal substances, and finally synthesized hormones.[26]

The adrenogenital syndrome, as CAH had been widely known before the 1940s, had long occupied the minds of physicians interested in understanding the physiology of the adrenal glands and the mechanism of sex. It could be caused by a prenatal adrenal hyperplasia (this form later came to be called congenital adrenal hyperplasia) or by a renal tumor that developed later in life. The first recorded case of "hermaphroditism" thought to be caused by the adrenogenital syndrome dates back to the mid-nineteenth century. In 1865, the Italian anatomist Luigi De Crecchio published a curious case of a strange "apparenze virili in una donna"—a manly appearance in a woman.[27] De Crecchio had been called to assist in the autopsy of an Italian man, Giuseppe Marzo, who had died at the age of forty. The autopsy revealed a uterus and fallopian tubes, a vagina opening into the urethra, a prostate, no palpable testicles, and a six-centimeter penis. Giuseppe's physiognomy was that of a male. De Crecchio also noticed that his adrenal glands were almost as large as the kidneys.

The first description of the adrenogenital syndrome (AGS) under that name was published in 1905, describing a sudden onset of precocity and hirsutism in a ten-year-old girl that were caused by an adrenal tumor.[28] By the early twentieth century, dozens of case studies had appeared in the medical literature, many focusing on the sudden virilization of female patients suffering from adrenal tumors. Authors agreed that their findings indicated a connection between the adrenal glands and a person's sex. But how could the adrenals cause sex anomalies? After all, there were already two other glands thought to govern sex.

Up until the late nineteenth century, sex gonads were understood to determine masculinity and femininity.[29] Anyone who possessed ovaries was thought to be a woman, no matter her appearance or character, and anyone with testes was a man. The chemical messengers that originated from gonads were soon named sex hormones, with male sex hormone being the secretion of the testes and female sex hormone being the ovarian secretion. By the 1910s, the idea of gonads as agents of sex difference had been transformed into a concept of sex hormones as chemical messengers of masculinity and femininity. Despite a shift from gonads to the secretions of gonads, scientific conceptualization of hormones as sexed substances remained unchanged. Sex hormones were seen as the missing link between genetic and physiological models of sex determination. In the early decades of the twentieth century, scientists argued that sex determination was regulated by genetic factors and sexual differentiation by hormonal factors.[30]

The biology of sex hormones mapped neatly onto long-standing and widespread ideas about social differences between the sexes.[31] The most prominent case in point is, without a doubt, the work of Eugen Steinach. In 1910, the Austrian physiologist had attributed the idea of sex antagonism to hormones. In his view, the organism was a system of competing forces: male and female gonads secreted opposite, antagonistic hormones. Biological sex shaped every cell and thought of a human being. He showed through transplantation experiments with guinea pigs that the male gland stimulated traits that were inhibited by the female gland and inhibited those stimulated by the female gland (and conversely).[32] Steinach's theories resonated with public claims that women's biological destiny was the opposite of men's and that their roles were entirely shaped and restricted by their biology.[33] Consequently, equal political rights and equal access to education were not only against nature; they were unhealthy to women and their offspring. Historians have shown how this turn to a biology of incommensurable differences was triggered by the emergence of feminism and the extension of white middle-class women's roles as well as their entry into public spheres.[34]

The relationships among science, medicine, and sociocultural conceptions are not straightforward, with one reinforcing the others. Rather, social causes and biology coexisted at times in uncomfortable bonds until overwhelming contradictions caused a paradigm shift. It is tempting to see the clinic and the lab as spaces in which social norms and ideologies were confirmed and consolidated; however, the history of hormone research shows more complex relations. The idea of sex antagonism, for example, had been called into question in biology before significant cultural changes took place. When endocrinologists found that both sexes produced both sex hormones—a fact illustrated dramatically by Bernhard Zondek's 1934 finding of large amounts of estrogen in the urine of a stallion—researchers adjusted to the idea that the balance of sex hormones "made" an individual male or female.[35] By the end of the 1930s, the body had become ambisexual for physiologists and biochemists, and the secretions of sex glands were no longer seen as rigidly sex specific.[36]

The dismantling of sex antagonism meant that the gonads lost their primacy as the main organs of sex determination. They were crucial to the production and maintenance of the sexual body, but they were part of a larger glandular system that produced and maintained the hormonal balance. In particular, it became clear that the anterior pituitary gland had a complex reciprocal relationship with the gonadal hormones. In 1932, Carl Moore and Dorothy Price introduced the notion of end-organ negative feedback, in which gonads lost their primary position and became simply players in an orchestra, with the pituitary gland acting as conductor.[37] This meant a break with dualistic concepts of male and female as mutually exclusive categories, and a turn toward hormonal bisexuality. Male and female sex hormones were defined as closely related chemical compounds—differing in just one hydroxyl group—in the larger family of steroids. This radical remapping, however, happened mostly in the lab; in the clinic—and in the public—sex antagonism largely lived on. Clinical use of sex hormones did not necessarily follow the reformulation of sexual physiology. The new theories of hormonal bisexuality did not revolutionize the clinic, where sex hormones continued to be used purely empirically or in light of the older sexually polarized models of gonadal function.

The conceptualization of the adrenal glands was shaped by debates about sex glands and hormones. Before the 1930s, some authors had perceived the adrenal glands as male in nature, with the power to virilize women and to neutralize the feminizing influences of the ovary. Researchers were puzzled that the precocious puberty triggered by AGS always had "the character of a male puberty" and was not sex specific.[38] Their reasoning was firmly rooted in the still prevailing idea of binary and antagonistic sex hormones. The ovary was hermaphroditic at an early stage, one physician argued, and its testicular parts were connected to the adrenal cortex.[39] These fetal testicular cells could in some cases also be included in the adrenal glands and would develop into virilizing tumors. Due to their testicular origin, and within the logic of sex antagonism, one might expect virilism to develop in these patients with adrenal growth. The relationship between the adrenal cortex and sexual development seemed to offer a genuine explanation of the clinical presentation of AGS. As sex antagonism gave way to universal bisexuality, the adrenal glands emerged as something like a third gonad. By the 1930s, the certainty that the adrenal glands were male in nature had begun to waver. Hyperplasia or tumors of the adrenal cortex had different effects, depending on sex and age of onset. The adrenal glands were now seen as ambisexual, able to bring out the normally suppressed characteristics of the opposite sex. In congruence with the idea of universal bisexuality, it was thought that all women were partly male and that adrenal tumors of hyperplasia allowed a woman's innate partial masculinity to emerge.[40]

Studying Hermaphroditism at the Johns Hopkins Hospital

The study of hermaphroditism was not new to the Johns Hopkins Hospital. In the 1930s, Hugh Hampton Young—the hospital's head of genitourinary surgery from 1898 onward, who oversaw the development of the James Buchanan Brady Urological Institute and served as its director from its founding in 1915 until his retirement in 1942—gained prominence with his studies of the adrenal glands and AGS. In 1937, he published the first American treatise on the surgical treatment of hermaphroditism, *Genital Abnormalities, Hermaphroditism, and Related Adrenal Diseases*.[41] As a surgeon, Young approached hermaphroditism with a focus on genitals and anatomical structures. For his monograph, he collected hundreds of case histories from his clinic and from the literature, accompanied by photographs of ambiguous organs and medical illustrations of his surgical techniques and innovations. His interest lay squarely in the relationship between genital development and adrenal hyperplasia, the adrenal's "amazing effect on the female organs, the defeminizing of women and the development of virilism," and the development of a surgical solution for these cases.[42] As a urological surgeon, Young did not consider biochemical therapy but instead proposed partial and total adrenalectomy—the latter the surgery Lawson Wilkins tried as a last resort on the infant Mary, as we saw at the beginning of this chapter—procedures that yielded little success and left physicians struggling to keep patients alive through adrenal substitutes.

Young's monograph and clinical practice highlight the problems that clinicians faced in cases of hermaphroditism. A patient's sex was "diagnosed" by the presence of a male or female gonad, but physicians took the hormonal, gonadal, anatomical, and psychosexual conditions into account when deciding the "true" sex of a patient, with the conviction that everyone should clearly belong to one sex or the other. Studies of Young's clinical work through his patient records and case notes show how it was shaped by two factors: one was his relationship with each individual patient and his observation of that person's character and wishes; the other was the maintenance of social norms such as marriage and heterosexuality, a consistent concern in cases of "ambiguous" sex.[43] In his writings, gonads might have been the ideal signifier of "true" sex, but clinical decisions were often based on additional factors. In this "era of idiosyncrasy," doctors made decisions of sex assignment case by case, based on their discipline and experience.[44] Young's approach to hermaphroditism was shaped by his conceptual notion of the sexed body and by his practice; he was, first and foremost, a surgeon. His decisions for treatment of so-called hermaphrodites were determined by the identification of the "true" sex of the patient and the practicalities of surgical treatment to implement this decision.

Young's diagnosis of "true" sex involved a complex set of calculations grounded in anatomy and physiology. Though he still understood the gonads as the central elements in determining sex (at least in theory), the unambiguous identification of hermaphrodites' gonads proved troublesome. Furthermore, the direction in which a patient would be surgically altered was often born out of a careful weighing of the signs and signals of body and of personality. This followed from the understanding that gonads had a double function, both parts of which had profound effects on apparent sex: as reproductive organs producing eggs or sperm, and as glands secreting hormones that shaped sexual anatomical characteristics and behavior.[45] In Young's view, treatment and sex correction decisions rested largely on "the perceived hormonal (rather than reproductive) interpretation of gonadal function" (63). Consequently, the surgeon's decision in the determination of the hermaphrodite's "true" sex was based on what was perceived as the behavioral manifestation of hormonal secretion. Young read from personality backward into the body. Psychological traits, appearance, behavior, and sexual desires were interpreted as outcomes of hormonal influences. Sexual characteristics of the body were interpreted as visible signs of hormonal influence. Most of all, the life a patient was leading, or seemed capable of leading, was taken as evidence of hormonal status. It was this that ultimately influenced treatment decisions and the direction that sex surgery would take (90–93). This approach was quite different from the treatment recommendation later developed in Wilkins's clinic.

Congenital Adrenal Hyperplasia

A year after Young published his treatise *Genital Abnormalities*, Wilkins encountered his first (tragic) case of congenital adrenal hyperplasia (CAH) in a young boy. On October 11, 1938, D. W., a boy of three years and seven months, was referred to the Pediatric Endocrinology Clinic at the Harriet Lane Home for Invalid Children. His parents had traveled to Baltimore from Florida hoping to find help for their child. D.'s development was delayed, and from an early age he had been very difficult to feed because of "a poor appetite, and peculiar likes and dislikes of certain kinds of food."[46] He was sexually precocious; he developed pubic hair when he was only five months old, and he grew rapidly in height and weight. Only "seven days after admission he suddenly died,"[47] and upon autopsy D. was diagnosed as having had CAH. In a tragic twist, the postmortem diagnosis revealed that the child's death might have been prevented. He had "self-medicated" to compensate for the life-threatening salt loss typical of the condition by eating salt in large quantities at home. "During the two and one-half years previous to his entrance to the hospital," Wilkins wrote, "he must have kept himself alive by eating large amounts of salt. In the hospital he was not given free access to salt but was given the regular ward diet, which contains the normal amount of salt and, as a result, died suddenly." D.'s parents were devastated and expressed the hope that they would help Wilkins in his studies "and perhaps some children in the future."[48]

After the fatal case of the little boy from Florida, Wilkins pursued systematic research on the condition, focusing on patients at his clinic, connecting with other experts on adrenal diseases, and experimenting with different substances in the hope of finding a cure. Though surgery continued to play a role in treatment strategy, Wilkins represents a shift toward endocrinology. By the time Young retired in 1942, patients with CAH had been coming to the Pediatric Endocrinology Clinic rather than Young's Urological Institute, a clear shift from an anatomical to a hormonal perspective. Patient records reveal that parents traveled with their children to Baltimore from other states, referred by colleagues who knew of Wilkins's expertise. Between 1936 and 1949, only 14 of the clinic's patients were listed under the category of CAH in the diagnostic roster—6 males and 8 females. The number of CAH patients increased rapidly once Wilkins started treating patients with cortisone in 1950. By 1956, he had already admitted 80 patients with CAH—20 males and 60 females.[49]

The "Push of Nature"

In treating CAH, Wilkins was concerned with two interconnected issues. One was to prevent death and address symptoms such as accelerated growth and sexual precocity in all children; the other was to address the virilizing effects CAH had on female patients. By the late 1940s, no effective treatment was yet available for CAH. After all his years of experimentation, Wilkins knew very well that no hormonal treatment had been successful. Estrogen had no effect on the adrenals in such cases, he stressed.[50] Throughout the 1940s, he had experimented with many drugs to try to stem the virilization of his CAH patients.[51] He tested a wide range of androgen analogs, each differing from natural testosterone by one or two small chemical groups. His proclaimed goal was to find a compound that would compete with the patient's natural androgens without itself being an androgen, thereby inhibiting the virilizing effects of the patient's own hormones. In 1948, Wilkins began to experiment with adrenocorticotrophic hormone (ACTH).[52] Produced and secreted by the anterior pituitary gland, ACTH increases the production and release of corticosteroids and cortisol from the adrenal cortex. Wilkins hoped that ACTH would regulate the hyperactive adrenals, bringing natural steroid levels into the normal range, yet results were not promising.

Wilkins did not favor adrenalectomy. Young had tried the surgical removal of up to one and a half of the adrenals.[53] But, Wilkins lamented, this procedure had yielded poor outcomes. Not only did virilization continue, but also in cases of subtotal adrenalectomy patients had to be sustained "on extensive adrenal hormones with great difficulty and expense." There was simply no adequate replacement therapy, and practitioners were driven "almost crazy in trying to keep these poor people alive afterwards."[54] Cases like Mary's show the high risk these young patients faced from such heroic surgical interventions.

These worries about keeping children alive were coupled with apprehensions about what kind of life girls with CAH should lead. More precisely, the specific symptom of pseudohermaphroditism in girls forced physicians like Wilkins to address the question of sex. In turn, these concerns reveal the inconsistencies in debates about sex. Wilkins's concerns are best summed up in a panel discussion, "The Adrenal Gland in Health

and Disease," at the annual meeting of the American Academy of Pediatrics in late November 1948.[55] At the panel, the discussion after
Wilkins's presentation on CAH soon turned to the clinical options available to physicians. "How should we handle these patients who are female pseudohermaphrodites?" he asked his audience. The physicians, in
turn, wondered what they should do if they encountered such patients.
Wilkins could only reply that the treatment of patients with symptoms
of pseudohermaphroditism was "one of the most difficult and discour-
aging problems [they were] faced with." He complained, "We are unable
at the present time to do anything to combat the excessive androgen
push these patients suffer and that causes the virilization of the female."
He added, "It is a most pathetic sight to see these girls gradually become
more and more virilized as time goes on" (548).

None of the surgical or hormonal avenues had yet proved effective in
curing the metabolic imbalance and/or halting and reversing the clinical
symptoms of the condition. The "push of nature," Wilkins noted, was
stronger than the remedies at hand. His suggestion about how to handle
the situation seems surprising at first: he recommended to his fellow
physicians that they ignore the girls' chromosomal and gonadal female
sex and "let them be male." Wilkins was aware that this advice might
seem controversial to some of his colleagues. Other specialists might
disagree with his assessment, he admitted, but all he could say was it
might be best to let the young girls grow up as boys, since they would,
in his opinion, look too male to be able to live as women. If the patients
were, however, already older and had been raised as females, he was
"very much opposed to reversing things and turning them into males"
(548). Patients should continue to live as girls and women, despite their
male appearance. In these cases, physicians sometimes tried to modify
their patients' bodies rather than change their assigned sex. Nathan
Talbot, director of the Pediatric Endocrinology Clinic at Massachusetts
General Hospital, had suggested in 1942 that girls with "adrenal cortical
hyperplasia," another term for CAH, receive orally administered dieth-
ylstilbestrol, a synthetic form of the hormone estrogen, which would
cause "development of the female secondary sexual characteristics and
improvement in psychological outlook."[56] Hugh Young and Hugh Jewett, Young's successor at the Brady Urological Institute, also prescribed
stilbestrol. Mostly, this led to breast development even in small girls, but
it did not at all address the underlying condition.

It seems at first glance surprising that Lawson Wilkins, in a discussion
with other physicians, would so casually abandon the dogma of biological sex. This discussion reveals on different levels how complicated sex

had become in the previous decades. First, it shows that it was at least imaginable for a pediatrician of Wilkins's stature that children could be raised in a sex different from their biological one and that they could adapt (or learn) to live more satisfying lives in their assigned sex than their biological one. Even though this recommendation was based on the limitations of medical intervention, it suggested a belief in and reliance on medical technology to make the chosen sex assignment convincing. Second, it reveals imprecise and inconsistent practices and recommendations. Physicians had several ways of determining sex. They could examine a child's external genitalia, palpate for internal reproductive organs, do a biopsy to determine gonadal sex, and pay attention to a person's psychological sex based on identity, behavior, and sexuality.

Physicians like Wilkins also adapted their diagnosis of sex based on their clinical experiences with such patients. A closer look reveals that Wilkins's recommendation had developed out of his clinical practice, where medical norms of sex were deeply entangled with his concept of development.[57] His assignment of sex depended on whether he saw a case as pathological or as a variant of development. In cases of what he saw as common variations in development of "maleness" and "femaleness," Wilkins took a wait-and-see approach. Whether a child was to be considered normal or not was often just a matter of timing. Children developed at different speeds, and development of physical and "psychic" traits varied with each child. When it came to variations in "maleness" and "femaleness," Wilkins generally cautioned against radical hormonal interventions, because they threatened the child's well-being and development far more than these normal variations. "Unfortunately," he warned, "serious and sometimes permanent psychologic maladjustments are frequently attributable to the attempts of parents to force a 'different' child into a standard mold" (147). Variation was a natural part of development; it was pressuring a child into a stage of development that did not fit his or her own biological norms that caused psychological problems.

In cases where deviation from sexual norms was based on an underlying pathology, Wilkins did recommend medical interventions, even though he knew that therapeutic options were limited and mainly surgical. Simply put, living with anatomical differences could lead to maladjustment. In cases where there was no underlying pathology, natural patterns of development would balance out in the end. In cases with an underlying pathology, such as congenital adrenal hyperplasia (CAH), the anatomical differences would not diminish but accelerate, not only endangering the child's health but also threatening adjustment and thus presumably the happiness of the child, adolescent, and adult. Wilkins's recommendations suggest that what mattered most to him was that his patient could live up to the social expectations of masculinity and femininity rather than biological preconditions.

Wilkins suggested that psychological health or adjustment was influenced by the experiences of somatic differences (147). Before him, Young had believed that femininity and masculinity resulted from hormonal influences and that these characteristics could be used to deduce a person's hormone levels.[58] Wilkins's concept of the hormonal body was more sophisticated, based on recent developments in endocrinological research. His cautious therapeutic approach was therefore also based on a new understanding of sex hormones that had replaced the concept of antagonistic male and female sex hormones with a more complex feedback model in which the pituitary gland featured prominently.[59] This shift was accompanied by a break with a dualistic concept of male and female as mutually exclusive categories and a turn toward hormonal bisexuality.

In his 1950s textbook, Wilkins differentiated between two groups of patients: "sex reversals," where hormones feminized or masculinized children (for example, girls with CAH), and "intersexes" due to genetic or intrauterine influences in early fetal life. In both groups, his approach spoke of his clinical pragmatism and of what he saw as the limitations of medicine at the time. If the child was still an infant or preadolescent, Wilkins thought that "the physician is called upon to decide whether it should be raised as a boy or a girl."[60] In young intersex children, this decision should be based "upon the character of the external genitalia as well as the nature of the gonads."[61] The verdict on sex depended on how the genitals would lend themselves best for adaptation according to a "phallic standard": If the phallus was long enough (and testes present), male genitalia should be constructed. However, if the genitalia were so "feminine" that they could not be converted into "the male type," then testes should be removed.[62] When confronted with adult intersex patients, Wilkins continued Young's practice of going with habitus and psyche. "When intersexes do not seek medical aid or advice until adolescence or adult life," Wilkins wrote, "one should be guided by not only the nature of the glands and the external genitalia, but also the general habitus, psyche, and secondary sex traits of the patient. The removal of gonads which are opposed to the general habitus and sexual desire of their possessor is justifiable."[63] Confronted with the fait accompli, Wilkins thought it more important to achieve what he perceived as normality than to hold on to the ultimate signifier of sex—the ovary or the testis.

The same pragmatic advice was given for the treatment of female pseudohermaphrodites when the condition was caused by congenital adrenal hyperplasia. If the diagnosis was made in early infancy, the practitioner in theory had more leeway. The decision again was whether to raise the child as female or male. According to most contemporaneous definitions of sex, these children were considered female. "Most physicians have advised that these patients be raised as girls and have attempted to develop feminine characteristics by surgical and hormonal treatment," Wilkins wrote. Those physicians based this decision on the fact that gonads and chromosomal sex were female. Wilkins, however, considered the attempt to raise such girls as females futile, noting that "the unfortunate patients continue to become more hirsute and muscular, and more masculine in their general habitus and behavior." He recommended the complete removal of the clitoris in girls raised as girls, since it would later become "a source of extreme embarrassment and erotic stimulation." To the objection of some that this procedure might "deprive that patient of future sexual gratification," he responded that it was "justified because it removes some of the tensions and problems which cause serious difficulties."[64] He did not elaborate what those difficulties were.

Wilkins's approach made the fixability of intersex genitalia a central focus of sex assignment and recommended the shortening or removal of a large clitoris in girls with CAH who were already raised in the female sex. But clitoridectomy was not a new procedure. US physicians had performed clitoral surgeries on women since the mid-nineteenth century to either preserve or restore appropriate sexual behavior, as the historian Sarah B. Rodriguez has shown.[65] What this long history of clitoral surgery reveals is that medical experts absolutely "knew the clitoris to be a unique and powerfully sensitive sexual organ, the 'electric bell' of female sexual instinct."[66] Its presumed role in women's sex lives was, however, deeply shaped by medical conceptions of (sexual) health and by cultural notions of women's roles and duties. Procedures such as the removal of the entire clitoris (clitoridectomy), the removal of the hood of the clitoris (female circumcision), the removal of smegma, and the breaking up of clitoral adhesions were framed as therapeutic and prescribed to curb masturbation, combat homosexuality or hypersexuality, and enhance women's capacity for orgasm (with their husbands). Since the late nineteenth century, masturbation had been one of the primary reasons for clitoral surgeries. Physicians thought that an unhealthy (i.e., irritated) clitoris provoked women to obsessive masturbation; the prescribed treatment was clitoral surgery to remove what caused these

irritations. The medical concern was to restore health, and yet it was underwritten by the conviction that these treatments directed patients toward "proper," socially desirable sexual relations with their husbands. In
addition to sexual ill health, sexual deviance and racial otherness were
read onto the body. An atypically large clitoris was considered a sign of
hypersexuality or lesbianism, though doctors were unsure whether the
size of the organ was the cause or the effect of these sexual practices. It
was also considered a marker of racial difference in African American
women.

Surgery on pseudohermaphrodites was conducted under similar assumptions. Earlier physicians mostly had responded to what they perceived as sexual anomalies with social prescription; but by the mid-
nineteenth century, surgery emerged as "a second possibility for managing
hermaphroditism," even though only in the late nineteenth century did
this second possibility become a viable option due to surgical innovations
such as antiseptics and anesthesia.[67] In their attempt to establish their
patients within a dimorphic anatomical and social norm, physicians pon-
dered proper sex roles as well as proper sexual activity. An enlarged clitoris
might lead to masturbation, penetration, and homosexual behavior, or
just general confusion in terms of a person's true sex. Of course, the latter must be established first, as the same organ could, depending on the
choice of sex, be a small phallus or an enlarged clitoris.[68]

Thus, following Wilkins's recommendation of raising CAH girls as
males, a large clitoris was a small phallus. "When one is faced with the
choice of procedures in early infancy, it is possible that the pathway toward masculinity may be the easiest and best to follow," Wilkins proclaimed in his textbook. The patients' secondary sexual development
would be "controlled by the predominance of androgens in spite of
the fact that they are genetically female." Ovaries and uterus could be
removed—though Wilkins did not think it essential, since the organs'
development was arrested or atrophied.[69] He recommended that an operation on the clitoris be performed in an effort to make it more functional as a penis. In addition, he recommended administering additional
testosterone at puberty.

The suggestion to choose the sex to which a patient could socially
adapt was an important revision of previous convictions that physicians
should determine and insist on a patient's true sex. Other doctors at
the time would have suggested raising these children as girls; after all,
laparotomies would clearly show that they possessed ovaries and uteruses. True, biological sex had become more complex over the previous
decades. While many physicians still regarded testes and ovaries as the

sole determiner of a person's "true sex," others came to realize that other organs could contribute to a person's sex characteristics. Clinicians like Wilkins also knew that a person could look or behave like a member of the sex opposite to his or her gonads or sex chromosomes; what they called habitus and "psychic" traits did not always cohere with what a laparotomy (or later the Barr body test) might reveal. Scholars have called the decades before 1955 a period of idiosyncrasy, in which sex was often assigned on a case-by-case basis.[70]

In the late 1940s, medical and scientific practitioners were still debating the mechanics of biological sex determination and weighing which sex characteristics would eventually determine a person's true sex. However, even if a true sex could be uncovered, they realized it might not end up being the best sex for the person in question. What is more, even if one were female according to one's gonads and chromosomes—as in the case of girls who had CAH—their appearance (and possibly psyche) would, according to Wilkins, still be male. This would make it next to impossible to fulfill the social expectations of being a woman as they existed at the time: feminine appearance, marriage, and motherhood. A virilized woman with CAH who had lived as a man, looked like a man, identified as a man, and desired women should not be forced to live as a woman, he thought, even though she had ovaries. The clinical decision was not to find the true sex of the patient but to choose the "better" one—the one that allowed children to grow up without conflict and to fulfill their social roles.

It is not surprising that physicians like Wilkins felt competent to discuss marriage as part of a medical treatment plan. Marriage had become a part of physicians' professional domain in the early twentieth century. The historian Elizabeth Reis has shown that already in the 1910s, doctors weighed in on marriage suitability.[71] These recommendations grew with physicians' increasing participation in the eugenic movement, as doctors became experts on decisions about who should and could marry and have children.[72]

Treatment decisions reflected social expectations of what it meant to live as a man or a woman as much as the limits of medicine—there was simply no treatment available for CAH, and the physician could only try to keep the child alive and treat the effects of the excessive androgen production. "The only hope at the present time," Wilkins complained at the 1948 conference, "is that perhaps someday someone can find something to have an antagonistic effect upon adrenal androgen, some anti-adrenal drug, somewhat similar to anti-thyroid drug."[73] That day arrived less than a year later with the introduction of cortisone.

Cortisone

In June 1949, the same month that Mary died of complications from her adrenalectomy, Wilkins's desired "anti-adrenal drug"[74] appeared, although it did so for a very different condition, in a different form than he imagined, and under difficult circumstances. That month, Dr. Philip Hench at the Mayo Clinic in Rochester, Minnesota, announced that cortisone had successfully relieved fourteen patients suffering from severe rheumatoid arthritis.[75] The substance itself had been isolated in 1935 as compound E, later renamed cortisone.[76] Cortisone and its dramatic effects—including enabling wheelchair users to get up and walk—were celebrated as a modern medical sensation. The *New York Times* gushed, "The hormones seem to perform what can be described only by that much abused word, 'miracle.'"[77] Another *Times* article from August of the same year, on the possibility of harvesting the tropical plant *Strophanthussarmentosus* as "a potentially unlimited source of cortisone, [the] new miracle drug for treating arthritis, rheumatic fever and possibly some other degenerative diseases," was titled "The 'Elixir of Life.'"[78]

It may seem surprising that cortisone would come to play such an important role in the conceptualization of gender at Hopkins. After all, it is a substance that did not carry the same burden of assumptions about sex that estrogen and androgens did. It was decidedly not associated with gendered assumptions about its sex-specific properties. Yet the material circumstances of its introduction, its reception, and its effects shaped Wilkins's assumptions about how medical intervention was crucial for finding the proper sex for his CAH patients. The drug was introduced at the center of what historians of medicine describe as "the shift in emphasis from infectious to chronic diseases that occurred in post-war medical and pharmaceutical research."[79] Like insulin, which had been introduced in the treatment of diabetes more than two decades earlier in 1921, it turned out to be no cure despite its dramatic effects, and it needed to be taken continuously, producing at times severe side effects.[80] It was a product of World War II and its immediate aftermath. In explaining the initial lack of interest from pharmaceutical manufacturers, the chemist Edward C. Kendall, who in 1935 had first isolated compound E from bovine adrenal glands, remarked in his Nobel Prize acceptance speech that "for many years there were few who believed that any product of the adrenal cortex would find a place in clinical medicine other than in the treatment of the relatively few patients who had Addison's disease."[81] This changed with the US entry into World

War II in 1941, when "the medical departments of the army and navy approached the National Research Council of the United States with the request that the hormones of the adrenal cortex be made available"—in the hope that these substances would help increase air force pilots' resistance to oxygen deprivation, enabling them to fly at higher altitudes.[82] The small quantities of cortisone available in the immediate postwar era were an outcome of the resulting program to manufacture corticosteroids synthetically.

The perception of cortisone as a wonder drug was based on its dramatic therapeutic effects on patients with rheumatoid arthritis. Hench, according to the historian Viviane Quirke, had been fortuitous in choosing a dose that would produce the dramatic effects which "would capture the attention of his fellow physicians and the press."[83] Its scarcity also shaped the manner in which cortisone was sought out, distributed, and perceived. When the drug's manufacturer Merck & Co. synthesized compound E in 1948, it did so in an exceedingly complicated procedure involving thirty-seven steps just to get a few grams.[84] In July 1949, the production costs were 10,000 USD per gram, and a daily dosage of cortisone was as much as 1,000 USD. By the end of the year, the price of cortisone had sunk to 200 USD per gram—still a very high price at the time.[85] In 1950, pharmaceutical firms Merck and its competitor, Armour, distributed cortisone (and adrenocorticotrophic hormone) only to a "small network of academic consultants."[86] Over the next few years, physicians tried out cortisone as a therapeutic for a variety of medical conditions and diseases, including schizophrenia and depression because of the euphoric responses it triggered in patients. Only after the chemist Percy Julian successfully synthesized cortisone from soybeans could it be mass produced. This breakthrough made possible the large-scale production of cortisone and lowered the costs of the drug significantly.[87]

Restoring the Proper Sex

Lawson Wilkins joined in this great enthusiasm in late 1949. At the time when cortisone became available, he was trying different steroid hormones to see what therapeutic effect they might have on his patients with congenital adrenal hyperplasia (CAH). His first goal was simply to find out whether cortisone would have any effect on a patient's condition. It was at the end of the same year that he first tried cortisone on one young patient, referred to only as P. R. in his published results, and within just two months he sent the results out for publication to the *Bulletin of the Johns Hopkins Hospital*.[88] Cortisone, he hoped, "if given in quantities adequate for or greater than the normal need of the body, might suppress the endogenous activity of the adrenals including the hypersecretion of androgen" (249). The fifteen-year-old girl, whose medical condition had been followed at Hopkins for eleven years, was—after a ten-day control period—treated with cortisone for fifteen days. The rare substance had been provided by Merck and was injected into the girl at six-hour intervals.

The results seemed most promising. The girl's 17-ketosteroids (17-KS) level decreased sharply, an indication of lowered androgen. It remained at a low level throughout the treatment and did not rise again until ten days after treatment had been stopped. The girl's 17-KS level mattered, because CAH was diagnosed not only by studying the appearance and development of a child but also by measuring the 17-KS level in the patient's urine. A high level of this substance was seen as evidence of a high level of androgens. Its decrease was an indication of therapeutic success. During the trial's short period, there was no improvement in the clinical presentation—that is, no change in the patient's virilization. Nevertheless, Wilkins was cautiously optimistic "that this drug may prove of therapeutic value" (252). The next step would be, he thought, to determine the minimal dosage needed to suppress androgen secretion.

Wilkins's evolving research strategy was straightforward and shaped by clinical needs. After he had tested whether cortisone had any effect at all and whether it was harmful to the patient, he tried to determine dosage and delivery. He had to find the minimal dosage necessary to bring about an antivirilizing result without causing too many side effects. Finally, Wilkins tested cortisone on all the specific symptoms of CAH to see whether it had an effect on them. Throughout the trial, one question lingered in every stage of the research: Would cortisone be a cure for CAH? To answer this question, Wilkins would have to follow patients over a longer period of time. For the moment, once the cortisone therapy was discontinued, patients' 17-KS levels returned to their former high, and without daily dosages of the drug, all symptoms returned.

Cortisone showed significant results in all patients. Determining the correct dosage, however, was an individualized process of maximizing the reduction of symptoms and minimizing side effects. Patients were divided by age and sex into subgroups according to the definition of the syndrome and the manifestation of its symptoms.[89] After all, not only was the definition of the symptoms sex specific, but the treatment goals also differed according to sex. One group consisted of older female patients whose symptoms manifested as pseudohermaphroditism.[90] Here, along with the decrease of 17-KS, the study of the clinical effects on sexual and somatic development was of the most interest. Would cortisone diminish the patients' virilization and trigger a process of feminization? Both could only be observed through long-term study and could only be fully evaluated after patients had been studied continuously for five to seventeen months.[91]

"Diminishing virilization" was measured through decreased hair growth and diminished facial acne, all indications of lowered androgen level but difficult to quantify and measure. Aside from the chemical evidence of the androgen level in the body—also measured only indirectly through the 17-KS output—it was difficult to quantify virilization. Simple observation, Wilkins thought, "left no doubt" of a definite decrease in the girls' growth of body hair.[92] For some time, Wilkins and his team tried to measure progressive devirilization by shaving and weighing axillary hair, but they soon had to acknowledge that this method was problematic. "We do not have great confidence in this as a quantitative method because of various technical difficulties," he conceded.[93]

Wilkins and his team both expected a decrease in virilization and tried to promote feminization in their female patients—regardless of their ages. By feminization, they meant the start of sex-specific adolescence, including breast growth, vulvar development, changes in the vaginal smear, and finally another sign of feminization—regular menstrual periods. These "treatment successes" would eventually necessitate another form of medical intervention; previously, girls with severe forms of CAH had never menstruated. Now, with cortisone, many girls had their menses for the first time. The blood flow required an outlet, which sometimes had to be surgically constructed.[94]

Another group of patients consisted of young girls and babies with pseudohermaphroditism and electrolyte-regulating defects.[95] With this group, cortisone was lifesaving; most of these patients had been admitted to the hospital in states of dehydration, and the most pressing tasks were to combat the electrolyte defect and ensure survival. Wilkins also studied the effect on somatic growth and development, and he looked for any sexual changes, though not much was to be observed at such an early age. Most girls had a large clitoris and pubic hair, with the latter diminishing during treatment. Dosage was crucial. In one child, for example, Wilkins achieved "normalization," but she started to develop signs of overdose; she became obese in spite of a low-calorie diet, and she developed a "moon face" similar to patients with Cushing syndrome.[96] Once more, this confirmed to Wilkins the necessity of finding the right dosage, a tricky task in a growing child whose needs were ever changing. His goal was to avoid inhibiting growth or causing Cushing-like symptoms while using a strong-enough dose to trigger a therapeutic effect. Once the child was "well maintained" on cortisone—defined by a chemical value (low 17-KS) and by appearance (less virilized, less precocious)—the patient was supposed to be under lifelong medical supervision. If treatment meant hospitalization and control, the maintenance phase was a long leash. The parents were supposed to administer cortisone orally or intramuscularly; regularly send urine samples collected over twenty-four hours; and take the child to the clinic once a year for evaluation to measure hormone levels, evaluate development, and assess the child's social adjustment through psychological interviews.

As time passed and these children grew up, patients themselves would become increasingly responsible for their medical maintenance—a peculiar disciplining of the self that included monitoring body and mind constantly. The implicit goal of a patient's long-term treatment was to ensure social adjustment according to the social norms of the time; occasionally it became a strange pursuit of happiness where becoming healthy was substituted for being happy and normal enough, passing as one's assigned sex and erasing all visible differences—even those which were not sex specific, such as height. Considerable work was invested in effecting a "normal" gender identity that fit the contemporaneous (heterosexual) standard of male and female.

For Wilkins, the treatment was a success. On March 30, 1952, the *Washington Post* ran a short two-column article titled "Cortisone Helps to Restore Sex Balance."[97] A day earlier, Wilkins had announced during an American Cancer Society–sponsored tour of cancer centers that "the hormone cortisone restores proper sex to help some girls who turn masculine, or boys who develop sexually too early." When injected into "youngsters," the article explained, "their own adrenal glands get lazy and stop making the excess doses of male hormone." He made a point to mention that the hormonal treatment had to be continuous lest the "masculinizing troubles return."[98]

In the end, cortisone turned out not to be a cure for CAH, but it became part of a lifelong management strategy for the chronic condition. A cortisone-based treatment required individualized establishment of the right dose in each patient as well as monitoring and reevaluation over time; this had a profound impact on patients' lives. Like the management of diabetes through insulin, treatment with cortisone restructured the daily lives of patients and their families.[99] Children came in yearly for evaluations and adjustments of dosage, and the clinical experience became a consistent part of their lives. During these evaluations, behavior and adaptation to the sex that had been chosen for the child were evaluated and measured in conjunction with chemical analysis of urine and blood, examinations, X-rays, and measurements of height and weight.

―――――――

Wilkins's Pediatric Endocrinology Clinic was a place where the idea that individuals could (and in some cases should) live in the sex that was not their biological one had been practiced before the psychologist John Money and his colleagues formulated the concept. The clinic was an intimate space where decisions about patients' health and care, about their body and sex, were made daily. Wilkins, like other physicians at the time, struggled with the realization that for some of his patients, their biological or "true" sex might not be the best choice. This recognition was shaped by his institutional setting, the particularities of the condition he was treating, the availability of some and absence of other medical technologies and therapies, and a concept of health that encompassed both the biological and the social. To restore health to an organism meant much more than to cure a disease; it denoted the ability to function in the world in terms of both biological and social norms. Wilkins's clinical experience shaped his decision to abandon the insistence on determining his patients' "true" (chromosomal or gonadal) sex and recommend finding the sex that was better for them and in which they could live convincingly. He did so amid the tension of treating potentially life-threatening adrenal pathology, clinical dissatisfaction with the practice of determining sex on the basis of sex glands, the maintenance of social norms such as heterosexuality and marriage, and a concept of health that favored adjustment and paid attention to development.

Wilkins became a decisive figure in the transformation of sex and the formulation of what we today refer to as the sex/gender binary: the differentiation between an individual's biologically determined sex and that person's environmentally shaped gender. His clinical experience with children with CAH led Wilkins to a pragmatic reformulation of sex—one based not on anatomical features alone but on social cues of a prognosis of functionality. His reasoning was not shaped, at least initially, by new social theories about culture and personality but instead by his experience as a pediatrician. This experience included a disease-centered clinical practice and its relevance in studying rare conditions, institutional traditions in treating patients, and a shift from one sub-specialty to another that indicates a reconceptualization of medical approaches and changes in medical definitions of sex.

Both before and after cortisone, Wilkins based his treatment decisions on the greater importance of social role over biological markers of sex. Previously, CAH children with acute metabolic symptoms had died, and those who lived had become more virilized and precocious over time. With no treatment, they had often simply been let be; the girls grew up looking increasingly "male"—or, if assigned as boys, they were allowed to follow the "push of nature." The boys became sexually precocious and grew into short adults. Cortisone enabled Wilkins to make interventions to restore what he conceived of as his patients' "proper sex." Their "adjustment" to their "proper sex" was paid for by the necessity of lifelong management, which transformed clinical practices and patients' experiences. Both of his recommendations—first, to follow "the push of nature" (suggesting that CAH girls live as males) and second, to restore one's "true sex" (suggesting that CAH girls be treated with cortisone and live as females)—were rooted in the same understanding of gender. In both instances, gender was something that could be "made"—supplemented by surgical shaping of the body.

Wilkins never abandoned his conviction that life outside the two, and only two, sexes—male and female—was impossible and undesirable. But the choice of sex was not determined by a person's "true" and biologically defined sex but instead by the sex that would be "better" for that individual. Indeed, other doctors before Wilkins had already suggested that choosing somebody's "obvious sex" (or gender) might be preferable to forcing them into their "true sex."[100] The question of what the "better" sex was remained deeply entrenched in the social convictions of the time. Wilkins considered it psychologically and socially necessary that his patients be able to live convincingly in one sex or the other. It was feared that sexual ambiguity or contradictions might impair a person's psychological health and happiness. In the end, Wilkins ignored his own advice not to "force a 'different' child into a standard mold." For him, managing his patients' sex was part of a treatment plan to restore health. What constituted health, however, was in the eye of the beholder.

Hope

Thus, beyond medicalisation, medicine has shaped our ethical regimes, our relations with ourselves, our judgment of the kinds of people we want to be, and the lives we want to lead.

Robert's most visible symptom was his (sexual) precocity: he was tall and muscular, and by the age of three his genitals had resembled those of an adolescent. He was admitted to Wilkins's clinic for suspicion of adrenogenital syndrome. We have seen in the previous chapter how the pediatric endocrinologist Lawson Wilkins diagnosed children as having congenital adrenal hyperplasia (CAH), suggested what sex they should be raised in, and introduced his new treatment with cortisone. At first sight, Robert's story seems exceptional. His sex, determined as male, was never in question. Cortisone seemed to have little to no effect on his symptoms of precocity. In this, his case was an unusual one compared to the "girls" with CAH described in chapter 1. Yet his story is extraordinary only in these details, not in the emotions at play and the ways in which the clinical encounter enveloped Robert and his family. Through his patient record, we can trace the medicalization of his life and the hope and despair that structured his and his family's lives.

Robert's story suggests how the clinic's medical interventions and innovations resonated with families who sought help for their children. It allows us to explore what led parents to take their children into this space and how these families experienced a wide array of social interventions aimed at the whole family. It reveals the sense of emergency that structured many encounters with CAH. It also illuminates prevalent faith in medicine as an institution, especially at an elite place such as the Johns Hopkins Hospital, and the promise—in Robert's case unfulfilled—to provide relief with diagnosis, treatment, and cure.

Not surprisingly, clinical encounters with infants and children revolved around the family. Parents took their children into the clinic and negotiated meanings of health and illness, of care and cure, of normal and pathological with the clinical team. Parents, mostly mothers, spoke for their infants and children, and clinical care was aimed at alleviating the parents' alarm and anxieties as much as the child's suffering. "The control of the clinical encounter between child, mother, and physician lies at the heart of the pediatric discourse," the medical historian Jonathan Gillis writes, and mothers' assessments of their children are detectable throughout the clinical record.[1]

Robert's life and that of his family had been unmoored by displacement and the search for treatment until they anchored their hope on the Hopkins clinic.[2] He was born in 1946 in Europe, where his symptoms of precocity—excessive growth and bone age, sexual maturation—were first noted and treated. Robert's parents moved to a city in the American Rust Belt in 1949, hoping for a better life and better medical treatment for their child. They were at first completely financially dependent on a charity that supported refugees. In the spring of 1949, his mother stopped by the office of Dr. Miller, an acquaintance of Wilkins's, at her local children's hospital seeking help.[3] Miller wrote to Wilkins, saying that he had acknowledged Wilkins as "the first endocrinologist" in United States but indicating that he found her presumptuous for wanting the best, even though the charity would have to pay for it. He thought she lacked a "realistic attitude." Robert's mom was persistent, however, and in August a colleague of Miller's, Dr. Smith, wrote to Wilkins, asking him for diagnostic advice and suggesting he see the boy.

On the occasion of Robert's first admission to the Johns Hopkins Hospital the next month, Mrs. Good, the social worker who was the primary person responsible for assisting the family, suggested that Robert's mother had Hopkins in mind all along:[4] "It is understandable that at this time, both parents will experience an emotional crisis. Since the time when they knew their child was different from other children, they have been trying to get help for him. In Europe they were told, 'If you could only get him to the Johns Hopkins Hospital in Baltimore'; when they got to this country they were again told that the doctors here were the only ones who could help him." Her eight-page report about the case also suggests the stakes: the mother was worried that the boy's trouble might break up her marriage due to the "constant tension tending to set them all on edge."

In the late 1940s, public trust in medicine was strong. The period from 1945 up to the 1970s is often retrospectively referred to as the golden age of medicine—a time associated with high esteem for the medical profession and high expectations of medicine's ability to treat disease effectively with new technologies and techniques.[5] Between the development of sulfa drugs in the 1930s and the introduction of penicillin in the 1940s, many felt that all disease was potentially curable. Death from infectious diseases was in sharp decline in 1949, and diagnosis became a step toward a process of normalization; it identified the cause at heart and held the promise of healing. Government and philanthropic organizations were investing heavily in medical institutions for research, education, and patient care. While this romantic image of a golden age of medicine—often invoked by medical practitioners themselves—has been shown to be fractured, incomplete, and at times inaccurate, it resonates strongly in many of the patient records of the Harriet Lane Home for Invalid Children (HLH). Robert's parents, who while still in Europe had been told they would find help at the Johns Hopkins Hospital for their son's condition, may have been particularly susceptible.

Robert's medical records preceded him at Hopkins, stating that the cause of his sexual precocity "could not be determined with certainty." In fact, it never would be; although his symptoms pointed to CAH, he lacked several key markers, such as a high level of 17-ketosteroids (17-KS) and indeed adrenal hyperplasia. His record includes a translation from a European clinic summarized in English as well as multiple patient histories taken at two clinics in the United States that the family had visited before Hopkins. The physician at one of these clinics corresponded with the Hopkins Pediatric Endocrinology Clinic, and these letters appear in the file.

Letters in the file also document that before Robert's arrival, it had taken several exchanges to establish that the charity caring for the family would fully cover the child's treatment. In early fall, a letter from the admitting officer at the HLH assured the parents that the home was aware of the medical costs being a burden and that "our doctors will bear that in mind while he is a patient here." However, Wilkins wrote to Mrs. Good that he had arranged to have Robert admitted "for a complete study of his case." This would require weeks of hospitalization and maybe an exploratory operation. Wilkins wrote, "I trust that if the parents bring him they will be willing to leave him for as long a period as we consider advisable."

Wilkins tried to diagnose Robert's underlying pathology through examination, tests, and finally, in October 1949, an exploratory laparotomy—surgically opening the abdomen and examining the bodily cavity for the presence of sex organs. Concerns for Robert's physical ailment were amplified by anxiety about his psychological adjustment to the "exuberant state of affairs down below." Within a few days after his admission, Dr. Leo Kanner, an Austrian psychiatrist and physician who had directed the HLH's child psychiatry clinic since 1930, saw Robert for an evaluation. Before Wilkins hired his own team of psychiatrists and psychologists, Kanner had been one of the psychiatric experts on whom he relied for evaluations. Upon examining Robert, Kanner "believed he [was] easily at his age level" and in fact had "the probability of superior endowment" in terms of intelligence; the psychiatrist attributed any difficulty to the recent immigrant's "language difficulty." The next day, Dr. C. H. Waskowitz arrived at a similar assessment using the Stanford-Binet test.

Woven into the medical record of Robert's life in the clinic was a dense fabric of social intervention that dealt with the parents' anxieties as much as with their social predicament. Easing the family's pain and despair would become a dominant theme in the medical treatment of this child. The clinic recommended that the family settle in Baltimore to have access to ongoing psychological help for everyone. When the clinic interrupted the estrogen therapy that had been started in Europe, it was the parents' response to Robert's acne, increased pubic hair growth, restlessness and irritability, persistent erections, and frequent masturbation at night that prompted the doctors to resume it, albeit at a lower dosage. His parents were not only worried about their child's health and future but also recovering from their traumatic wartime experiences and trying to settle in a foreign land.

On the day of Robert's admission, Mrs. Good met with his mother to address the mother's angst upon the request of the admitting service.[6] According to the referring administrator, the mother "was in a highly emotional state and was in need of someone with whom she could discuss the meaning of her son's hospitalization." Mrs. Good's report indicates that the mother grasped the social worker's "hand with both of hers" when they were introduced and "then held my arm as we went to the Social Service booth. . . . When she was seated she asked my permission to smoke and took a few eager pulls at her cigarette which did serve to calm her a bit." Robert's mother poured her heart out to the social worker. Mrs. Good noted that the mother was desperate for somebody who could help her "handle her own feelings during the course of [Robert's] hospitalization so that she could help him get the most from his care here." Robert was less than three years old, but between three other hospitals his mother estimated that he had spent about twenty-four months of his life in a facility. Mrs. Good wrote that the mother "thought her own anxiety . . . [was] going to make it hard for her to facilitate [Robert's] adjustment on the ward. She thought that perhaps she shouldn't visit him because he always became so upset when she left yet at the same time she didn't see how she was going to stand not seeing him because she had to be assured he was alright." "Her thoughts were constantly of him," Mrs. Good wrote, "and she realized that the reassurance she got from seeing him did give her some relief from her tenseness."

Mrs. Good offered to meet with the mother regularly and said that she could assist her in understanding the hospital policies and medical routine as well as with any misunderstandings that might arise due to language difficulties. Mrs. Good would also see Robert regularly to "help him adjust to the hospital and his medical care," and she would report his state to his mother when she was unable to visit him herself. In contrast to Dr. Miller's disgruntled criticism of the mother's apparent sense of entitlement to the best treatment for her son and her persistence in getting it for him, Mrs. Good noted that the mother was "hesitant to ask special privilege or bring herself to attention of those in authority." She described her as "a tense and anxious mother who seems to have invested a great deal of her emotional energy in worrying about this child and who has a definite need to be dependent on someone during the time evaluation studies are being done on her child." She saw the mother's traumatic experiences during World War II and her son's uncertain present and future as the main causes for her state.

In her report, Mrs. Good also evaluated Robert himself. Like Kanner, she attributed difficulties, in this case emotional, to "language difficulties," although she seems to have felt his command of English was stronger than Kanner did. She also referenced "many hospitalizations and changes in his environment." She described him as "an attractive, very alert, observing child" who appeared to be about seven. He was "powerfully built, walks with a swagger, has the facies of an older boy."[7] "When talking with him," she wrote, "it is difficult to remember that you are really talking with a very young boy of not quite three years of age." She added, "Discounting the language difficulty that he still has, we would assume that he is a child of superior intelligence." "On the ward" he was, she observed, "inquisitive, restless, and friendly."

Robert's voice is barely present in the record—partly a result of his young age. As in other cases, his parents had not told him why he was in the hospital. The reasons the social worker listed are quite telling. For one, "his parents did not know what to tell him" for lack of a definite diagnosis. But there was more: "They [did] not want him to think he [was] different from other children and, consequently have been at a loss as to how to explain their placing him in the hospital and leaving him except for occasional visits." "They have tried very hard," Mrs. Good wrote, "in [Robert's] social contacts to protect him from the knowledge that he is different from other children his age." How such protection affected him is lost to history, but the record suggests that parental anxiety and medical management had an effect on Robert. By October, it was noted that the child "[had] become quite a behavior problem." He was mimicking the boy with mental disabilities in the bed next to him, one physician wrote; he "screams, wets himself, stools in bed, has a constant scowl, 'chip on the shoulder.'" At this point, he had been in the hospital for three weeks—without having been told why—and the team of physicians was still trying to pinpoint his pathology.

As with his mother, Mrs. Good's assessment showed more empathy than the physicians'. The long stay had proved wearisome for the young boy, and not knowing what was wrong or why he was being subjected to constant examination distressed him. "[Robert] has been confused and somewhat distressed by the ward procedures," Mrs. Good noted in her report, "and one day when they wished to use him on rounds again, he went to the play teacher and asked 'Are they going to look at me again?' The examinations of his genitalia do excite and stimulate him sexually and he reacts by restless, excited behavior." She continued:

Certainly a lot of things have been done to this child, his parents have had to leave him for long periods of time and return to him. He has had long stay in hospital and is subjected to the many painful procedures which accompany diagnostic studies with no understanding of why these things are being done to him. It is hard for him to accept his parents' departure each day because I think he is never sure that they will really return. Also, while they are here, they protect him a little bit from the routines of the hospital. When they go, he is left alone to cope with a situation which he does not quite understand.

When Robert was discharged in early November 1949, medical personnel could offer the family very little, only "dietary instructions" and "reassurances." Reassurance may sound like peculiar medical currency—in fact, while seldom acknowledged so openly, it is always part of the medical repertoire. However, the inability to provide for themselves and the lack of a home compounded the parents' medical worries about their child. The mother could find no rest, and the charity arranged for her to receive medical care.

Upon his discharge, Robert's parents were determined to "attempt to bring the boy up as a normal child within the limits of his disease." They planned a permanent move to Baltimore with the help of the charity, which wrote Wilkins, asking "if it will be necessary for [Robert] to be seen at regular intervals" and whether staying in Baltimore would have "any benefit for him and his family." Mrs. Good discussed it with the doctors "in the light of the family's background and attitudes"; they said it was not "necessary from a medical point of view," but that there would be "value in the family's utilization of their emotional energies in establishing the home which this child needed rather than using them in the search for non-existent medical alleviation of their problem." The charity nonetheless funded the move to Baltimore.

Not "necessary from a medical point of view" is a telling phrase in this context. What became necessary for the "well-being" of the child is found on the margins of the record, not really "medical" yet still deeply entangled with medicine. After Robert's discharge in November 1949, the parents' anxieties about his appearance and sexuality continued. Mrs. Good recorded that the father said he had been unable to eat, sleep, or work during the hospitalization and that the mother had ongoing trouble eating and sleeping "because of her worry over the family's total situation and particularly the finality of the studies being done on [Robert] here." Even though many of the family's problems lay outside the realm of medicine, Mrs. Good proposed "that perhaps a definitive medical statement regarding [Robert's] difficulties and what might be expected from them and the opportunity to establish a home near enough to the hospital that its nearness would give them security might be one way of facilitating this family's adjustment in this country." Under the rubric "meaning of illness to family," she wrote, "Now they have come to the end of the journey, so to speak. Always before, there was the hope that something could be done if they could get to a certain place, now they are at that place awaiting a decision which may remove all hope from them and which will mean that they must accept the child as he is and learn to live with him." Mrs. Good summarized Wilkins's prognosis in a 1949 letter to the charity organization:

It is expected that when an adult, [Robert] will have the physical potentialities for holding a job and leading a normal life. Studies of children who have similar difficulties are in progress and the medical profession is hopeful that some day it will be able to offer real help to such children. When this help does become available, Dr. Wilkins would be interested in having [Robert] benefit by it. . . . Dr. Wilkins feels that [Robert]'s problem is now a social one and that any plan which would facilitate social adjustment is desirable.

The next year, Robert's mother began to consider how he would fare in school, and she again consulted the clinic. In recording this meeting, Mrs. Good noted that the mother "was very anxious to make a school connection of some kind" and also that she seemed "less tense and introspective in her conversation." The family no longer depended on the charity organization, though they still were struggling to make ends meet. Robert was doing well; the mother described "him with pride as a typical American boy—he plays cowboys, is interested in wild west movies, is enthralled with television which he watches in neighbor's home."

Many letters and notes were exchanged among the mother, Mrs. Good, Dr. Kanner's clinic, Wilkins, and the charity organization on how to school Robert. Robert's mother wanted the four-year-old to start school not only because she thought he "needed such an experience" but because both parents had to work during the day. The parents had also started to lie about his age, increasing it by a year, to facilitate this plan. The mother wanted Robert "to have something more advanced compatible with his size and with the age which she and [her husband] had given him." Again, Mrs. Good thought that this went back to "their real problem of being unable to accept this child as he is." Robert was tested and evaluated once more, and the doctors at Hopkins finally recommended to the board of education that the child be placed in school "above nursery school level." Both child and mother were scheduled for "continuing psychiatric interviews."

With this, Mrs. Good closed her case. "As there was no further service to be rendered by Social Service," she wrote, "the case is being closed, to be re-opened at the request of the mother or the doctors." Robert continued to come to the clinic for annual evaluations and examinations—though not for treatment—until 1960. During his last visit, schooling again was addressed; this time Robert himself had turned to John Money to ask about special college preparatory courses, and again the clinic got actively involved in assisting him. Robert's last trace in the record is a photograph dated 1970; the record has no further written notes on his relationship to the clinic.

Happy and Well Adjusted: The Psychologization of Sex in the 1930s and 1940s

In 1937, S. M., a seventeen-year-old white single woman, was admitted to Massachusetts General Hospital in Boston. She complained of absent menses and undeveloped breasts. The young woman "had always considered herself a female, physically and mentally healthy."[1] She was, however, quite worried that "she could not get married and have children," and she hoped that with medical intervention "she could become a normal girl" (311). The treating physicians examined the patient and performed a laparotomy, a microscopic examination of the biopsied tissue, and hormonal studies, which soon determined that she had male pseudohermaphroditism, "a condition in which the sex glands are male in spite of the presence of many female secondary sexual characteristics" (310). She felt a hundred percent female but was genetically male.

By the late 1930s, US physicians had become quite familiar with such rare but interesting cases of sex contradictions and were convinced that they alone had the expertise to diagnose a person's true sex. In theory, a person's sex was determined as the presence of either a testis or an ovary, but there was an increasing unease about what the right decision was in such cases. Even Hugh Hampton Young, urologist and surgeon at the Johns Hopkins Hospital who published the first American monograph on hermaphroditism in 1937, often felt compelled to recommend letting certain patients remain in the sex that they were living in, even if it contradicted their gonadal sex.[2] In the case of S. M., who was diagnosed as anatomically male but psychologically female, medical practitioners introduced a new method into their diagnostic inventory: they relied on psychoanalysis and psychiatric analysis to determine psychological sex. They also reached a different conclusion than they might have previously and argued that psychological sex, acquired in the course of growing up, trumped anatomy. Whether this was indeed "the first case of verified male pseudohermaphroditism studied psychoanalytically,"[3] as the authors claimed in 1942, mattered less than their remarkable conclusion that "based on the psychoanalysis, . . . the young woman in question had an emotional and psychosexual development typical for females."[4] Her environment and upbringing as a girl had determined her psychological sex, and her physicians recommended that she remain a girl.

This and similar case histories published in the 1930s and 1940s shared an insistence on the importance of psychiatric and psychological evaluation and the inclusion of a new group of experts—psychiatrists and clinical psychologists—in the diagnostic process. In this chapter, I show how the psychologization of American society and the popular acceptance of the paradigm of adjustment and maladjustment shaped the clinical engagement with sex assignment. These cases reveal the implicit acknowledgment that psychological sex could differ from anatomical sex as well as the assumption that environment, social situation, upbringing, and cultural patterns could determine a person's psychological sex. This was a remarkable shift from earlier concerns about morality and sexual deception in cases where the sex of a person was doubted or deemed contradictory.[5] Even more so, with the development of new surgical techniques and safer anesthesia as well as new findings on the effects of sex hormones, the human body had become increasingly malleable. Thus, many physicians argued that it could be adapted to a person's psychological sex.[6]

A Turn to the Normal

By the mid-twentieth century, most Americans would agree that to be normal meant to be well adjusted and happy and that people's upbringing, environment, and culture played a big role in the formation of their personality. The idea that someone could be well- or maladjusted and the importance of adjustment to one's social group was pervasive beyond psychological textbooks, appearing in educational manuals, government policies, and the popular press. College students took courses on "maladjustment."[7] A psychiatrist reminded "his fellow Catholics" in a manual on maladjusted children that "nature needs to be nurtured to be receptive of Grace."[8] The *New York Times* applied the language of adjustment when it warned that personality maladjustment caused motorists to be "accident-repeaters."[9] In Arthur Miller's 1949 play *Death of a Salesman*, to be not just liked but "well liked" was a quality of great importance to the main character, Willy Loman.[10] This shift toward the social took place in different sites over the first half of the twentieth century, most significantly in psychiatry and the new cultural anthropology. Even scientists who insisted on the biological determinism of instinct considered nurture and environment important factors in human behavior and adjustment.[11]

The *maladjustment* model of mental disorder was the core conceptual model of psychiatry in America, from mental hygiene to the rise of a new public health role for psychiatry. The Rockefeller Foundation, for example, gave it its highest priority status for medical funding in the 1930s and 1940s. Psychiatrists became less concerned with the insane and those interned at state asylums. Instead, they turned their gaze to psychologically troubled individuals and dysfunctional social structures and relationships.[12] Building on a Darwinian concept of adaptation, the new psychiatry argued that mental health was contingent on individuals' proper adjustment. With the shift from a model of mental disease to one of mental disorder, psychiatrists were increasingly concerned with "not just insanity but *maladjustment*—that is, an individual's inability to adapt to his or her social environment."[13] The adjustment/maladjustment paradigm, in which adjusting to one's environment became the ultimate measure of a person's mental health, dates back to Adolf Meyer, who was psychiatrist-in-chief at the Henry Phipps Psychiatric Clinic at Johns Hopkins from its opening in 1913 until 1941.[14] His concept of "psychobiology" understood mental illness as failed adaptation rather than a distinct brain disease. He proposed that "the pathological processes underlying mental disorder took place not exclusively at the level of brain tissues or metabolism but also at the level of adaptive behavior and individual experience."[15] The goal of this new dynamic psychiatry was "to integrate the patient's life experiences with physiological and biological data."[16] Every individual was a singular experiment in nature, so knowing the patient's history was absolutely crucial for the physician. This new understanding of mental health transformed the specialty and its institutions.

By the 1950s, the language of adjustment had long since entered into popular discourse in the United States. The American public was ready to embrace this new approach to mental health and increasingly request scientific advice for all kinds of personal concerns and complaints.[17] Between World Wars I and II, applied psychology grew progressively important; its practitioners argued that they could assist Americans in adjusting to an increasingly complex society. By the end of World War II, the vocabulary of adjustment and maladjustment had permeated every aspect of American life. Educators, policy makers, politicians, and middle-class families used the language of adjustment to address urgent political problems as well as issues of everyday life, family, and work. Children and their development became an important focus of US politics.[18]

A Psychoanalytic Perspective

With the psychological turn, the medical focus in physicians' encounters with hermaphroditic patients shifted. By the 1940s, a focus on the psychological aspects of human sexuality had been added to long-standing debates about biological sex determination (sex chromosomes vs. hormones and gonads) in the approach to hermaphroditism.[19] In case reports, psychological or psychoanalytic analysis gradually became as important as medical examination, laboratory tests, and exploratory surgery. Reporting on a single exceptional case, psychiatrists and psychologists pleaded with medical practitioners to take their patients' psychological sex into consideration—rather than just focusing on anatomical features of true sex. Physicians and psychologists assessed the dreams, fantasies, desires, and ambitions of their hermaphroditic patients, describing them as male or female in stereotypically gendered ways.

This shift toward psychological sex was paralleled by significant changes in medical technology, surgery, and birth practices. Starting in the 1880s, physicians endorsed surgery as an appropriate intervention with growing insistence.[20] The introduction of asepsis and anesthesia had made surgery a more accessible and popular tool in the diagnosis and treatment of hermaphroditic patients—a development linked to the changes in surgical technology as much as to concerns about homosexuality.[21] Physicians worried that the "ambiguous" sexual status of their patients could, even unbeknownst to them, involve them in homosexual coupling, and surgery gave them the "ability to reestablish hermaphrodites within the boundaries of dimorphic sex, both physically and behaviorally."[22] New technologies such as anesthesia also made it easier to access and examine the bodies of people whose sex was doubted. In her analysis of nineteenth-century case reports of hermaphroditism in Europe, the historian Geertje Mak has shown how difficult it was at times for physicians to examine the bodies of those whose sex was in question.[23] Adult women often refused to have their genitals inspected by a male physician. This changed at the end of the nineteenth century when anesthesia became one of the available techniques "to overcome a patient's shame and pain" during a physical examination of the body.[24] Another factor was the growing number of hospital births. Physicians were increasingly present at birth and therefore diagnosed ambiguous sex at an earlier age; they dealt with parents and infants rather than with adult patients themselves.[25] They would increasingly build on the "data" from adult cases to promote early intervention. Assigning the right sex was an ever-increasing concern and cause of uncertainty.

By the 1940s, physical examinations of patients with intersex traits and "corrective" genital surgeries had become so routine that some psychiatrists and psychologists felt it necessary to caution their colleagues to delay procedures such as clitoridectomies or the removal of testes or ovaries until patients had undergone an array of psychological tests, psychiatric examinations, or psychoanalysis. They did not reject surgeries on principle but rather urged the primacy of psychological over biological sex. The majority of patients who underwent "corrective" surgery were teenagers or young adults who had already adapted to a sex role and wanted their psyche aligned with the visual appearance of their genitals. In such cases, psychiatrists thought that to insist on adjusting their bodies to their gonadal or chromosomal sex could have dire consequences such as serious psychological problems, maladjustment, and as they stressed again and again, unhappiness.

This insistence on psychological expertise in determining a different form of true sex and the privileging of a notion of psychological true sex over an anatomical one reflect the extent to which American society had become psychologized. That many practitioners so easily accepted that children became male or female regardless of or in spite of their biological sex was an expression of the new focus on the environment and on culture that dominated US social thought in general and the social sciences in particular.[26] This shift is obvious in the report on S. M. that the psychiatrist Jacob E. Finesinger, the gynecologist Joe V. Meigs, and the physician Hirsh W. Sulkowitch published in the *American Journal of Obstetrics and Gynecology* in 1942.[27] The first author, Finesinger, had been trained at Johns Hopkins University and Medical School, where he received a bachelor of arts degree in 1923, a master's degree in zoology in

1925, and his medical degree in 1929. After he became a resident in neurology at Boston City Hospital, he pursued graduate training in psychiatry at the Boston Psychopathic Hospital. He also studied psychoanalysis in Vienna and conditioned responses in Ivan Pavlov's Russian laboratory. Finesinger's time in Vienna left a deep impression on him, and he was known to acknowledge his debt to the father of psychoanalysis by commenting wryly about clueless colleagues: "We can't all be Freud!"[28] He remained in Boston as a faculty member at Harvard Medical School and at Massachusetts General Hospital until 1949, when he moved to College Park to become professor and head of the Department of Psychiatry at the University of Maryland.[29]

The 1942 article about the young woman who wanted to become a normal girl insisted on the importance of psychiatric and psychoanalytical analysis in patient treatment.[30] Even though S. M. had always considered herself a female, her doctors assessed her as biologically male. Examinations and tests revealed the "body contour of a thin boy," testes that did not, however, produce sperm, a large clitoris that "could easily be called a small penis," and a female-appearing vulva (311). A laparotomy could not locate a uterus, fallopian tubes, or ovaries. Yet all the physicians agreed that she had been reared "as a female, had feminine interests, and passed as a female." Finesinger's psychoanalytic study of the young woman set out to solve this puzzle, and he found that "the patient's early emotional development was typical of that found in females" (316). Her feminine behaviors, dreams, and ambitions included a childhood interest "in dolls, fine dresses, and in playing house" and later "in sewing, cooking, and in housework." The direction of her sexual desire was another clue to her psychosexual state: "During puberty she showed interest in boys, went to dances, and here too assumed the conventional feminine role," and she "had typical phantasies of being married and having a family" (311). Of course, since she was biologically male these fantasies could have been read as homosexuality and thus pathological. After all, sexologists had argued since the mid-nineteenth century that male sexual inverts (or homosexuals, as they later came to be called) displayed feminine behavior and characteristics, including the desire for other men.[31] It was the psychological determination of S. M.'s feminine psyche that transformed what would have been understood as homosexual desire into stereotypically gendered female behavior.

This determination was a departure from the point of view of practitioners who specialized in "hermaphroditism," such as the surgeon and urologist Hugh Hampton Young at Johns Hopkins's Brady Urological Institute. Young read from personality backward into the body and would thus have considered this patient a male who manifested female behavior and sexual desire because of female sex hormones.[32] The Massachusetts General doctors' reasoning was quite different. Their psychiatric and psychoanalytic analysis suggested instead that the patient's psychological sex was not in fact contingent on her body and that "factors other than the anatomic and glandular ones played the predominating role in [her] emotional and psychosexual development." By contrast, they wrote that "factors other than the anatomic and glandular ones played the predominating role in the emotional and psychosexual development."[33]

Finesinger and his colleagues were uncertain what it was exactly that produced this peculiar discrepancy between anatomy and psychology, but they proposed that "environmental and situational factors (reared as a girl, identification with mother, relationship to father, etc.) in the patient played the predominating role in her psychosexual and emotional development" (316). They suggested that S. M.'s relationship with her father, who had been cruel and abusive to her mother, might be one cause. The patient identified with her mother, and after her mother died giving birth to a younger sibling when S. M. was only nine years old, she "developed anxiety in relation to her father," fearing that he "would injure her just as he had beaten the mother" (315). Based on the psychological profile, Finesinger and his colleagues decided that she should continue living as a girl, and they proposed medical and surgical intervention to turn her into a more presentable woman. She was prescribed "large doses of estrogenic substances to stimulate breast development," and it was advised that later on a surgeon should attempt to construct a vagina for her (316). Rearing trumped anatomy in this case, but a convincing anatomical presentation was still essential for S. M. to continue her life as a woman.

Five years after he deemed the seventeen-year-old a girl, Finesinger saw a similar case. This individual was fifteen, and she, too, had been admitted to Massachusetts General Hospital "complaining of the absence of menses, lack of breast development, and a low-pitched voice."[34] J. E. S. "had always considered herself female" and was by her own account immensely distressed when—three years earlier—"she noticed a change in her voice which gradually became deeper and more masculine," and her clitoris "began to enlarge until finally she was ashamed to appear in a bathing suit" (1219). Physicians performed a physical and a laboratory examination, an assessment of her mental status, and an exploratory laparotomy, all of which suggested that she was male.

As revealed in the report on the case that Finesinger published in 1947 with his colleague, the gynecological surgeon Francis M. Ingersoll,

J. E. S. was sent to the psychiatric unit to decide "the true nature of her sex"—indicating not only a shift in the meaning of *true sex* but also in the expertise deemed appropriate for its determination. This issue could, according to Finesinger, be best decided by psychiatrists and psychologists. During the patient's seven admissions (presumably between 1943 and 1947), he concluded that her personality was definitely feminine. During her second admission, psychiatrists interviewed her twenty-eight times, using among other assessment instruments the Wechsler-Bellevue intelligence test, the Rorschach and thematic apperception tests, the Bernreuter Personality Inventory, the Minnesota Multiphasic Personality Inventory, and the Terman-Miles Attitude-Interest Analysis test. To obtain more details about J. E. S.'s fantasy life, they used free association. J. E. S. confirmed that she had always considered herself a female, and "during adolescence she fantasized [about] going out with boys to dances and had romantic ideas about marriage." During masturbation, she visualized "having intercourse with her future husband." This desire for intercourse with a male was interpreted as further evidence for her femininity. Finesinger stressed that in these fantasies she assumed "the passive role, and identifies with her mother and other females"—presumably to avoid any connotations of homosexual desire (1221–22).

Finesinger collected "facts" about J. E. S.'s family life, her upbringing, her personality, and her and her family's thoughts about her "problem." These details as well as the personality tests all showed "a deviation in the direction of femininity." J. E. S. identified with her mother, whom she idealized, and showed "no need for competing with males." Female qualities were listed as "neatness, orderliness and compliance." She also rejected "striving and masculine attitudes." All tests agreed that her personality was "definitely feminine." The wishes and opinions of family and of the patient herself also played an important role in assessing her sex. Her parents thought that since she had been reared as a girl, she should remain a girl. Her father even stated that "it would break my heart" if her sex were changed. But they left the authority to make this decision to the medical experts. They pleaded that their daughter remain a girl, yet they expressed their willingness to move to a new neighborhood if their daughter "returned home as a boy." J. E. S. herself wanted to be a girl and begged "to be made into one" (1222).

Whether or not the preferences of the patient and her parents played a role, as with the case of S. M., doctors determined that "the patient's predominant feelings and orientation were feminine," and therefore they set about making her anatomically more feminine. They prescribed stilbestrol, a "synthetic estrogen" first manufactured in the laboratory in 1938, to initiate menstruation and breast development (1223).[35] Doctors also decided on surgical intervention. They amputated J. E. S.'s "enlarged clitoris" without any acknowledgment of the consequences of this drastic procedure, but they retained her undescended testicle "in order to avoid castration which might have precipitated the disturbing physical and mental symptoms of the menopause."[36]

The article about the case included four "before and after" images linking psychological sex and successful adjustment to her appearance and ability to pass as a woman. The first one had been taken in 1943 and showed the patient naked, with a white bandage draped around her belly and genitals and with her chest exposed. The description read: "Patient in November, 1943. Note male physique and lack of breast development before treatment." Next to it was a photograph of her genitals taken in 1946, "showing perineum, enlarged clitoris, female urethra, intact hymen and introitus" (1219). The final two photographs had been taken in April 1947 after the decision that J. E. S. remain a girl had been made and after she had been treated with stilbestrol (1223). One image depicted the naked patient with the comment, "Note enlarged breasts and darkened areolae after stilbestrol therapy." Next to it, another image showed the patient fully dressed in female attire. Its caption read: "Note acceptable female appearance after therapy." According to her physicians, J. E. S. shared this assessment of her femininity. The report notes: "After three years of stilbestrol, her breasts developed. This pleases her. She is also grateful for the operation which removed her clitoris. 'I'm glad it turned out the way it did, I'm more suited for a girl'" (1222). Indeed, many patients may have shared the pervasive norms that underwrote these drastic interventions, unsettling though they may seem to today's reader.

The 1947 article also included a plea for doctors who came across such cases to acknowledge the importance of the psychological factors involved in them. Step by step, Ingersoll and Finesinger laid out the new marriage of psychological sex and surgery. They noted that "the appraisal of the patient's psychosexual behavior as determined by psychiatric investigation" should play a primary role in diagnosing sex. They specified that psychosexual behavior could contradict a person's structural and endocrine features. Because "situational and cultural factors played the significant role in the patient's emotional development," they proposed that all patients have access to surgical "transform[ation of] the external genitalia to fit the psychosexual behavior of the patient" once psychiatric assessment determined "sexual and social orientation" (1224–25).

"A Beautiful Experimental Situation"

As psychologists and psychiatrists increasingly inserted their expertise into diagnostic processes for individuals with intersex traits, they also used these cases to explore human sexual psychology. They asked: What was the process in which a person became masculine or feminine? How could one study the cause-and-effect mechanism of psychosexual development in humans? Hermaphrodites, they figured, were ideal experiments in nature, clues in the quest for an answer to what made individuals into men or women. The group had been the focus of many studies in the early twentieth century; as Albert Ellis wrote in 1945, "In the case of hermaphrodites we often have a beautiful experimental situation all set up for us, and all that we need to throw added light on the question of normal and abnormal sexual behavior is to observe the sexual psychology they display."[37]

What distinguished Ellis's work from that preceding it was its focus on sexual behavior to assess psychological sex.[38] His landmark study had begun as a term paper when he was a graduate student in clinical psychology at Columbia University. Ellis was interested in the question of whether homosexuality was inborn or acquired. His paper, which he published in *Psychosomatic Medicine* in 1945, examined eighty-four cases of hermaphroditism from the medical literature. Ellis was intrigued "that most hermaphrodites whose sexual direction was known were heterosexual in spite of their physiological and hormonal anomalies." Based on this, he argued that "familial and cultural teachings" strongly influenced the direction of the human sex drive.[39] Most of the time, hermaphrodites assumed "a heterosexual libido and sex role," meaning one based on attraction to the sex opposite from the one in which they were raised. Ellis consequently argued that environmental factors, rather than "direct hormonal or other physiological factors," caused heterosexuality or homosexuality in hermaphrodites.[40] Ellis, who used the common term *sex role*, had determined that sex was social. The power of the human sex drive might be contingent on physiological factors such as hormones, but, he argued, "the *direction* of this drive does not seem to be directly dependent on constitutional elements" (119, emphasis in original).

Ellis's study was remarkable. He split up sex into various characteristics: upbringing, body build, external sex organs, internal sex organs, gonads, hair growth and distribution, menstruation, sperm production, sex hormone production. Then he examined how each factor shaped sexual direction (i.e., orientation) and sex role. After comparing these social and somatic factors, he concluded that "in general, there was almost perfect agreement between the sex roles and the libidos displayed by these hermaphrodites—in spite of the fact that there was little agreement between sex roles and libidos on the one hand and any of the somatic characteristics investigated on the other" (116). Individuals raised as males predominantly had a masculine libido and sex role, and those raised as females had a feminine libido and sex role. Physiological factors, it seemed, were "not decisive in determining the masculinity or femininity of pseudohermaphrodites" (118).

Sexual direction was central to Ellis's analysis. At the time, the question of whether sexual inversion was "constitutionally" rooted or due to psychogenic causes was a live debate within psychiatry. In the first decades of the twentieth century, Sigmund Freud's psychoanalytical perspective had been among the most influential, challenging older ideas about degeneration as the cause of homosexuality. For Freud, heterosexuality was the normal outcome of proper psychosexual development. All children experienced a homosexual phase on the way to adult heterosexuality, and humans' instinctual, constitutional bisexuality allowed for both homosexual and heterosexual desire. Exclusive male adult homosexuality could have many causes but was essentially the outcome of an arrested psychosexual development and instinctual fixation that had set in before the transition to normal heterosexuality. Freud eventually postulated in his "Three Essays on the Theory of Sexuality" that an unresolved oedipal phase and intense attachment to the mother could cause male homosexuality.[41] Not all psychoanalysts agreed with Freud's thesis. For example, Sandor Rado, a Hungarian psychoanalyst who emigrated to the United States in the 1930s, rejected Freud's claim of universal bisexuality and postulated an overwhelming environmental force and phobic response to the opposite sex as a cause of homosexual behavior.[42] In the mid-1950s, Albert Ellis, who frequently lectured at the discussion groups of the homophile organization the Mattachine Society, argued similarly that "exclusive homosexuality could be explained only as a phobic response to the opposite sex and a compulsive fixation on members of the same sex."[43]

In his 1945 article on the sexual psychology of human hermaphrodites, Ellis argued that people were generally heterosexual for two reasons: one was anatomical and the other cultural. "Usually, the possession of the secondary sexual characteristics and external sex organs of one sex makes it physically more convenient and pleasurable for the possessor to have sex relations with members of the other sex," he proposed.

"Cultural patterns of living then reinforce these physical tendencies and heterosexuality results."[44] While the first part of this reasoning might be ascribed to a lack of imagination or experience—pleasure is, after all, in the body of the beholder—the second argument highlights the growing focus on cultural patterns in shaping how psychologists thought about masculinity and femininity.[45]

In his analysis, Ellis proposed a new connection between body and mind, that of appearance and psychological sex. The more convincingly these individuals passed as either sex, the more they were accepted as such and thus adjusted to their sex role and sexuality. Though he had concluded that most hermaphrodites were attracted to the sex opposite from the one in which they were reared, he attributed any departure from this—including "homosexuality, bisexuality, or psychosexual immaturity"—to distress from "having attributes of the sex other than that in which he or she has been raised, and of being conspicuously 'queer' in his or her and others' eyes because of such anomalies."[46]

The body still mattered, but in quite a different way from its role in the previous psychiatric model. It had become subordinated to psychological adjustment and a means to achieving normal development. What determined a person's sexuality and psychological sex? People had certain expectations of how a male or female body was supposed to look and developed a self-image based on their body's appearance. The experience of being perceived as male or female shaped their psychosexual development. This had important practical implications. For one, bodies could and should be shaped to minimize any "queerness" and thus consequent maladjustment. But the necessity of making psychologists part of the medical approach to hermaphroditic cases was just as big a shift. Ellis's plea reflects this: those "to whose lot the firsthand study of hermaphrodites invariably falls," he wrote, must consider it hereafter "their scientific duty" to see that "all hermaphroditic individuals who may come to their attention" receive the benefit of "thoroughgoing psychiatric and psychological investigations, in addition to the usual physiological ones."[47]

"With Respect to What Their Best Future Happiness Will Be"

The adoption of the psychologization of sex and the adjustment/maladjustment paradigm seeped into the clinic, where physicians considered psychological aspects of hermaphroditism and wrestled with the question of what constituted sex in conducting their practice. During the

Ninety-Ninth Annual Session of the American Medical Association in San Francisco in June 1950, the urologist Frank Hinman Jr. gave a talk on the treatment of and sex assignment in girls with congenital adrenal hyperplasia (CAH). The son of the first trained urologist in the state of California, Hinman had studied at Johns Hopkins Medical School under Hugh Hampton Young and had received his MD at Hopkins as well. He became a resident of urology at the University of California, joined his father in private practice, and engaged in urological research and education. In 1951, he was one of the eight founders of the Society of Pediatric Urology. In 1958, he became the Chief of Urology at San Francisco General Hospital.[48] Hinman's main research interest lay in bladder defense mechanisms, but at the 1950 AMA meeting he read his paper about an aspect of intersex: "Advisability of Surgical Reversal of Sex in Female Pseudohermaphroditism."[49]

Hinman's talk offers an interesting comparison to Lawson Wilkins's contemporaneous approach. He had even consulted with Wilkins at Hopkins in January 1949 on the case of a two-year-old girl diagnosed as having CAH and facing increasing masculinization, and he had taken the latter's advice. Wilkins explained that if the patient in question had been older and already been reared as a girl, he would have suggested keeping her in the female sex. In this particular case, however, he suggested choosing the male sex, because "raising her as a boy would present fewer problems in later life." If Hinman pursued this path, Wilkins recommended "that the ovaries and uterus might later be removed." The child was "discharged to be raised as a boy, named Allen rather than Anita," and the birth certificate was changed by affidavit and "without difficulty."[50]

Like Wilkins, Hinman was not ready to completely overthrow the dogma of gonadal sex. He had, he assured his audience, "no quarrel with the use of gonadal sex as the basis for treatment of male pseudohermaphrodites." Yet he shared with Jacob Finesinger and his colleagues a conviction of the importance of psychiatric evaluation in sex assignment.[51] He also aligned with their positive view of surgical interventions, proclaiming that "most children with intersexual external genitalia can be converted into acceptable boys or into acceptable girls by appropriate surgical measures," indicating not only the availability of such surgical procedures but also their general acceptance. He was, however, ready to ignore gonadal sex in females with CAH based on the specificities of their symptoms. They faced progressive masculinization after birth, and they developed the "secondary sex characteristics of a boy" as well as a "deep voice, a somewhat masculine physique, a beard and hairy body and a receding hair line."[52] Thus, they should be raised as boys.

Hinman counseled his fellow physicians to consider all "surgical, endocrinologic, psychologic, moral and legal" aspects of sexual ambiguity.
In his discussion of five patients with CAH at his clinic whose gonads
indicated they were female, he wondered whether they might be better
off living as men. It was urgent that physicians be aware of this option,
to avoid the practice of clitoridectomy at an early age and consequently
forsake the possibility of a sex reversal to male. "The purpose of this
paper," Hinman voiced empathically, was "to prevent needless phallic
sacrifice" (423). These girls could be raised as either masculinized females or sterile males with ovaries. Even if they were raised as female,
he advised physicians "to defer clitoridectomy until puberty to be certain that the factors favoring ultimate feminization will still be present"
(428). Despite this caution, Hinman's expectation that surgery would
necessarily, sooner or later, be part of the treatment of such cases is another indication of the surgical shift in the treatment of patients with
intersex traits.[53]

The cases Hinman described were of patients between the ages of
three and a half and eighteen years, whose parents first sought treatment for them during their infancy. This timing was crucial, as Hinman
argued that by the age of two, enough signs would have manifested
themselves to enable a near-final assessment of what surgery would be
ultimately advisable. Correspondingly, physicians like Wilkins recommended diagnosing intersex conditions early so that competent and
knowledgeable physicians could decide which sex to assign.[54] "And it
is at this age—before irreversible social and psychic changes have taken
place—that the decision as to sex must be made, to be determined,"
Hinman argued.[55] Surgically, it would be possible to construct a phallus out of a clitoris "so that at puberty the boy will have a serviceable
penis." As for appearance, these girls would continue to virilize and look
increasingly male.[56] Hinman gave his talk just as cortisone was being
tested as a possible treatment for children with CAH, but he mentioned
this new treatment option only in passing, referencing Wilkins's case
report published months earlier.[57] If cortisone was deemed safe for use,
it would be most useful for girls who had already been raised as girls, he
noted. "Whether it should be administered to children with strong masculine social and psychologic trends might be questioned," he added.[58]

When Hinman turned to the psychological aspects of raising a girl in
the male sex, he told his AMA audience that he supported the general
agreement of psychologists and psychiatrists. Hormones were responsible for the "quantity of sexual drive," but "psychologic and environmental forces" shaped the direction of that drive. He argued that the

cases reported in the literature suggested that his patients and any other girls with CAH assigned as male would adjust well to masculinity. Sexual direction served as indicator of proper adjustment to sex. He cited Albert Ellis's claim regarding the heterosexuality of pseudohermaphrodites, assuring doctors that part of the adjustment would include choosing "women as sex objects." Age was also crucial, as "a person seen early enough (before the age of 2 or 3 years) will fit best in the sex in which he has been arbitrarily raised."[59] Hinman's statement reflected general agreement about the first two to three years being formative in child development. His consideration also implicated the subtle shift from accepting patients' psychological sex as their "true sex" to arguing that children will adjust to the sex in which they had been "arbitrarily raised." In short, Hinman acknowledged a shift in clinical practice from accepting that children's psychological sex was shaped by their environment to considering the possibility of controlling the outcome of psychological sex development.

Hinman stressed that his recommendations could support patient happiness. Indeed, he addressed the question of any moral objections to accepting a person's social sex over the biological one by saying that his advice was both pragmatic and compassionate. He did acknowledge the existence of objections by the Catholic Church. The success he had promised in making the patient sexually attracted to females would be the driver of this objection. Since the church believed that a person's "actual or genetic sex" never changed, this aspect of CAH treatment would lead to a female desiring another female (427). Representatives of the Episcopal Church, on the other hand, saw no religious factor involved, but they recommended "the person be given the fullest opportunity for spiritual integrity and development." Hinman noted that religious objections to following psychological sex could easily end in tragedy, the most prominent example being a well-known case observed by Hugh Hampton Young. In his monograph, Young described how a priest had forbidden a young man to marry his fiancée because he was biologically female (though raised in the male sex), and the young man had consequently died by suicide (428).[60] In addition, Hinman advised that "for his own protection, the physician should of course have written permission from both parents and be assured of their full understanding and consent," although he did not believe there could be serious legal objection to the practice he proposed (428).

The brief discussion that followed Hinman's talk suggests he had a receptive audience. No one objected to his proposition that upbringing and environment, rather than anatomy, determined a person's psychological sex. Rather, his colleagues agreed that the happiness of these patients was at stake and that a prognosis of happiness trumped any biological prerogative. "I think," one audience member agreed, that Hinman "makes a good point, that [patients] should be considered with respect to what their best future happiness will be, and probably a great many of them will be much happier if raised as males than if raised as females, even though they are genetically females" (429). A prognosis of future happiness would continue to serve as justification for medical and surgical interventions.

To Be Happy and Well Adjusted

Lawson Wilkins's team in the Pediatric Endocrinology Clinic at Johns Hopkins's Harriet Lane Home for Invalid Children started developing standardized recommendations for diagnosing sex in the late 1940s. They did so based on Wilkins's clinical experience with patients with CAH as well as their increasing reliance on the authority of psychiatrists and psychologists. Some of the HLH patients and their families visited his clinic multiple times over many years, and as the children grew up in and through these clinical encounters, they participated in the creation of a psychological profile not just of the child but of the family unit. The latter was considered an important environment in which adjustment and psychological health was both assessed and manufactured. Patient records show that what seems consistent and well thought out in published case studies was in fact an inconsistent patchwork and constant adaptation. They reveal the actual work invested in diagnosis, sex assignment, and consequent assessment of psychological health to determine whether children adjusted well to the sex they were living in. Within multiple visits, clinicians adapted to what seemed the best strategy at the time.

Carol's case is a fitting example for the shifting landscape of sex. First, the psychiatric evaluations of her case concerned the entire family unit for determining proper adjustment (and sex roles). Second, the interventions to match her appearance to the sex she was being raised in (which happened to be her gonadal and chromosomal sex) yet again displayed the conviction that clinicians could (and should) choose the sex that seemed best for the child's prognosis of adjustment and happiness. And finally, in her file we find that her mother's understanding of happiness and a life well lived was incommensurate with the clinicians' definitions of adjustment and health.

Born in the fall of 1941, Carol was Wilkins's patient from twelve days after her birth until his death in 1963.[61] As an infant, she was diagnosed as having the non-salt-losing and thus non-life-threatening form of congenital adrenal hyperplasia. Contrary to the advice he would later give Frank Hinman Jr., Wilkins advised the parents to raise her as a girl after a laparotomy revealed internal female reproductive organs. He focused his clinical care on the somatic manifestation of her condition, such as virilization and accelerated growth, but he also took pains to assess whether she developed "normally" in terms of her sex assignment. During the twenty-three years that Carol visited the clinic at least once a year, Wilkins and his colleagues evaluated her level of adjustment as part of their medical evaluations. Her behavior over the years was noted in the record next to her physiological values and closely followed during each admission as Wilkins and his colleagues observed her appearance and her (inconsistent) gender performance. In 1944 they wrote, "She is a very bright, active, precocious child. Appears quite intelligent. Her appearance and actions [seem] to be quite feminine." The following year, Wilkins thought she had a "very feminine appearance." He assessed Carol's gender at every visit, noting in 1948 that she was a "tomboy" and that "she still will p[l]ay as easily with boys' toys as with girls['], which causes her mother some concern." "The child in general," he wrote, "is hyperactive, rough in her play and has a rather deep voice."

Between 1945 and 1950, Carol was psychologically evaluated twice, although Wilkins paid ongoing attention to her gender expression through her behavior. Both evaluations provide insights into the psychologization of everyday life, the concerns about well-adjusted families bringing up well-adjusted children, and the importance of gendered norms. The first occurred in 1945, when Wilkins recommended that a psychiatrist see the four-year-old and her parents to discuss "the neighborhood problem." Carol's condition had put her at the center of "much sexual attention" by little boys. "One of the neighbors has called on the mother to get more detailed information about [Carol]'s condition," Wilkins wrote, and he advised the parents to move to a new neighborhood. The Hopkins psychiatrist Dr. Jacob H. Conn assessed Carol's psychological state and concluded that "the problem is a very complex one including endocrinological, psychological and social factors." Conn, a 1929 graduate of the University of Maryland Medical School and a private practitioner, had been affiliated with the Johns Hopkins Hospital since 1931.[62] He was also a hypnotist and a child psychiatrist who had developed a method of play interview to deal with phobias in children. He interviewed both Carol and her parents, evaluating the whole family unit for emotional stability. Dr. Conn's report was integrated into the consecutive notes in Carol's patient record that cover the years between 1944 and 1946 alongside notes on treatment for pharyngitis (August 1945: "Treatment: bed, fluids, aspirin"), administration of worm medicine (March 1946), and general examinations (April 1946: "Has been very well except for colds. Ravenous appetite, Very active. Bowels okay." "Child continues to grow and virilize at rapid rate").

Although Conn concluded that Carol exhibited "no serious neurotic behavior pattern," he was less sure about her parents. In his interview with the mother, Conn learned that she had initially not told her husband about their daughter's diagnosis for fear that he might die by suicide. The mother's account of her husband's emotional state cast doubt on "her own stability," Conn noted. Five years later in her second psychological evaluation at Hopkins, she would still remember this moment, and she told the psychologist:

At the time I went to Dr. Conn—well, maybe I ought not to tell you—but when I left his office I thought he thought I was practically insane, I didn't go back. . . . At the time [Carol] was born, I didn't tell my husband. It had just been a year since his mother's death. During that year that the baby was coming, he was so disinterested. Then along came the baby and he fell right in love with her. He'd never had anyone dependent upon him. I did not tell him [about Carol's diagnosis] until the second baby was born. Dr. Conn thought I was just a little short of crazy.

Conn described Carol's mother as "a very determined over-protective type of person who must 'plan' for everyone with whom she comes into contact." She was indeed well trained and educated, and even though she had become a stay-at-home mom and housewife, Conn thought that she was still "the head of the family."[63] But, he wrote, "as far as I can determine [the mother] was very pleased with the psychiatric interview."

The suspicion of an overbearing mother underlying Conn's assessment was widespread in the mid-1940s. Blaming mothers for maladjusted children was certainly not new, and ensuring proper gender and sexuality had long been at the center of these concerns.[64] In 1942, the author Philip Wylie coined the term *Momism* in his book *Generation of Vipers* to complain about mothers' supposedly excessive protection of their children and the smothering of especially the male child, which would inevitably result in a generation of weak and dependent men.[65] By 1945, Wylie's depiction of middle-class and middle-aged women as domestic tyrants became the most compelling and publicized aspect of his book—even though, as the historian Rebecca Jo Plant shows, the author was actually reacting to the obsolete ideology of moral mother-hood that had been dominant during the interwar period. Nevertheless, many contemporaries across the political spectrum appropriated his "anti-maternalist" critique. Although Wylie himself lacked scientific credentials and was known as much for writing fiction as nonfiction, popular media such as *Look* magazine ran excerpts of the book. It influenced psychiatrists and social scientists, who began "to appropriate and expand on the concept in works of their own, lending it a semblance of scientific credibility."[66]

Beyond mothers, social scientists, psychologists, and psychiatrists alike worried about what was wrong with the American family in the mid- to late 1940s. Families were "personality factories"[67] and crucial for producing well- or maladjusted American children. In this environment, advanced by the same confidence in psychiatric expertise that drove the turn toward psychological sex, the new field of family therapy emerged in the 1950s. The family unit became the new patient, expanding the attention on the mother-child relationship.[68] It is not surprising, then, that Conn focused on sex roles in the family. After all, Carol was supposed to learn these from her parents, and since there was already concern whether a virilized girl with congenital adrenal hyperplasia (CAH) could fulfill a feminine role, the reversal of roles in her family was seen as problematic.

When Wilkins started treating his patients with cortisone in 1950, Carol was among them. The second psychological evaluation of her and her parents followed the beginning of this treatment, and it involved three separate doctors. The notes on this evaluation total seven pages and feature many direct quotes. Doctors St. Clair, Gaits, and Putkoski (which department they were from is unclear) first interviewed the mother and the father separately. The parents' masculinity and femininity were at the center of their concerns, specifically the suspected role reversal. Carol's mother, they noted, "gives the impression of a human adding machine, and a rather domineering and masculine one at that. She talked quite profusely and at times would cut short one sentence in order to start on another. She fidgeted with her hands and gloves and seemed quite tense." The father, they thought, seemed weak and emotionally unstable. This family portrait, consisting of direct quotes from their interview, reveals as much about the value system of the Hopkins physicians as about the family.

Carol's case also reveals how the practice of observing and determining a person's psychological sex could slip into engineering the proper sex. This was in a way the natural outgrowth of the acknowledgment

that psychological sex was shaped by the person's environment and upbringing. While Wilkins's advice to Hinman in 1949 suggests that he
may have been wishing he had suggested that Carol be assigned the
male gender at birth, his handling of Carol's case shows that by 1951
the availability of cortisone, and thus the option to halt and reverse
virilization, made both Wilkins and his colleagues feel that the female
sex would be the best choice. The team evaluated the appearance of
eight-year-old Carol (dark complexion, deep and masculine voice), her
behavior (assertive and bossy), and her choice of toys (a Roy Rogers pis-
tol). Carol told her parents that she was actually a little boy. She also
stated that she was in love with a girl in sixth grade, Mary Rose,[69] and
that she would marry her because "she has long hair and she doesn't like
any boys—just me." After studying her behavior, the team of psychiatrists assessed that Carol was "more of a little boy than a girl." Reluctant
to change her sex assignment at the age of eight and convinced that
she would become more female in the course of cortisone treatment,
the doctors recommended that better adjusting her body to her sex of
rearing would improve her psychological adjustment: "In conference
it was felt that plastic surgery to create a satisfactory vagina for [Carol]
should be considered and that psychotherapy with [Carol] and both
parents should be undertaken." Her masculine tendencies, they hoped,
would disappear once her body was made to better fit her sex of rearing and her family unit was properly therapized. Proper adjustment to
sex role and sexual direction (i.e., attraction to men) would follow. The
doctors considered her masculine tendencies to be a reversible result of
conflicts between an assigned female sex and living in a male-appearing
body. They were convinced that such resolution would ensure her future
happiness.

But Carol's case shows how the treatment goal of happiness was very
much in the eye of the beholder. Both her physicians and her parents
claimed that her health and future happiness were their main concern. Yet the psychological interview reveals that health and happiness
meant different things to these groups. Carol's mother worried about
her daughter and her future—after all, before cortisone became available as treatment, Wilkins had told her that Carol would never marry
or have sexual intercourse. Dr. TeLinde, the gynecologist at the time,
had disagreed with this assessment, but Carol's mother mentioned that
"Dr. Wilkins said no and he's always right." She told the team, who interviewed her, "Dr. Wilkins advised me not to have any more children,
and he told me she would never be a marriageable woman." Carol was

the eldest in the family, and Wilkins had indeed recommended that her parents not have more children because they might also have CAH.

Two of Carol's younger brothers did have CAH, but her mother expressed no regrets. "I feel it's terrible to have no one close to you," she said, suggesting that a daughter doomed to spinsterhood had all the greater need for siblings. "After all, [my husband and I] won't live forever. Anyway I went ahead. Both of the boys have this adrenal condition." Carol's mother was operating with a different currency of what counted to make life worth living. If the medical prognosis was loneliness, then her concern trumped Wilkins's worries about heredity and disease. However, she said, she was worried that her sons could never become fathers and that Carol would never marry. "I'm more worried about [Carol]," she added, because her daughter "has pseudo-hermaphroditism. She'll never be able to get married." In fact, those physicians who had recommended, as Hinman had, assigning people with Carol's medical profile to the male gender identity sometimes put marriageability at the center of their recommendations. A woman who would not be able to marry might be hard-pressed to support herself; male sex assignment would be a practical solution.

Measuring Adjustment

Whereas Carol's mother saw her children's future happiness as a reflection of multiple factors, practitioners like Lawson Wilkins saw appearance as a benchmark for proper adjustment and future happiness. In cases of children with CAH, he worried that male-appearing girls would have a hard time becoming socially integrated; after all, how could a girl who looked like a boy live a normal, happy, and well-adjusted life as a woman? His treatment of Karen reflects the full expression of this view.

When Wilkins first saw Karen in his clinic in 1947, she had already led a life full of medical intervention, having been a patient of Hugh Hampton Young's at the Brady Urological Institute since shortly after her birth in 1934.[70] There had been uncertainty about her sex at birth, and after a laparotomy confirmed the presence of female reproductive organs (in 1939!) and thus her already assigned female sex (and the diagnosis of CAH), Young operated on her genitals to form a separate urethra and vagina. During this procedure, he also amputated her clitoris, which in his estimation was too large (i.e., male appearing). Then in 1942, Young performed an adrenalectomy of her left adrenal in a failed attempt to combat the symptoms of CAH. The same year, he prescribed stilbestrol with the rationale that it would have an antagonistic reaction to the high presence of virilizing androgens, thus counteracting their impact on Karen's appearance.

Wilkins evaluated fourteen-year-old Karen as having a peculiar mixture of male and female attributes. As a result of Young's stilbestrol prescription, she developed breasts. But Wilkins noted that she was also excessively hairy.[71] Even though he generally rejected estrogen as treatment for CAH, he continued her prescription, because he thought she seemed to respond well to it. The decision to continue a hormonal treatment with no therapeutic effect other than feminizing certain features of a patient was an expression of the rather murky terrain involved in treating Karen. The point of the stilbestrol, in Wilkins's view, was to encourage feminine development and to counterbalance the physically "masculinizing" effects of androgens. She had in fact had breasts since the age of seven because of the hormone treatment.

In Wilkins's assessment, Karen was well adjusted overall. She was doing "satisfactorily" in school and getting along well with her peers, and, he added rather cryptically, "there have been no sexual difficulties." Sexual behavior was another measurement of proper adjustment, and though he never defined or explained what he meant by "sexual difficulties," his notes in other patient records suggest that such difficulties included exhibitionism, paying too much attention to one's genitals, frequent erections (impossible in Karen's case, given her surgery), and masturbation. More important for her adjustment, in Wilkins's view, was that she could socially pass as a woman. "Her condition is unusually presentable for a female pseudohermaphrodite of this age," he wrote, and "in fact, in her clothes she could pass for a normal girl of 16 to 18 years." Passing—that is, to convincingly appear as one's own sex despite somatic contradictions—included her demeanor, her appearance, her behavior, and her personality, all of which were expressions of successful socialization as a girl and/or woman.[72] Wilkins noted, "Her disease certainly seems to have produced a minimum of psychological problems. She seems well adjusted and quite happy."

––––––

By the late 1940s, a widespread psychologization of American society and a popular acceptance of the paradigm of adjustment and maladjustment had long since become part of the medical evaluation of sex, shifting how medical practitioners approached the question of determining a person's true sex. Not only did psychiatrists profess to have the skill set to determine psychological sex, but they also argued that it was a better indication of the sex a person should live in than any biological sex characteristics. They recommended that psychiatric evaluation and psychoanalytical studies become essential components in the assessment of sex in intersex patients. If these individuals' psychosexuality contradicted their anatomy, it might be the better approach to adjust their body to their psychological sex through surgery and with the prescription of hormones. For many clinician-researchers, these recommendations seemed intuitive and convincing.

Nevertheless, clinicians' approaches to what actually constituted sex between the early 1940s and the early 1950s seem inconsistent at times. In their case studies, they describe slightly different constellations of the interaction between nature and nurture, psychological sex and the body, and doctors and their patients. For Jacob Finesinger it mattered much, for example, that his teenage patient, diagnosed as male pseudohermaphrodite, said she was female and wanted to remain a girl. Frank Hinman Jr., who pleaded that his colleagues include a psychiatric assessment of a patient's sex before making any irreversible interventions and who stressed the importance of environmental factors, nevertheless also claimed in the same breath that gonads were the sole determiner of sex in cases of pseudohermaphroditism. Negotiations and measurements of sex in Wilkins's clinical records reveal that he expected psychological sex to follow sex assignment. For him, it mattered little that Carol said she wanted to be a boy and behaved like one (as determined by mid-century measurement of behavior and toy choice) or that Karen's femininity was that of a young woman several years beyond her actual age. Yet all these case studies share the acknowledgment that psychological sex could differ from anatomical sex and the assumption of a malleable body which could be adapted to a person's psychological sex. The goal of medical intervention in intersex cases was no longer determining an unobtainable true sex but assuring that these patients would become well-adjusted individuals.

Coming of Age

We sometimes find even our own bodies opaque. We may be sick without knowing why, or in what way or how seriously. We may be sick, even without a sense
of sickness.

In the previous chapter, we met Karen, whose life had been
full of medical intervention from the day she was born in
the fall of 1934, weighing a little over seven pounds, as
the first and only child of her parents.[1] I have described
her psychological evaluations, her clinical visits, and the
evaluation of her adjustment. This chapter addresses how
Karen experienced her condition, as she grew up always in
negotiations with the clinic. Like most girls with congenital adrenal hyperplasia (CAH), Karen lived a life of intense
medical management and surveillance but for a long time
was told little about her condition. Thus, as she grew up
inside and outside the clinic, she had few tools with which
to make sense of clinical encounters and medical interventions, many of which focused on questions of her sexual
anatomy, gender role, and sexuality. How did Karen experience a life mediated by medical intervention and by the
attention given to her body? In the following, I have tried
to reconstruct Karen as a person from the records of her medical life by following disjunctions, errors, resistances, compli-
ances, and the few notes about the life she might have led
outside the clinic.

At first, there is no voice. Just a baby, whose sex was
debated when she was born. The attending doctor noted
her genitals and thought that her clitoris was enlarged, but
since "there was a definite vaginal opening," he eventu-

ally pronounced the baby a girl. For the next two years, her parents raised Karen as their daughter. But in 1936 when she was twenty-seven months old, they became worried about the appearance of her genitals and took her to the Johns Hopkins Hospital. During the examination, doctors saw a "penis-like clitoris" and proclaimed it was "impossible to say whether the child [was] male or female." Only a laparotomy would tell, but Karen was too young in their opinion for such a procedure. On top of that, they were almost certain that she had adrenal hyperplasia. As she had no life-threatening symptoms, the doctors advised the parents to bring their daughter home and return the following year.

Karen's medical record extends thirty-one years until 1967, when she—for reasons not noted in her patient record—stopped visiting the clinic. Before that time, Karen had experienced medical examinations, evaluations and tests, relationships with doctors and nurses, and symptoms of CAH, including those obvious to her and everyone around her and those unnoted by anyone other than her physicians. Doctors closely studied and monitored her health, her body, her genitals, her appearance, and her behavior. As Karen grew up, however, her voice increasingly inserts herself into the record, and her story reveals both the opacity of her illness experience and the porosity of the border between the clinic and the world that surrounds it. This is her story in the patient record.

The Hopkins doctors did not recommend laparotomy until Karen reached the age of four and a half years. Thus, for more than two years after her initial visit they were still not 100% sure about her sex despite repeated examinations, although they generally thought Karen was female. Her parents considered her a girl and raised her as a daughter. The diagnosis of CAH required a confident confirmation of sex, but there were other factors as well. The urologist Hugh Hampton Young, Hopkins's eminent expert on hermaphroditism and adrenal hyperplasia at the time, performed the exploratory procedure "to confirm once and for all female sex." He took tissue samples from what he thought was her ovary and, according to the record, "did a plastic operation to form a separate vagina and urethra." He also amputated Karen's clitoris—an intervention of drastic consequences yet noted in the surgical report without any further comment.

Karen's patient record reveals much about Young's medical motivation and sense of success. Fourteen days after the operation, he wrote with apparent satisfaction, "With the legs in normal position the vulva looks absolutely normal." However, he noted, "it is only 2 weeks since operation and it is not thought wise to insert a finger or make a vaginal

KAREN

examination. The immediate result of the operation seems to be splendid." Young advised that Karen's vagina had "not been instrumented or dilated since operation as it was thought better to wait and let [the family physician] do this at home." She was discharged fifteen days after her operation and scheduled to return in five months. Her record claims she "had a smooth convalescence." Yet there are traces that indicate otherwise, including notes in her record that the little girl was "hard to manage."

A year and a half later, in 1941, Karen and her parents returned for another admittance to Hopkins to "check on her unusual pseudohermaphroditic condition." Her parents thought their daughter was doing quite well. She was described as "a healthy looking, well developed and well-nourished white girl." Karen, now six, physically resisted the medical examination. She was, it is noted in the record, "not cooperative at all" and "would not permit examination [of her labia] by palpation." Upon their visual inspection, her physicians noted that there was "no clitoris" and that the "hair growth of pubic hair [was] rather excessive and follows male pattern." During this admission, Karen underwent another procedure. This time, Young performed a "bilateral exploration of the adrenals and the removal of the left adrenal," a common surgical approach to adrenal hyperplasia at the time.

With her sex confirmed, her genitals "fixed" to fit a particular version of her confirmed sex, and the attempt to combat her adrenal hyperplasia through surgery completed, Karen had undergone the last of her major operations. Medical interventions continued, however, and in lieu of therapies, these focused on chronicling her development and measuring and enhancing her femininity. In 1942, the synthetic estrogen stilbestrol was prescribed to feminize the seven-year-old girl, and her doctors considered this prescription a success, noting "some development in her breasts and the progress of virilization seemed to be arrested." Karen took the drug for the next five years, and her body was carefully monitored during that time: her height and weight, her 17-ketosteroids level, her increasing hirsutism, and her bouts of acne that doctors sought to combat with an increase in her stilbestrol dosage.

Hugh Hampton Young retired in 1942 and died in 1945. By this time, patients with CAH had started going to Lawson Wilkins's Pediatric Endocrinology Clinic. In 1947 at the age of thirteen, Karen met Wilkins for the first time, and he would continue to be her physician until his death in 1963. Karen, now in eighth grade, was assessed once again at the facility: She was doing "satisfactorily," and, the doctor's note continued, "she gets along well with other children and does not seem too much concerned about condition." She was tall for her age and precocious, all signs of CAH. Wilkins described Karen as muscular, with hair growth on her abdomen, thighs, and legs. In the record we also find a note that, due to the stilbestrol, there was "a rather surprising amount of breast development."

When she was a teenager, Karen's femininity was at the center of medical attention. "Throughout all this time the girl has been brought up as a normal girl," her doctor wrote. Her social integration was carefully followed, and it seemed important to note that in her second year of high school, she participated "in all teen age activities and gets along well with one and all." In January 1948, Wilkins described her as "intelligent," "well mannered," and "unusually presentable for a female pseudohermaphrodite of this age." "In fact," he mused, "in her clothes she could pass for a normal girl of 16 to 18 years." Throughout the whole year, Karen's life was structured around repeated and extensive hospital visits and long absences from home, friends, and school. She alternately resisted and complied with the doctors' prescriptions: "During this period she was on a constant calculated diet which she took fairly well but there were frequent refusals [emphasis in original, with pen]."

At the age of fourteen and after twelve years of medical encounters, Karen started taking cortisone. Treatment with "Compound E" was still experimental at the time, and for this reason she was admitted for two months to Wilkins's clinic for observation. "Karen is a pseudohermaphrodite," Wilkins wrote. "Although she still exhibits marked evidence of virilism, when dressed she is unexpectedly feminine in her appearance and manner and a remarkable adjustment to the problem appears to have been made." His hope was to reduce the "adrenal cortical hormone from the endogenous source" and consequently reduce her "virilism." Wilkins considered the cortisone trial a success: Karen's 17-KS were substantially lowered. There were no changes in her physical exam. That is, she did not look less virilized. Karen, it seems, was becoming "healthier," though she may not have perceived any change.

No one had yet told Karen what it meant that she had a condition called CAH. She knew "little of the implications of her condition and understands this hospitalization is another attempt to initiate the menses." Amenorrhea served as an explanation for her constant presence in the hospital, for the tests and procedures that spilled into her daily life in the form of collecting urine samples, and for the need to take daily dosages of cortisone. At fifteen, an age when most of her peers were menstruating and going through puberty, she had "never been told of her endocrine disturbance and no problems have arisen concerning this

except for some questions as to the reason for her failure to menstruate."
When in January 1952, at the age of eighteen, her menses finally com-
menced, it was noted in the record as a moment of medical triumph:
"Phone conversation with [mother] revealed that on Wed. [Karen]
started to menstruate. Bleeding has continued until the present times
using two napkins a day. In the first day of menstruation [Karen] had abdominal discomfort." The dates and intervals of her menstruation were
added to the many measurements that were already taken on every visit.

Increasingly, Karen's life and wishes occupied more space in the record. For example, in 1950 one doctor arranged "that some plan be made
for providing activity for Karen during the time she is in the hospital."
This was the first time the record specifically addressed her long stays in
the hospital and the effects those might have on her. A worker from social services talked to Karen about what she wanted to do during her stay
and described her as an "agreeable, friendly girl who seems to be most
accepting of her hospitalization." She was "perhaps a little more mature
than most sixteen year olds" due to her frequent hospitalizations. Otherwise, Karen's interests were "typical teen age—the traditional football
game in her community, worry over school work, interest in getting 'experience' that will help her when she gets a job." The teenager was eager
to shake up her hospital routine, or, as the social worker put it, "[Karen]
was most pleased by the interest shown by the staff in helping her pass
time and expresses this. She said that it was boring hanging around the
ward all day with nothing special to do; if there was some way she could
use her typing it would help her keep up with her class [which she was
taking in high school]." The social worker arranged meetings with the
person in charge of all volunteer activities and then left it to Karen to
"work things out." She started working in the volunteer activities office,
where she read to patients and wrote letters for them in the afternoons.

Karen's relationship with the clinic and its occupants gradually shifted,
however. Sometimes she objected to yet another examination. In June
1942, the attending doctor was far from pleased with her attitude. "Examination was very limited," he wrote in the examination notes, "since
[Karen] was extremely cantankerous about being examined [emphasis in
the original, with pen]." In Karen's teenage years, what had been previously described as her being occasionally "difficult to manage" (1939)
and "not cooperative at all" (1941) turned into frequent reluctance to be
subjected to the pedantic examinations and objection to the display of
her body for teaching purposes. By the age of sixteen, she seems to have
become increasingly impatient with the whole routine. The intern, who
examined her meticulously, wrote in his notes: "She is quite reluctant to

undergo the proposed study, and treats all questions and proceedings as unnecessary but inevitable. When approached on other matters, she is quite relaxed and pleasant."

Other times, the clinic became a surprising ally in Karen's quest for independence and selfhood. In 1952 the eighteen-year-old, still an only child, was trying to gain some independence: "Her home life is said to be overprotected by her father and mother, and the patient is not able to express her hopes and fears to her mother. It is hoped that a change in environment will be beneficial." Not all clinical relations were the same. Karen was getting along with some medical personnel better than others and formed alliances of trust with some and not others. She increasingly voiced her preference in these medical encounters, evident only in short notes in the record: "[Karen] came today for examination but is very nervous and says she is always nervous unless examined by Dr. Wilkins [emphasis in the original, with pen]."[2]

After the hope that cortisone would be a cure for CAH turned into the certainty that it was to be taken for life, Karen continued to come to the clinic into her adulthood. She returned for evaluation of her cortisone dosage and for tests and measurement once a year. Over the years, she gradually gained independence. In 1953 at the age of nineteen, she started working at her first job. Four years later, as she pursued further professional training, she was renting "a room in a private home." In 1959, she started a new job with higher qualifications based on her training, "about which she is quite happy," and moved to the YWCA.

Karen's independence again shifted her relationship with the clinic. Control was at the center of this relationship. In her childhood, her doctors had communicated with her parents to ensure that she was taking her medicine and controlling her weight. As Karen started to live independently and away from home, she took over her own medical responsibility. Her doctors now communicated directly with her, at times growing frustrated with the lack of medical control they could now exert over her. For example, she kept forgetting to take her medication. In 1954, Wilkins wrote, "She admits that she occasionally forgets a pill." He thought this was the main cause of her irregular menses, yet all he could do was remind her and complain about her carelessness. In 1956, Karen again admitted that she forgot "at times to take her cortisone, particularly at night." In 1961, an impatient underlining in the record indicates that she was still forgetting to take her medication: "It has been emphasized to her once more the importance of taking her cortisone regularly [emphasis in original]."

Doctors turned to Karen's parents to compel compliance but with little success, although her mother wrote letters to her physicians reporting on and inquiring about their daughter's irregular menses. In 1962, after finding Karen's 17-KS level too high, doctors even wrote to the mother of the then twenty-eight-year-old, urging her to make sure "that she is taking the medication in the prescribed amount and manner." The mother replied as if the responsibility of communicating with Karen lay with the doctors: "If [Karen] was not taking cortisone regularly, she was urged to do so." Karen kept forgetting to take her pills on the weekends—as the doctors complained in 1964—thereby affecting the regularity of her menstruation and, in their view, the success of the treatment.

Another point of conflict was Karen's weight. Weight gain was a side effect of the cortisone treatment, and her doctors wanted her to lose weight. Karen, however, refused to adhere to the diet doctors had prescribed for her "obesity." On every visit her weight was taken, her obesity noted, and her adherence to the diet or lack thereof observed. This led to a litany of comments on her appearance:

In 1952 at 147.5 lbs.: "Although [Karen] has lost 8lbs, she is still considerably overweight and of short stocky build."

In 1953 at 156 lbs.: "Is not adhering to her diet. Shows generalized obesity."

In 1954 at 151.5 lbs.: "Has not dieted consistently. . . . She is still of very broad, chunky build with excess obesity. In spite of this she presents a fairly attractive appearance, dresses well and has a distinctly feminine figure."

In 1955 at 140 lbs.: "[Karen] present a splendid appearance and has lost sufficient weight to have a rather good figure although still stocky."

In 1956 at 148 lbs.: "Her weight fluctuates from time to time and she is careless about her diet. . . . She looks <u>unusually</u> fine [emphasis in original, with pen]. Her face is much more feminine and attractive. Her complexion is good. Skin looks soft and pink (with the aid of cosmetics)."

In 1957 at 167 lbs.: "She admits that she is lackadaisical about restricting her diet."

In 1960 at 168 lbs., in her last medical encounter with Wilkins: "She is fairly attractive young woman in spite of her obesity."

In 1961 at 160 lbs.: "She is somewhat overweight but attractive."

In 1962 at 149 lbs.: "She is on medication to reduce appetite and is continuously decreasing intake in an effort to lose weight."

Perhaps Karen's priorities were simply different from those of her doctors? After all, she seemed "quite satisfied and pleased with her condition" (1957), and at every visit she expressed pleasure in her work. Doctors were undaunted, however. In 1964 at 184.5 pounds, the doctors noted that her weight gain was caused "by excessive eating particularly sweets." They added, "[Karen's] disease <u>is well controlled on her present</u>

medication. Her only <u>problems seem to be emotional</u>. Her obesity seems to fall into this category too. She was encouraged to diet as before [emphasis in original, with pen]."

Karen's life and the offerings of medicine seem to have become incommensurable. Karen was out in the world, she had moved away from her parents' home, she was working, sharing an apartment with a roommate, and she was training for better positions, "about which she [was] quite happy." If the treatment goal was to make Karen healthy—in the sense of being able to live in the world—then her very being in the world also got in the way of treatment. Life had a normality of its own; it included working, eating, sex (1964: "She has coitus without complaints"), friendship (1964: "She continues to maintain the same apartment with a <u>roommate who accompanies her today</u> [emphasis in original, with pen]"). All of these were in constant negotiation with the demands of medical normality—that is, taking medication, controlling one's diet, and strictly following medical instruction.

Life is full of loose ends, and quite appropriately this is how Karen's record ends—with no closure (for the historian) and just a single note. A single lab report from 1967 states her 17-KS level as 15.3—elevated, which indicates she might still have been skipping her cortisone pills. A note was scribbled to repeat the test a month later, but no further record of Karen is found in the archive.

THREE

Culture, Gender, and Personality

In 1947, twenty-six-year-old John Money boarded the S.S. *Rangitiki* to sail from New Zealand to the United States. His plan was to spend a year as a fellow at the Western State Psychiatric Institute in Pittsburgh under the supervision of the chief psychologist, Saul Rosenzweig.[1] Born into a poor and religious family, the ambitious young university lecturer had exhausted the educational options of his home country after earning a double MA from Victoria University College in philosophy/psychology and education. Money was part of a worldwide postwar influx of scholars into the United States for education and training unavailable in their home countries.[2] In addition to his time in Pittsburgh, he ultimately studied at Harvard University's newly founded Department of Social Relations, writing a dissertation that served as a blueprint for his later ideas about a learned gender role. Although he had intended to return to New Zealand for a university career, he instead moved to Baltimore to work at the Johns Hopkins Hospital in 1951, and he lived in that city until his death in 2006. Money joined Lawson Wilkins's team to work on a study evaluating the psychological health of patients with intersex traits, which resulted in his developing both the concept of a learned gender role and long-lasting management protocols for intersex patients.

John Money is a curious figure in the history of the inception of gender in the second half of the twentieth century;

he has been cast as a well-intended innovator and as an evil, experimenting mad scientist, depending on how and when his story has been told.
Was he "the leading sexologist in the world,"[3] a pioneer in the frank and
unprejudiced study of intersex, transsexuality, homosexuality, and erot-
icisms, and a psychologist who had a manner with his patients that was
"benevolently paternal rather than dogmatically patriarchal"?[4] Or was he
Dr. Evil, responsible for a ruthlessly normalizing approach to intersex
case management that led to countless genital surgeries, and a callous
careerist who experimented on children to prove his own theories of
gender malleability?[5] Much of the scholarship is an artifact of the debate
between these two points of view. Money himself worked without ceas-
ing to cement his role at the center of the story of gender; he could not
have imagined the tidal change in public opinion that turned him into
a monster in the early twenty-first century. Yet there is perhaps a third
way to think about John Money. If we understand his scientific practice as an authentically historical phenomenon rather than weighing its
contribution against present understandings, it becomes obvious that
this eccentric figure typified a particular branch of behavioral sciences in
the 1940s and 1950s. More than anything else, Money was a product of
the scientific and cultural environment of his time. Cultural relativism
and an emphasis on the role of environment, on development, and on
learning were all strong currents of thought already at work in the US
social and behavioral sciences, and these ideas shaped his research program, methods, and theories. In other words, his regarding sex roles as
learned had become neither new nor controversial by the late 1940s—at
least not in the social sciences.

In the following, I show that Money's interest in cultural patterns and
the role of the environment in shaping behavior was a product of the
previous three decades, in which social scientists convincingly and pas-
sionately argued that culture and environment trumped biology as determining factors in behavior. Anthropologists debated and challenged
biological notions of racial difference starting in the 1910s, and by the
1930s most social scientists studying human nature had shifted from be-
lieving in a biological explanation of human action to considering culture, experiences, and environment as the primary basis of differential
human behavior. Alongside race, sex (and sexuality) had also become
an area where cultural explanation trumped biological ones. Money's
transition from New Zealand graduate student to US psychologist occurred at a moment of a profound shift in which an increasing insistence on social determination and belief in the importance of fostering
the right American personality through child development and social

engineering became prominent. How, then, was a culturalist notion of behavior and personality adapted to clinical psychology and the patient interview? Or more precisely, how did an acceptance of norms as socially constructed intersect with the assessment of psychological well-being?

Cultural Patterns

To understand the intellectual institutional milieu and moment in which John Money pursued his graduate studies in the late 1940s, we must first focus on the previous three decades, when a new way of thinking about behavior and human nature made its mark on the US social sciences. The culture and personality school, often referred to as cultural relativism, was a loose network of social scientists who, beginning in the 1920s, explained differences in human behavior through a focus on culture. Many of the scholars in this subfield, most of them anthropologists, outright rejected biological theories of race, sex, and sexuality and pointed to different "cultures" as the origins of very diverse patterns of human behavior. Culture, and thus behavior, was learned and passed on from one generation to the next.[6] Most of these scholars shared a specific interest in race, sex roles, and sexuality, and saw themselves as "cultural critics who brought anthropology to bear on the political and social controversies of their time."[7] By the late 1920s and early 1930s, the historian Carl Degler asserts, culture had triumphed over biology—if only mostly in the social sciences.[8]

The critique of biology as the determinant of human behavior and capabilities first emerged from a critical engagement with race. Throughout the nineteenth and into the twentieth century, scientists and physicians had sought to produce empirical evidence to support and justify arguments of the racial inferiority of people of color and the superiority of the white race, a practice referred to as scientific racism, racialism, or race science.[9] Franz Boas, a German-born US anthropologist, ushered in a new culture- and history-centered, relativistic school of anthropology which became dominant in the twentieth century with an exhaustive critique of scientific racism and of the discipline's universalizing assumptions about what constituted humans. Boas declared that there were no significant innate differences between races and civilizations, and he argued that differences in physical appearance did not equal any significant differences in mental or social capacities or functions. Any social disparities between one people and another derived from culture and history, not biology.[10] The culture and personality school of anthropology was highly influential in shaping perceptions of race and human difference in the first half of the twentieth century, to the point that in 1949, the United Nations Education, Scientific and Cultural Organization (UNESCO) issued a statement on the concept of race that aligned with Boasian anthropology.[11]

In the 1920s and 1930s, a new generation of female social scientists followed Boas's call for cultural comparison. They used their studies of other cultures to question the universalized sexual norms and sex roles of their own Western culture and to expose the apparent faultiness of the measurements of sexual difference and their consequences. In doing so, they newly addressed the question of differences between the sexes by exploring how environment shaped behavior. This was a serious shift in assumption: social environment or culture, not biology, was the source of differences in male and female behavior. By the late 1920s, the view had prevailed among social scientists and psychologists that, despite biological differences, especially those concerning reproduction, socialization largely drove behavioral and functional differences between the sexes.

In 1928, a young female anthropologist did for sex what Boas had done for race. Margaret Mead, one of his students at Columbia University, published a study of sexual practices in Samoa and made a case that Samoan sexuality was as culturally specific as was Western understanding of what constituted a proper and natural sexuality.[12] The observation of sexual practices and values in non-Western societies was an implicit critique of Western sexual norms, and her study of Samoan culture offered a contrast between the mal-effects of the puritanical American family and (obviously romanticized) seemingly freer and healthier practices among Samoans.[13] Mead's stressing the relativity of norms and institutions was a call for tolerance and open-mindedness toward other cultures, but she also meant to show American youth that their feelings of sexual guilt were culturally specific and far from "natural," and that other societies offered competing value systems.[14] This highlights an inherent tension in the cultural relativism approach: to argue that all cultures were equally valid and to utilize these cultural differences to point out problems in one's own society.

Mead also addressed the cultural specificity of "sex roles"—masculinity and femininity—in her work. In 1935, she published *Sex and Temperament in Three Primitive Societies*, in which she argued that even though all societies "institutionalized the roles of men and women," differences in sex roles did not necessarily follow the same patterns everywhere.[15] That children in all societies could be raised in such cultural uniformity to conform to these sex roles indicated the strength of social conditioning. After World War II, Mead once again turned her attention to sex roles, this time including a focus on America.[16] In *Male and Female*, she asked how men and women were to (re-)consider their maleness and their femaleness in the twentieth century during a time of postwar cultural renewal.[17] She engaged extensively with biological differences, specifically in regard to sexuality and reproduction, and she drew from animal behavior to argue that humans were being created by and through culture. For example, in a chapter titled "Human Fatherhood Is a Social Invention," Mead argued that the role of fatherhood is culturally acquired and not biologically grounded, because among the great apes to which humans were closely related, fathers played no significant role in raising children.[18] "For our humanity rests upon a series of learned behaviours," she wrote, "woven together into patterns that are infinitely fragile and never directly inherited."[19]

From the mid-1930s on, Mead focused increasingly on the mechanisms of personality development and the role of child rearing and childhood experience. She was particularly inspired by the neo-Freudian school, which shaped the popular reception of psychoanalysis. In trying to adapt Freud's theories of the structure of human psyche to the insights of cultural relativism, neo-Freudians like Karen Horney, Erich Fromm, and Erik Erikson connected the study of "culture" with that of personality and the valuation of social determinants with individual aspirations. They stressed the role of culture and social forces in shaping an individual's personality rather than innate, biologically determined urges.[20] Mead's growing interest in child rearing was not unusual. In the late 1930s, anthropologists, psychiatrists, and psychoanalysts paid increasing attention to the impact of early childhood experiences on personality development, and by 1944 they had frequently collaborated in studying these questions.[21]

During World War II, the US government and the public were concerned with what had caused whole nations to embrace fascism and to commit genocide. Cultural relativists, who had previously argued that different cultures produced different values, faced the question of what it meant if those values were fascist or authoritarian. If culture was passed on by learning and experience, how could a given society ensure that these pitfalls be avoided? Finally, could America learn from the horrors of totalitarianism and guarantee its ability to raise American children to become democratic citizens?[22] Mead had already turned her gaze on the United States in 1942 and published one of the first national character studies, an analysis of American culture, in which she reiterated the argument that personality formation was primarily determined by the culture inhabited by the individual.[23] While the book was a quickly written account meant to contribute to the war effort, it foreshadowed Mead's and other cultural relativists' insistence on the existence of a specific American character and emphasis on child development, both factors that would become increasingly important after the war.[24] Mead, for example, insisted that postwar planning had to root out undemocratic social behaviors through proper development and child rearing.

After World War II, the culture and personality school took another crucial turn when growing concern for child rearing was complemented by growing interest in social engineering. In the 1920s and 1930s, cultural relativism had abandoned biological definitions of social categories such as race, gender, and sexuality, and rejected the biological determinism of eugenics. A mainstream phenomenon in the United States during the first half of the twentieth century, eugenics aimed to improve the future human generations through the selection of desired heritable characteristics. Eugenicists shared the belief that certain groups should be encouraged to reproduce, while those with undesirable genetic traits should be prevented from having children.[25] Cultural relativism discredited biological determinism, but this did not end the effort to improve the human race. Nor, more precisely, did it discourage the effort to make Americans immune to the threat of fascism and, more important in the beginning Cold War, communism. Margaret Mead, fellow Boasian Ruth Benedict, and others contributed to this Cold War effort by writing about the emergence of authoritarian cultures and personality and by studying child development to avoid these pitfalls.[26] They penned studies about the national character of Germany and Japan, and they claimed that by focusing on how children were reared one could obtain an analysis of the character of adults.[27] This signified a shift away from the relativist principle that all cultures were equally valid and that cultural differences had to be tolerated. Ethnographic observations, they argued, could be applied to establishing a democratic personality in American youth.[28] Not heredity but learning and rearing were essential for producing the right kind of citizens.

Yet a focus on culture could be as deterministic as a focus on biology. The historian Joanne Meyerowitz suggests that culture and personality approaches produced a particular form of social engineering, "replac[ing] race with culture and nature with nurture . . . reject[ing] eugenics (or the biopolitics of childbearing) and promot[ing] instead a biopolitics of child rearing."[29] Though the direction of this social engineering was in theory not determined, national concerns during the Cold War shaped its direction to endorse existing norms and boundaries, social adjustment to a cultural status quo, and consequently binary sex roles. Conventional sex roles mattered, as they established women's roles as mothers, those primarily responsible for "transmitt[ing] culture to their children through early personality-shaping interactions."[30]

By the mid-twentieth century, the biopolitics of child rearing had come into full bloom. These concerns were high on the agenda of the Midcentury White House Conference on Children and Youth held in Washington, DC, in December 1950, the fifth in a series of meetings hosted by the president of the United States since 1909. The forty-eight hundred delegates, among them Mead, set out to debate the questions, "How can we develop in children the mental, emotional, and spiritual qualities essential to individual happiness and responsible citizenship? What physical, emotional, and social conditions are necessary to this development?"[31] No other time period had seen such an intense focus on appropriate child rearing and applied scientific and medical expertise to ensure a well-adjusted youth of America, producing a productive and similarly well-adjusted adult population and thereby securing the democratic future of the country.[32]

Becoming a US Psychologist

John Money undertook his journey from New Zealand to the United States right at the postwar moment when cultural relativism shifted toward social engineering and when the attempt to create one unified and collaborative social science out of many disciplines was institutionalized at Harvard University's newly established Department of Social Relations. Born on July 8, 1921, in Morrinsville, a provincial town in the Waikato region of New Zealand's North Island, Money was the oldest of three siblings. His parents were not educated beyond primary school and were fundamentalist Christians—members of the Plymouth Brethren, a conservative evangelical movement. In 1927, the family moved to Lower Hutt, near Wellington, to improve their prospects, but within two years, when Money was just eight years old, his father died. To help support her family, his mother, Ruth, took in her own mother, two unmarried sisters, and paying boarders. Money spent the rest of his childhood in a predominantly female household in consistent poverty.[33] His childhood instilled in him a dislike of religious dogma and sexual prudery as well as a deep class-consciousness alongside his ambition to transcend his meager beginning.[34] Science would become his religion.

Economic constraints shaped Money's studies and would continue to structure his decisions throughout his education. After completing high school early at the age of sixteen, he attended the University of New Zealand in Wellington. In 1935, New Zealand's first Labour government had been elected, and in the country's new social democracy, university tuition was free of charge for those who qualified academically. At the time, however, no scholarships or student loans were available to cover living costs. Victoria University College, a teachers' training college near the university, paid its students a small stipend, so Money enrolled there in order to support himself while studying. He also enrolled as a part-time student at the university, taking evening courses. If he rushed, he could make it from the training college to the university in time for the 4:00 p.m. lectures; this was a time of day when no lectures in the natural sciences were offered. Forced to exclude the natural sciences from his degree, he turned to psychology as the only science he could study as an undergraduate, though at the time psychology was part of the Philosophy Department.[35] After Money earned a double master's degree in psychology and education in 1944, his professional and educational choices were limited. He could not continue his academic training, as no PhD in psychology was offered in New Zealand at the time, and his status as a conscientious objector during World War II barred him from using his teaching certificate to become a schoolteacher. Instead, in March 1945 he accepted an appointment as junior lecturer at the University of Otago in the southern city of Dunedin, where he taught "undergraduate psychology" and "supervised one of the two sections of the undergraduate laboratory course."[36]

Money was already determined to seek wider horizons. The budding psychologist felt cut off from the world and complained in letters to his family and friends that his access to the US psychological literature was limited. His mentor at Victoria University College and New Zealand's first professor of psychology, Ernest Beaglehole, had spent some time at Yale University in New Haven, Connecticut. There he had joined "the founders of psychological anthropology: Edward Sapir, Ruth Benedict, Margaret Mead and others in the 1930s."[37] His accounts left a lasting impression on young Money and helped steer him toward US psychology and anthropology.[38] He applied to several graduate schools in the United States, with the hope of receiving financial support.[39] Psychology at Columbia University in New York and the new Department of Social

Relations at Harvard were at the top of his list, as he was eager to study with a new breed of psychologists present at these institutions: experimentalists firmly rooted in the social sciences. Since Harvard rejected him and Columbia offered no financial assistance, Money decided to take an offer he had received from Saul Rosenzweig, chief psychologist at the newly opened Western State Psychiatric Institute in Pittsburgh, which was soliciting graduates in psychology from abroad to apply for residency training. This position provided room and board and a yearly stipend, which was "an amount sufficient to finance an extra year in graduate school," Money wrote to his family.[40]

The Western State Psychiatric Hospital had opened in September 1942, and in 1945, after opening an outpatient clinic, it was renamed the Western Psychiatric Institute and Clinic. Rosenzweig was well known for his undogmatic approach to psychotherapy, also known as the dodo bird hypothesis, the premise that "all methods of therapy—when competently used—could be equally successful."[41] He, too, had done his graduate training at the Harvard Psychological Clinic, along with Henry A. Murray, who in 1946 became a founding member of Harvard's new Department of Social Relations.[42] Money, who still had his eye on graduate school, took classes on Rorschach testing to become adept at psychological testing and to acquire credits for his PhD. During his year in Pittsburgh, he reapplied to the graduate program at the Department of Social Relations after having taken the Graduate Record Examinations in Pittsburgh.[43] A recommendation from Rosenzweig no doubt strengthened his application, and in September 1948 he became a graduate student there. Although Harvard only covered part of his tuition fees, he could not pass up his dream of joining the first interdisciplinary department of its kind in the United States.[44]

Social Relations

The provost of Harvard University had announced a major shift in the school's organization of the social sciences on February 1, 1946. The Department of Social Relations would be a new department incorporating the former Departments of Sociology, Social and Clinical Psychology, and Social Anthropology under the Faculty of Arts and Sciences.[45] The committee of prominent scholars who had called for the change said it was long overdue, as interdisciplinary research efforts during World War II had already "virtually obliterated distinctions that were already breaking down between social scientists engaged in the study of fundamental problems of social relations."[46] Harvard's Department of Social Relations was indeed more a child of World War II than of the Cold War. The mobilization of science and scholarship during that war had transformed the meaning and importance of interdisciplinary cooperation and fundamentally altered the nature of funding and the organization of academic research.[47] When the United States entered the war, new research possibilities emerged for the human sciences. Sociologists, political scientists, anthropologists, economists, and psychologists were called on to contribute to the war effort and used their expertise to examine army and civilian morale, the social structure of the Axis powers, propaganda, and enemy intelligence, among many other phenomena. From these joint efforts emerged the sense that, as the historian Joel Isaac puts it, "a new 'behavioral science' had taken shape, which, like the physical and biological sciences, could be a source of both fundamental laws and technological control."[48] Isaac describes Harvard as "an especially hospitable venue for the sorts of challenges that interdisciplinary behavioral scientists had to face" due to its specific research tradition and the wartime experiences of the department's founders.[49]

The sociologist Talcott Parsons, founding chairman of the new department, had a particular vision for the new social sciences: bringing together sociologists, cultural anthropologists, and psychologists to elucidate the basis of human activity and develop a general theory or general laws of social relations.[50] In the early 1950s, he was shifting from his voluntaristic theory of action to functionalism and systems theory.[51] He considered society to be a structure with interrelated parts such as norms, customs, traditions, and institutions. Individuals had expectations of other peoples' actions and experienced their reactions to their own behavior. These expectations were not arbitrary but resulted from accepted norms and values of the individual's society. As behaviors were repeated in multiple interactions and over time, these expectations became ingrained and an accepted part of a social structure, creating a "role" that a person took on. The resulting social relationships were constitutive of an actor's personality, and the family was the primary site of socialization. This understanding underwrote a conviction that personality was produced through social interactions and experiences.[52]

Instruction in the new department began in the summer term of 1946 and offered an undergraduate program in social relations as well as graduate programs leading to the master of arts and doctor of philosophy degrees in sociology, social anthropology, social psychology, and clinical psychology.[53] The sociologist Arthur Vidich, who started his graduate studies at the department in 1948, remembers the program as one in which "the social relations curriculum floated ideas in all directions." The department, he continues, "was full of intellectual confusions and contradictions and attracted a remarkable collection of professors, instructors and graduate students, whom Parsons organized into a loosely knit administrative unit."[54] The department's aim was "cross-fertilization" (617) across the four disciplines. First-year students enrolled in its proseminar, which was cotaught through weekly lectures by the senior faculty, with founder Parsons, the anthropologist Clyde Kluckhohn, and the psychologist Henry Murray dominating the department's interdisciplinary approach. Parsons impressed onto the new students the need to develop a common vocabulary in the social sciences and to overcome disciplinary differences, although the simple exposure to the wealth of disciplinary vocabularies did not necessarily lead to an interdisciplinary perspective (617). In practice, students mostly worked with the professors of their choice and discipline, but they formed interdisciplinary study groups to try to cope with the task of digesting multiple disciplinary vocabularies and vast reading lists (618).

Psychology and Social Relations

Social psychologists and neo-Freudians, who felt increasingly alienated in psychology departments modeled on the natural sciences, found a more welcoming home in the Department of Social Relations. Harvard's psychology department had focused on a very narrow interpretation of experimental psychology that included animal learning and psychophysics. Consequently, the formation of the Department of Social Relations allowed two researchers formerly ill-fitted to the natural science model to find a new home. Henry Murray was originally trained as a medical doctor and held a PhD in biochemistry, but after reading the works of Carl Jung and Sigmund Freud, he focused his research on psychology and psychoanalysis. He had entered the Harvard faculty through the newly formed Harvard Psychological Clinic, which he joined in 1926. His colleagues there did not share his conviction that psychoanalysis was a worthwhile object of study within the discipline, nor did they appreciate his rejection of psychological reductionism and his interest in psychoanalytical theories of personality.[55] This hostility and opposition between traditional experimental and the new social psychology caused a rift. While the main part of the faculty remained in experimental psychology, Murray and his colleague, the social psychologist Gordon W. Allport, joined the Department of Social Relations in 1946.[56]

Murray's and Allport's work played a major role in shaping the face of US psychology by adding subjects such as personality and abnormal and clinical psychologies to the academic study of psychology as worthwhile areas of research.[57] They were especially interested in personality development. In 1937, Allport had published a psychological investigation of *personality*, in which he explored the etymology of the term.[58] For him, personality was "what man really is": "the dynamic organization within the individual of those psychophysical systems that determine his unique adjustments to his environment."[59] Murray, too, had a distinctly interactionist conception of personality. He believed that it resulted "from the interaction of numerous factors, both internal and external to the individual, and manifesting itself through numerous processes."[60] To understand an individual, one had to assess that person's psychological needs as well as the environmental forces (or "press," to use Murray's term) that affected him or her.

In 1935, Murray and Christiana Morgan, an artist, writer, and psychoanalyst at Harvard University, developed the thematic apperception test (TAT), which became one of the most widely used projective psychological tests.[61] The TAT measured an individual's unconscious by asking the person to interpret a series of pictures.[62] Murray's psychodynamics of personality was part of a development, as John Money himself would later argue, that "swept over American clinical psychology in the postwar era," when clinicians and psychologists found broad applications for the TAT.[63] The comprehensive case study method Money learned in a course he had taken with Murray deeply influenced his clinical approach, and the TAT became a central test in his clinical repertoire.

Murray's psychology combined and included aspects of the culture and personality school. In 1949, he coedited the anthology *Personality in Nature, Society, and Culture* with Clyde Kluckhohn, another prominent figure in the new department, who combined anthropological and psychological thinking in his work.[64] In their introduction, the men claimed that the unique postwar focus on the relation of the individual to society brought together psychiatrists, psychologists, social workers, students of education, biologists, and anthropologists as contributors to this volume.[65] Among them were Margaret Mead, Geoffrey Gorer, Talcott Parsons, Gordon W. Allport, Saul Rosenzweig, and Ruth Benedict, all seeking answers to questions such as "How much of an individual's personality is fixed by his biological constitution? How much is personal life style influenced by the society's traditional designs for living (its 'culture')? Why are ways of behaving that are punished by one group rewarded, or at any rate tolerated, by another? Is individual deviance culturally defined, or are there absolute standards of psychological abnormality? What is the role of outstanding personalities and of other individuals in social change?" (xv) In answering these questions, Murray and Kluckhohn wrote, they rejected the conventional separation of individual versus society. "Personal figures," they argued, "get their definition only when seen against the social and cultural background in which they have their being." No individual alive was not part of any group or not influenced by norms and behavior. Traditionally, most social scientists were interested in similarities of personality, whereas psychotherapists and psychologists focused on differences; but de facto these matters were "inextricably interwoven": "In actual experiences, individuals and societies constitute a single field" (xvi).

An Inquiry

With a rich repertoire of ideas at hand, Money started working on his dissertation in 1950, with George Gardner of the Judge Baker Child Guidance Clinic in Boston as his adviser. Gardner was a pediatrician and psychiatrist, a clinical professor of psychiatry at Harvard Medical School, and the psychiatrist-in-chief at Children's Hospital Boston. Money had first met him when he wrote a term paper, "Psychosexual Development in Relation to Homosexuality," in Gardner's tutorial Fieldwork and Seminar in Clinical Psychology.[66] Initially, Money had planned to choose the same topic for his doctoral thesis, but then he became intrigued by a case of hermaphroditism after Gardner presented on it.[67] Like other clinician-researchers before him, Money found "hermaphrodites" to be "a living paradox" and hoped that studying them would allow him to compare "body morphology and physiology, rearing and psychosexual orientation."[68] For this comparison he needed cases, and Gardner not only provided Money with guidance for his dissertation but also introduced him to a network of well-known clinician-researchers. These contacts gave him access to their patient records and case studies, literature, and—most important—patients.

Gardner's network eventually connected Money with Lawson Wilkins. Also at this time, Gardner introduced Money to Stanley Cobb, chief of the Psychiatry Department at Massachusetts General Hospital in Boston, who was a leader in the fields of neurology and psychiatry in the 1930s and 1940s. Cobb, who had been taught by the psychiatrist Adolf Meyer, founded Harvard's Department of Neurology in 1925 and its Department of Psychiatry in 1934 with funding from the Rockefeller Foundation.[69] With his interest in focused mind-body issues and psychosomatic medicine, he famously claimed in his *Borderlands of Psychiatry* (1943) that he had solved "the 'mind-body' problem . . . by stating that there is no such problem. The dichotomy is an artefact," and he suggested stepping away from any either-or position—a point Money would pick up in his own study of the mind-body unit.[70] For now, Cobb was an important contact who gave Money a student appointment in his department, which legitimized his research presence in the hospital and allowed him access to its library. As he later wrote, this appointment gave him access to the "physicians responsible for the care of hermaphrodites in pediatrics, gynecology, endocrinology, and, at Children's Hospital, plastic surgery (Dr. Donald W. MacCollum)." Money also got to know Fuller Albright, who was, like Wilkins, one of the leading researchers in clinical endocrinology. Albright in turn recommended Money to Fred Bartter, who was conducting research on and developing treatment for girls with congenital adrenal hyperplasia (CAH).[71] Finally, Bartter introduced Money to Wilkins at the 1950 meeting of the American Academy of Pediatrics in Boston, where Wilkins gave an all-day workshop on pediatric endocrinology.[72] This network and chain of connections gave Money vast access to prominent clinician-researcher networks along the East Coast.

As a result, Money could draw from the vast material of 248 cases recorded between 1895 and 1950 for his dissertation, "Hermaphroditism: An Inquiry into the Nature of a Human Paradox" (submitted in 1952). Moreover, he interviewed ten patients and used his analysis of the interviews as case studies to fulfill the clinical requirements for his PhD.[73] As we have seen in previous chapters, the cultural and psychological exploration of sex roles and sexuality paralleled a longer medical debate about the nature of sex that was based on the study of so-called hermaphrodites, often referred to as experiments in nature. Like psychologists, physicians struggled with how to apply theoretical discussions about the nature of sex to their patients in the clinic. Even more so, psychiatrists and psychoanalysts increasingly argued, as we saw in chapter 2, that a person's psychological sex had to be included in the assessment of a person's true sex. Yet the actual mechanism by which psychological sex was formed remained speculative. Despite a theoretical definition of sex being based on the nature of a person's gonads, the period from the 1920s to the early 1950s was an era of idiosyncrasies in the medical management of patients with intersex. Many practitioners operated without a set standard for addressing patients with intersex traits and struggled to integrate new biological and psychological information and findings in their clinical encounters with these patients, a situation Money sought to resolve.[74]

The methods and lines of inquiry Money applied in his dissertation served as a blueprint for his subsequent studies at Lawson Wilkins's Pediatric Endocrinology Clinic, even though he did not use the term *gender* yet. He posed two basic questions, one about the orientation of psychological sex and the other about psychological health. First, he asked how individuals with various forms of hermaphroditism and genital anomaly adapted themselves to the sex in which they were reared, especially if their anatomy did not appear to conform to that sex. Was it their physiology or the impact of rearing that was ultimately enduring? He arranged the published cases according to body morphology (i.e., intersex traits) and then compared these sets of data with information on sex of rearing based on two variables, which he had named nonlibidinal orientation and demeanor (this would become *gender role* in his Hopkins study) and libidinal orientation (what we would call sexual orientation today). Using this comparison, Money deduced that although sex hormones determined the presence or lack of libido, the direction of this libido or "individual erotic preferences" was not based on "unlearned determinants" or on that "which is commonly described as constitutional or instinctive, organic or innate." "Sexual outlook and sexual behavior"—used in lieu of *gender*—was also not based on "unlearned determinants."[75] Based on these findings, he concluded that in most cases of hermaphroditism, rearing was the most important factor in a subject's identification as a man or a woman. Money argued that it appeared that psychosexual orientation had a "very strong relationship to teaching and the lessons of experience and should be conceived as psychological phenomenon" (5).

The second question Money addressed in his dissertation concerned the psychological health of patients with intersex traits, or, as he put it, the "mental health of these people who so often appear ludicrously dressed in the clothes of the wrong sex" (3). He claimed that these individuals made "adequate adjustments to the demands of life," seeking to debunk the prevailing idea that psychosexual conflict created psychopathology. Based on the evidence of the absence of psychopathology in the hermaphrodites he found in the existing literature and in his patient interviews, he reasoned that "traditional and contemporary theories which ascribe the origins of nonorganic psychosis and neurosis exclusively to psychosexual conflicts and problems must be suspect" (7). Throughout his thesis, he criticized the gonadal standard that had prevailed since the nineteenth century and the manner in which intersex individuals were treated. He argued that emphasizing gonads had made the microscope "a sort of tyrant," but that it did not always prognosticate pubertal and secondary sexual development accurately. He contended that practitioners and researchers had allowed "moralistic horror at the possibility of errors of sex leading to marriage between persons of the same sex" to lead their care, to the patients' detriment. He praised physicians who in recent decades had started to give "primary weight to the emotional disposition of a patient" (8–9). In other words, Money commended those who listened to their patients rather than blindly following a biological definition of sex.

Social Relations in the Clinic: Connecting Individuals to Cultural Patterns

If the first part of John Money's dissertation followed the familiar (medical) pattern of reviewing and analyzing (mostly published) case studies of hermaphroditic patients, the second part showed the clinician at work.[76] The ten clinical interviews he compiled for this section were an application of theory to practice, illustrating the integration of various theoretical concepts into an analysis of patients' adjustment to their sex roles and an evaluation of their psychological health. The group consisted of six teenagers between the age of 12 and 17, three patients who were in their twenties (20, 22, and 24, respectively), and one who was 37 years old. Each case study consisted of a description of the medical case file, Money's assessment of the patient's psychosexual history through interviews, the results of an array of tests, and finally Money's psychological appraisal. These clinical interviews disclose a range of particular concerns and convictions that underwrote Money's analysis. They are also intimate stories (many with direct quotes) from the ten individuals that document their daily struggles in living with intersex traits, specifically genital variations, and they reveal much about sexual attitudes and mores, the process by which sexual knowledge and medical diagnosis were translated into daily practices and family patterns, and the wishes and hopes of these individuals.

The clinical assessment of the ten patients included no fewer than four separate tests. One was the Wechsler-Bellevue Intelligence Scale, developed by the psychologist David Wechsler in 1939, which was the most widely used intelligence test in America at the time.[77] Wechsler's version provided an overall IQ and a separate IQ that included verbal and performance subtests; these included pictures and were more suitable for smaller children.[78] The ten patients also took the Rorschach test, which Money had learned to use during his time at Pittsburgh Western Psychiatric Hospital, and the draw-a-person test, originally developed by Florence Goodenough in 1926, which was often used to assess intelligence in small children.[79] Money used it to assess whether patients drew themselves as girls or boys. He also adapted Henry A. Murray's thematic apperception test. In addition to the pictures in the standard test, he included "ten pictures especially chosen to elicit stories of relationships between two people of ill-defined age and sex."[80] He certainly performed these tests to demonstrate his skills to his committee. But he also did so due to the growing importance of psychological testing in midcentury America.

Regardless of tests, the interviews with the ten patients, each lasting a minimum of six hours, provided the more significant material for Money's assessment of psychological health, and much of these conversations centered on sexuality. His own self-concept likely played an important role; he prided himself in addressing human sexuality in an objective, open-minded manner, his style partly modeled on his readings in the culture and personality school of anthropology, where the study of sexual practices has been an essential theme. Nevertheless, to approach the delicate subject of human sexual behavior in a detached "scientific" manner was still controversial in the 1950s. The biologist Alfred Kinsey had practiced another version of detached objective sexology when he conducted a large-scale survey about the sexual practices of Americans.[81] His work was scandalous, not only because it revealed a much higher variation of sexual practices among Americans than had been assumed, but also because it lacked any moral judgment. Every sex act (that led to orgasm) counted as valid. This shift from a qualitative to a quantitative model of sexuality, which simply measured what people actually did sexually, was considered a value-free objective approach by its supporters, yet the very choice of measuring sexual practice in a quantitative and detached way without categorizing it as normal or abnormal was a political move in itself.[82]

Money strongly agreed with Kinsey that religious prudery was the cause of much sexual ignorance and consequent suffering. Both men were informed by a historically specific notion of science as objective truth, and both felt that a strict religious and puritanical attitude toward sexuality had caused them suffering when they were growing up.[83] Money later wrote that growing up with the "antisexualism and the anti-masturbation hysteria of Victorianism" had spread "a sinister influence" over him and his generation of youth. So "profound" was this experience that it kept him, he admitted, "professionally and personally engaged in rectifying it."[84] In his letters and early publications, Money positioned himself as an advocate of rational thinking and planning, sexual education, and the expression of sexuality without religious guilt or prudish morality During his patient interviews in 1951, he found that many of them were, as he characterized conservative religious attitudes toward masturbation in a letter to his brother, "scared by all the old completely incorrect, horror stories."[85] They suffered from their lack of sexual knowledge and, in most cases, their ignorance of their medical condition.

Money considered sexual and anatomical knowledge important themes in evaluating the patients' mental adjustment. In all ten cases, he inquired about their level of knowledge about their own medical history and condition. He also solicited what they knew about sex, sexuality, and reproduction, and how they had acquired this information. In many cases, patients knew little about their condition or sexuality in general, and more often than not, Money concluded that they felt burdened by the confusion that their ignorance and the lack of a vocabulary to talk about these issues created. Children learned about sex and sexuality from their friends more often than from their parents; they were sometimes sent to talk to a priest, or they observed the facts of sexual reproduction among pets; three of the patients said they had learned about pregnancy by observing a cat giving birth to kittens.[86] Parents' neglect of this side of their education was connected to what Money in one case referred to as the "modesty and prudery" (37) in which some of the children were being raised, denoted as "stringent sexual morality" and described as "prudery which almost amounts to priggery" (174). The individuals he interviewed were often not just ignorant about sex but also felt that sexual desire or activity was wrong and sinful. "As a matter of fact, I still have the feeling that it's a bit nasty or dirty," one patient confessed (125–26). This was heightened by their anxieties about their genital and sexual status, about which most had not been properly informed.

Money's persistent recommendation that clinicians speak openly and in scientific terms to parents and children, present their condition as part of a natural development in need of medical assistance, and give children an age-appropriate vocabulary to discuss their bodies, sex, and reproduction reflects the opinions he expressed in presenting the ten cases in his dissertation. This insistence is rooted in his biography and in a particular conception of and belief in an objective notion of science, which does not question its own rationality but positions science in opposition to superstition, puritanism, backwardness, and antidemocratic tendencies.[87] Beyond patients' personal struggles, their lack of knowledge concerned Money because it limited the extent to which his interviewees could or would share and thus allow the assessment of their psychosexual adjustment. Patients' ability to converse about their sexuality was an important theme in these case histories, because Money's analysis of ego function and psychosexual role required them to discuss their sexuality and sexual fantasies.

The inability to speak freely about sexuality was even greater when it came to homosexuality. Money wanted his patients to openly discuss all sexual practices, but it comes as no surprise that during this period of moral panic around any form of sexual deviance, they were at pains to reject any suspicion of homosexual behavior. Homosexuality was widely debated in mid-twentieth-century America, a period often referred to as the Lavender Scare that led to the mass dismissal of homosexual people from government service.[88] Increasing visibility and the social and demographic changes during and after World War II paved the way for the emergence of gay communities and networks. Even more so, Kinsey's studies had shown that homosexual experiences were much more common in men than previously assumed. He measured human sexual behavior on a scale rather than as a binary. In explaining his 0–6 scale of sexual orientation, Kinsey argued that "males do not represent two discrete populations, heterosexual and homosexual. The world is not to be divided into sheep and goats. It is a fundamental of taxonomy that nature rarely deals with discrete categories. . . . The living world is a continuum in each and every one of its aspects."[89] His decision to consider all sexual acts valid was controversial and widely debated in the US press. Yet at the same time, in the long term these findings also normalized homosexuality as one of many sexual outlets and helped foster the emergence of a group or identity for gays and lesbians as an oppressed minority.[90]

Contrary to Kinsey, John Money upheld a binary understanding of sexuality in his psychological assessments; and even though he proclaimed a nonjudgmental attitude toward homosexuality, his clinical case studies nonetheless depicted same-sex desire as an observable sign of a failed adjustment to sex of rearing. In contrast, his letters from the time indicate none of the contemporaneous anxiety about homosexuality but rather an inclusion of homosexual practices in the repertoire of normal human sexuality. Very much like Albert Ellis in his study of sexuality, Money measured sexual orientation on the basis of sex of rearing, not on biological sex. Accordingly, in this logic if a patient lived as a man despite having ovaries and a female internal reproductive system, sexual attraction toward men rather than women was considered homosexual and a sign of maladjustment to the psychosexual role—regardless of their biological sex. Since the norms of manhood and womanhood required active heterosexuality, same-sex practices or desire were indicators of psychosexual maladjustment.[91]

The young men and women Money interviewed were highly fearful that any indication of homosexuality would cast doubt on their at times fragile status as males or females. A young man of twenty-four, diagnosed as female pseudohermaphrodite with a small penis and internal female organs, had been reared as male and undergone male hormone therapy. Money's psychological appraisal described him as fully masculine and concluded that "his life is an eloquent and incisive testimony to the stamina of human personality."[92] The young man was college educated, of "superior intelligence," and married to a woman, and he spoke openly about his sexual and medical knowledge and experiences. Encounters with homosexuality came up quite a lot during his conversations with the psychologist, and he seemed to connect them to doubts about his masculinity. There had been some experimentation with his brother during childhood, and he told Money that during college "that issue came really into focus." There were some "queer flabs around," and one acquaintance "knew an awful lot of the fairies around." "A couple of homosexual guys in the dormitory committed suicide," he recounted, and one night, as he was "lamenting about women," a guy propositioned him. In his narration, the young man's reaction was a strong one: "Gee, I about vomited on the spot." He was worried that there was something about him that attracted this kind of attention, and he thought he might have been attractive to "some joker" because he was not a "terribly hairy person" and because of his femininity, those things about him which were "less pronouncedly masculine."[93] Homosexuality in his narration was firmly associated with gender inversion of some kind.[94]

Another measurement of adjustment and psychological health stands out in two of the ten cases: the appraisal of the American character. The New Zealand expatriate felt confident in his letters to family and friends to pen pages on pages of "ethnography" about American culture.[95] In his case studies, he assuredly described the characteristics of a typical American youth. Far from being yet another peculiarity of Money's personality, this particular form of assessment is implicated in the mid-twentieth-century focus on social learning in the development of a well-adjusted personality and normative social roles.[96] The national project to define American culture and "American character" first became important to support the war effort in the 1940s but continued into the 1950s. During World War II, culture and personality anthropologists such as Margaret Mead, her husband, George Bateson, and Ruth Benedict had engaged in so-called culture cracking to quickly achieve an understanding of a national culture and to use that knowledge for the Allies' advantage during the war.[97]

In her 1942 book *And Keep Your Powder Dry*, the first of a series of new national character studies, Mead aimed to describe the essence of American culture.[98] Her assertion that something like an "American character" actually existed carried a lot of weight, even though the description of such character was rather commonplace: "moralistic, ambivalent about aggressiveness, oriented toward the future, and inclined to interpret success or failure an index of personal merit" (507). Mead also pointed out in her chapter "We Are All Third Generation" that the particular immigrant experience (in her view, most Americans were children or grandchildren of immigrants at the time) and assimilation process that all Americans faced were formative for the American character. The English anthropologist Geoffrey Gorer joined Mead in this assumption in his 1948 book *The American People*, another study of national character. Gorer and Mead argued that it was not the distinctiveness of ethnicities that underwrote the American character structure but the shared experience of being uprooted, of losing contact with the past and being faced with the experience of mobility and change (508–9). Just as the war effort fostered the search for and construction of an American identity, so the postwar period focused on ensuring that children developed the right kind of American character and learned to value democracy, freedom, and equality, guided by a "mixture of faith in the right and faith in the power of science."[99]

Money's reflections about the American youth and specifically American boyhood reflect the nation's ongoing investment in a normative American disposition. He felt completely comfortable assessing two of the patients in his dissertation as typical or nontypical American youth. One was a thirteen-year-old boy who had been reared as a girl until her sex was changed to male during a hospital admission at the age of two years and three months—by means of a name change, a new set of clothes, and a haircut. Money thought the boy was repressed and had mixed ego functions. The teenager had no sexual history and was training for the priesthood. His father had died in his infancy, and Money considered the boy's closeness to his mother to be the root of many of his problems. In his psychological appraisal, he wrote, "In summary, this young adolescent male who lived as a girl for the first two years of his life obviously was not, on first acquaintance, a thoroughly typical American boy, though there was absolutely no doubt that he was an American boy. There was nothing effeminate about him, but it did not require great discernment to appreciate that he was in the midst of an adolescent struggle with sex and the assertion of his manhood."[100] At the time, psychologists emphasized learning and conditioning in cases of boys who failed to acquire their proper male role. The fear of the "sissy" was especially predominant during the 1950s, and effeminacy in boys was coded for homosexuality. It was up to parents to guide these young boys to a masculine role and heterosexuality, and a mother's relationship to her son was more often than not considered to be the cause of deviation from sex roles and presumably appropriate sexuality.[101] In the case of the thirteen-year-old boy, Money concluded that the family constellation, particularly the mother, the boy's upbringing, and his genital anatomy, caused his maladjustment. "His hypospadias condition [i.e., a condition in which the opening of the urethra is not located at the tip of the penis], and probably the early change of sex almost certainly contributed to his problem," he mused. "His problem may well have existed, and is found not uncommonly in an anatomically normal [youth] exposed to the same family experiences and moral teachings."[102]

The second case was a young man of twenty years who was diagnosed as male pseudohermaphrodite and reared as male with a penis anomaly. In contrast to the thirteen-year-old, Money referred to him as well adjusted. He was heterosexual and masculine, Money assessed, with some anxieties during childhood. In his psychological appraisal, he concluded, "In summary, this young man of twenty appeared to have suffered no ill effects from a genital deformity which required that he sit to urinate for the first nineteen years of his life. He was almost a model of what the average citizen believes a healthy, well-adjusted American youth should be: confident, self-reliant and optimistic; versatile with automobiles and gadgets; enthusiastic about baseball and other sports; discreet but not backward in sowing a few wild oats and openhearted and generous."[103]

Both examples of "American youths" were white, and Money's description of them stands in stark contrast to his depiction of the two Black youths in his case histories.[104] One was a seventeen-year-old raised as male but diagnosed as true hermaphrodite with a masculine psychosexual role. For this case history, Money included many direct quotes from the interview to tell the story of a young man who, despite his difficult upbringing and awareness of his "sexual ambiguity," was remarkably well adjusted.

"This youth," he reasoned in his psychological appraisal, "is another living testimony to the impact of rearing and to the stamina of the human personality in the face of sexual ambiguity of no mean proportion." The young man, he continued, seemed generally aware of his situation and down to earth; "only in regard to a career was he inclined to build castles in the air, occasionally daydreaming of sudden aggrandizement without hard work" while showing low drive and little ambition. Money juggled a culturalist and a biological explanation for these character traits, assessing that "it may be that the lackadaisical folkways of the Negro South have been too deeply ingrained, but it is also possible that his relatively weak energy level is a direct function of weak sex hormone production."[105] While Money routinely used his patients' milieu to explain their psychosexual status and behavior, he explicitly applied racial stereotypes in his few case studies of Black patients.

This culturalist explanation of personality was applied even more in the case of the thirteen-year-old girl. The girl had been diagnosed as a male pseudohermaphrodite and raised as female. Money assessed her with good ego functions, despite referring to her low IQ, and with a feminine psychosexual role. She tested as "feeble minded," yet as her case story evolved, Money suspected that her behavior was caused by extreme anxiety and fright due to the unfamiliar hospital surroundings. A Black social worker became involved in the case, and as she gained the child's trust, the girl lost some of her fear, much to Money's surprise, it seems, as he pointed out in his assessment: "The subsequent change in the girl was little short of astonishing. It was the first time that she had received any direct information about the nature of her anomaly and the reason for the surgery she had been given." True to his convictions, Money decried the ignorance in which the child had presumably been kept and the fear that had been instilled in her. This was very much in line with his general loathing of ignorance and prudery, but again he used the child's cultural and racial background as a ready explanation for her troubles. "Her aunt and all her relatives inculcated such fears into her," he wrote. "In part they were a method at child training; for the adults wanted the child's anomaly kept secret. But they were also part of the family's folklore. The grandmother, a devout Southern Negro Baptist, was genuine in instilling a fear of men into the little girl, especially of white men."[106] It is hard to assess from his account whether Money, who had written letters detailing his critique of the racial injustices in the American South to his family and friends in New Zealand, considered that the violence her family encountered in the South warranted her grandmother's warnings.

Big Claims, Small Concessions

In 1951, when Money handed in his dissertation, he had been offered a full-time faculty appointment teaching psychology at Bryn Mawr College in Pennsylvania, a research assistantship with Henry Murray at Harvard, and a postdoctoral fellowship at the Johns Hopkins Pediatric Endocrinology Clinic. Money declined Murray's offer, as he was impatient to graduate. He later reflected that he "weighed the pros and cons of Hopkins and Bryn Mawr with fellow Harvard students and faculty advisers, until I was persuaded not to underestimate the prestige in American psychiatry of John Whitehorn, successor to Adolf Meyer, the founder of the Phipps Clinic at Johns Hopkins."[107] He negotiated with Bryn Mawr for a part-time appointment and moved to Baltimore in the fall of 1951.

That fall he also sent his dissertation to his adviser, George Gardner, who replied to him on October 31 that he was "very, very much impressed." There was one aspect of the thesis, however, that he found problematic. Gardner suggested that Money "modify or at least rephrase" the two conclusions on the final page. He objected to Money's formulation "that any theory of constitutional or instinctual determination of sexual orientation and behavior is discredited." He thought it to be "an unnecessarily blunt" statement. He suggested to "modify the phrase to read somewhat as follows: that 'in the light of our findings it would seem that all of our present day theories of constitutional determination of sexual orientation and behavior need careful reexamination.'"[108]

Gardner chose slightly stronger words in decrying Money's other conclusion. He wrote, "I am even more appalled, John, by the unnecessarily aggressive bluntness of your second conclusion: 'that theories of the psychoanalytic variety attributing some psychoses to emotional and psychosexual origins are discredited.'" Again he thought Money was overstating his findings. Surely, "some psychoses might be due to 'emotional and psychosexual origins,'" he insisted. He also objected to Money's claim that "theories which ascribe neurosis to psychosexual conflict are indefensible without further modification." Gardner suggested that Money rephrase this sentence as a suggestion rather than leaving it as statement. He then proceeded to include a more personal observation: "If I may be allowed a personal note here, John, it would seem to me that perhaps you, for whatever cause I don't know, may have a very, very low opinion of the importance of 'psychosexual conflict' and perhaps you did unconsciously set as your task to discredit all theories of atypical behavior that have even the flimsiest attributable origins in such conflicts." Whether this was the case or not, Gardner concluded, his "suggestions regarding the modifications of these conclusions would be more in keeping with the results which this very important and very excellent study demonstrate."[109] Money added the suggested nuance to his conclusion without changing his major claims:

> To summarize and conclude, the evidence of this review of 248 cases of hermaphro-ditism carries implications for two important aspects of psychological theory. The first has to do with the origins and determinants of libidinal inclination, sexual outlook and sexual behavior. . . . In brief, it appears that psychosexual orientation bears a very strong relationship to teaching and the lessons of experience and should be conceived as a psychological phenomenon. . . . On the whole, however, one thing is clear: tradi-tional and contemporary theories which ascribe the origins of non-organic psychosis and neurosis exclusively to psychosexual conflicts and problems must be suspect. They require re-examination, if not modification and revision.[110]

Money submitted his final version in December and received his PhD in social relations at Harvard University in the beginning of 1952. He was finally a psychologist who would work at the top research hospital in the country.

————

Though often depicted as an unusual and eccentric figure (and despite being of New Zealand origin), the psychologist John Money was to a large extent representative of a particular school of thought in the US social sciences that had emerged in the 1910s and 1920s. His early ca-reer serves as a prism to understand how ideas about common cultures and individual personality, many of them commonplace by the 1940s, were integrated into the clinical practices of intersex case management. Social scientists had started questioning the idea of a biological basis for most behaviors and stressed the plasticity of human behavior, arguing that what many scientists and physicians had considered natural male or female behavior was molded by culture rather than rooted in biology, as evidence from other cultures had shown. By the late 1940s, a new social determinism had encouraged the study of not just how children's personalities developed but also how one might foster the development of a particular personality (and avoid others).

When Money began his doctoral research on the psychological health and adjustment of individuals with intersex traits, he could build on three decades of culturalist approaches. He also entered an intellectual landscape in which social scientists thought increasingly about how to shape learning and development in early childhood to manufacture an American democratic personality. Binary and circumscribed sex roles ensured the proper transmission of American culture from mothers to children and allowed for the measurement of individual adjustment or maladjustment. Money's doctoral research, which served as a blueprint for much of his Hopkins work on gender roles, integrated these ideas about the role of child rearing and development, cultural patterns, a particular American character or personality, and binary sex roles with his faith in the objectivity of science. In his doctoral study, he proposed that his data showed that psychological sex followed the sex in which a child was raised and that the resulting anatomical contradiction did not negatively affect mental adjustment and psychological health. He also stressed the importance of frank conversations about sexuality, unimpeded by what he deemed puritan superstition, and of informing patients in an age-appropriate manner about their conditions and their sexual anatomy. When Money joined Lawson Wilkins's team at the Pediatric Endocrinology Clinic to study the effect of the newly introduced cortisone treatment on the psychological health of patients with congenital adrenal hyperplasia (CAH), he found a setting fruitful for expanding the observations from his doctoral research to a formulation of a set of recommendations that were deeply invested in the belief that behavior could be manipulated and shaped into proper gender roles.

FOUR

Making Boys and Girls: Gender at Johns Hopkins

For the general public, *gender* came into the world with a whimper, not a bang. To be precise, it arrived between parentheses, used as an alternative term for *psychologic sex*, as in "psychologic sex (or gender role)," in a two-page press release dated May 2, 1956. This is all the more surprising since it came alongside the bold announcement that masculinity and femininity were learned and not biologically determined. According to the press release, "*Not one* of the bodily factors determines a person's sexual outlook and orientation; . . . it is, on the contrary, determined by the kind of rearing that a child has."[1] The statement summarized the results of a three-and-a-half-year study of "children with disorders of the endocrine gland" from a psychiatric and psychological perspective at the Johns Hopkins Hospital by Drs. John Money, Joan G. Hampson, and John L. Hampson (Department of Psychiatry), in collaboration with Dr. Lawson Wilkins (Department of Pediatrics).[2]

This chapter follows "gender role," from its empirical origin in Hopkins's Pediatric Endocrinology Clinic in the early 1950s, through debates at interdisciplinary roundtables and conferences, to its presentation in a set of six strategic publications between 1955 and 1956. In 1950, as we have seen, the pediatric endocrinologist Lawson Wilkins introduced a treatment for congenital adrenal hyperplasia (CAH). Cortisone halted both the life-threatening aspects of the condition

such as salt loss and the in no way life-threatening ones such as the virilization of genitals and altered appearance in girls. Before the introduction
of cortisone (and before Money's new concept of gender), Wilkins had
recommended raising such girls as boys; some had already been mistaken
for boys at birth, and they would continue to virilize and look increasingly male. After cortisone became available as treatment, Wilkins recommended raising females—who were identified as such by their female reproductive organs and eventually by the Barr body test for chromosomal
sex—as girls. In both scenarios, physicians recommended surgical intervention that adjusted patients' genitals, gonads, and internal accessory
reproductive structures to the assigned sex. By 1951, Wilkins was in the
middle of a research project testing various effects of the cortisone treatment for CAH patients. He had already published a preliminary report
about the treatment's promise and had presented his results at the International Pediatric Congress in Switzerland in June 1950.[3] His next step
was to determine whether cortisone would be a cure for the condition or
part of a lifelong treatment regime (like insulin for diabetes).

Wilkins also sought to learn more about the psychological effects of
the cortisone treatment and its consequences. He wondered whether
doctors should, say, reverse the sex assignment of those girls who had
been, following his earlier recommendations, raised as male now that
cortisone was available as a new treatment.[4] To pursue such a study, he
needed a team. He found a psychiatrist practically next door: Joan Hampson. Born in 1922 in England, Hampson had received her undergraduate
degree from the University of Manchester and had come to Johns Hopkins Medical School in 1946 on a Rockefeller Foundation Scholarship to
study medicine.[5] When Wilkins hired her, she had just completed her
residency in psychiatry at the Henry Phipps Psychiatric Clinic, the building adjacent to the Harriet Lane Home, which housed Wilkins's clinic
at Hopkins. The clinic's founding director and the father of psychobiology, Adolf Meyer, had retired from his position as psychiatrist-in-chief
at the Phipps in 1941; his successor, John C. Whitehorn, served as study
supervisor along with Wilkins. Next, Wilkins chose a psychologist: John
Money, then still a graduate student at Harvard's Department of Social
Relations. Though the Harriet Lane Home had its own Pediatric Psychiatric Clinic, headed by the psychiatrist Leo Kanner, Wilkins selected an
outsider and a psychologist to work as Hampson's partner in the study.[6]
He also arranged for a grant to support the new team. He facilitated a
meeting between Money and Frank Fremont-Smith, medical director of
the Josiah Macy Jr. Foundation, who agreed to provide financial support
for "the psychological accompaniment of the new cortisone therapy."[7]

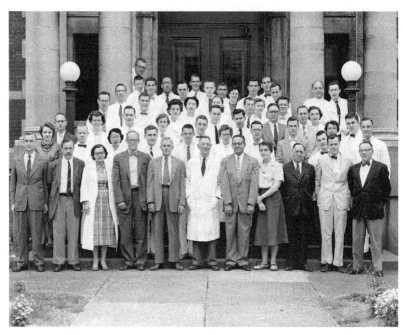

Figure 4 John Money, Joan Hampson, John Hampson (*on the left, first three rows*), and Lawson Wilkins (*center, first row*) at the annual group photograph of the Johns Hopkins Hospital Department of Pediatrics, Harriet Lane Home staff, 1956. *Front row, from left to right:* (1) Money; (2) Clark; (3) Ferencz; (4) Eisenberg; (5) Josephs; (6) Wilkins; (7) Gordon; (8) Guild; (9) Kanner; (10) Childs; (11) Livingston. *Second row, from left to right:* (1) Hampson; (2) Dodson; (3) Nakuamura; (4) Cavanaugh; (5) Bunnell; (6) Phelps; (7) Sidbury; (8) Hopkins; (9) Holman; (10) Norton. *Third row, from left to right:* (1) Hampson; (2) Avery; (3) Miller; (4) unidentified; (5) Kenny; (6) unidentified; (7) Perlman; (8) Cornblath; (9) Lauricella; (10) Zinkham. *Fourth row, from left to right:* (1) Jelks; (2) Hurwitz; (3) unidentified; (4) unidentified; (5) unidentified; (6) Levy; (7) Jacobsen; (8) unidentified; (9) Larson; (10) Nitowsky; (11) unidentified. *Fifth row, from left to right:* (1) James; (2) Kamin; (3) unidentified; (4) Wood; (5) Pauli; (6) David; (7) David; (8) unidentified; (9) Migeon. *Sixth row, from left to right:* (1) Smith; (2) Pinkerton; (3–7) unidentified.

Over a period of three and a half years, Money and Hampson, later joined by Hampson's husband, John (fig. 4), studied ninety-four patients at Wilkins's clinic. Discussions of case studies of individual patients and the shared experiences of physicians and surgeons played a significant role in structuring the argumentation the team put forward. Before the team published their findings in six papers, Money and Joan Hampson had attended several meetings to engage with other medical experts and scientists; the settings for these meetings included an inter-university roundtable conference at the University of Pennsylvania, a pediatric symposium on adrenal function in Syracuse, New York, and a sex research conference in Amherst, Massachusetts.[8] Transcripts of the discussions that took place among physicians, surgeons, psychologists, psychiatrists, and sex researchers allow us direct access to the responses, shared concerns, resistances, and alliances of those who took part in these formative conversations about gender.

The Girl Had a Testis: Biology versus Culture

Everybody agreed that ten-year-old Geraldine had at least one testis, but Joan Hampson could not have cared less. As she told the medical team from the University of Pennsylvania Hospital that had gathered for an interuniversity roundtable, "I am sure that by now it is abundantly evident that we at Hopkins do not put much weight in gonads per se."[9] It was an odd situation. Everyone in the assembly more or less concurred that this girl, despite "actually" being a boy, should remain a girl. Nevertheless, Dr. Paul György, Chief of Pediatrics at the University of Pennsylvania Hospital, was "a little taken aback by the revolutionary statement that gonads have nothing to do with sex." Gonads mattered, even though he, too, was convinced "that Geraldine was a boy and should be raised as a girl"—seeing no contradiction in his statement.[10]

György's consternation at the sudden insignificance of gonads in the determination of sex was understandable. Since the late nineteenth century, medical experts had insisted that in most cases of hermaphroditism a person's "true sex" could be determined via his or her gonads.[11] Yet the pediatric endocrinologist Lawson Wilkins, who confirmed the presence of a testis (and who was convinced that the patient's sex chromosomes would test male as well), knew from his clinical practice that the child's true sex might not be the best sex for her.[12] Additional factors such as the child's genital anatomy and psychosexuality had to be taken into account. Geraldine had a "testis, and a pretty good-sized phallus, which could have been made into a fairly normal phallus by a hypospadic operation. However, she also had a well-developed vagina which could be functional."[13] At birth, the decision could have gone either way (male or female) based on her anatomy, but after she lived ten years as a girl, the doctors believed that the decision of sex could not rely on these (inconsistent) biological factors alone. "Anatomic, gonadal, endocrinologic, and psychologic aspects" all played a role in cases of hermaphroditism, Wilkins argued, and in the end, decisions rested—more often than not—firmly on what he called "psychologic considerations" (775). His insistence on the importance of the "psychologic aspects" might have seemed unusual for a pediatric endocrinologist, but it was in fact shaped by his clinical experience with these patients. This experience had taught him to privilege adjustment over anatomy.

This friendly exchange among experts at UPenn was sparked by a clinical encounter in July 1953. The then nine-year-old Geraldine had come with her mother to the University of Pennsylvania Hospital with the chief complaint (in her mother's words) of a "growth on her privates" (771). When examined at Penn, it was thought that she had "a marked hypospadias with bilaterally undescended testicles." At first, the pediatricians at Penn "agreed that this patient had more masculine than feminine traits; hence, if she could be psychologically prepared for a change of sex, the hypospadias should be repaired and the testicles brought into the scrotum" (773). The mother was strongly opposed to a sex change, however. Dr. Rashkind, a physician at Children's Hospital of Philadelphia, described Geraldine as a child of "short stature and of markedly impressive muscular development." At her admittance in 1953, she was "attired in female garb, but strutting, walking more in the manner of a 'boy than of a girl.'" He continued to describe her as a "friendly, cooperative, very poised child who does not seem to have any degree of anxiety over her condition" (771). She had three siblings, two brothers and a sister.

This case history was fairly typical and shows the two main questions physicians were wrestling with at the time: What if the sex the person lived in was contradictory to the appearance of gonads and to their sex chromosomes? In such cases, which of the multiple and contradictory sex markers should determine a patient's sex? For ten years, Geraldine's mother had insisted that she had a daughter and had raised the child as such, despite the doubts that surfaced at the time of her birth. According to the case history, "At the time of delivery, the attending physician could not tell the mother just exactly what the sex of the child was. The mother, being strongly desirous of having a girl, decided to rear the child as a girl. She named the child Geraldine in her own admission for the contingency that if ever the child should turn out to have been a boy rather than a girl, the name could easily be shortened to Gerald" (772). For Wilkins and his colleagues, this narrative described a common scenario in such cases: a tentative sex diagnosis at birth by an overwhelmed physician, a parent strongly committed to one sex over the other, and consequent biological development that contradicted the sex assignment at birth.

At first, the experts at the University of Pennsylvania Hospital diagnosed this girl as a boy; but unsure of this diagnosis and its consequences, they sent Geraldine to the Johns Hopkins Hospital to be examined by Lawson Wilkins and the gynecological surgeon Howard Jones. John Money and Joan Hampson also interviewed the child during her visit. In January 1954, both teams met in Philadelphia to discuss their findings. At that time, Money and Hampson had already interviewed forty-four patients for their psychological evaluation of hermaphroditic patients during Wilkins's cortisone study, and they were in the process of preparing their findings for publication. While their recommendations were still somewhat cautious, their basic findings were already in place.

Wilkins, who was the most senior and renowned member of the team, prepared the floor for Money and Hampson by setting up the pragmatic problem they were facing: If this girl was male by all the standards of the time, then what were they to do about the fact that he had been raised as a girl for the last ten years? In other words, which aspects of the case should govern their decision? (779) And could the girl be a boy if she did not have a penis? "If we are going to raise an individual as a female in spite of male gonads and a male chromosomal pattern merely because there is no penis or anything that could be made into a penis," Wilkins said, "we must be certain to what extent the whole psyche and psychiatric pattern of the individual is dependent upon hormones, upon gonads, and upon chromosomes and to what extent they are dependent upon environment and the method of rearing" (783). This was of course the very question that Money and Hampson were in the process of investigating at the clinic and which was widely debated among practitioners at the time.

For the team working at Hopkins under Wilkins's supervision, the boy was without a doubt a girl and should remain one. After interviewing, observing, and testing Geraldine, Money and Hampson were convinced that she was "psychologically . . . entirely a girl" and thus should remain living as such. Her mannerisms ("posturing, gesturing, position of limbs when sitting and talking, inflection and rhythm of speech") were entirely feminine, and after ten years as a girl, any change in sex would lead to problems in her social role. If she changed to living as a boy, Money asserted, she would not be able to live convincingly as male; rather, she would give "the impression of a very sissified male homosexual" (782). Homosexuality, or in this case the impression thereof, was far from a desired outcome in 1950s America and implicitly and at times explicitly shaped the decision-making process in sex assignment.

Though often considered a sign of maladjustment, in this instance it was understood that homosexuality could be produced by an involuntary gender inversion caused by a change in sex assignment.

Rather than being the prime motivation for firm sex assignments, however, the avoidance of homosexuality was folded into a normalizing process where somatic features, behavior, and psychic status were controlled to achieve an intelligible biological and social norm. In Money's case studies, the danger of inadvertently producing a homosexual through forced reassignment of sex served as an argument for sticking with a child's assigned sex despite biological contradictions. Homosexuality in this instance served as both proof for an environmental theory of sex and a caution against sex changes based on gonads or sex chromosomes. If children learned their gender roles, this process included heterosexual orientation. To change the sex of children to make it match with their anatomy consequently led to gender inversion in behavior and desire. Historians of this period have observed a change in tone and have pointed out an intensification of anxiety about homosexuality in the years just before Money's introduction of gender role; they have argued that the fear of, or perceived threat from, homosexuality was instrumental in the development of treatment standards.[14] Wilkins certainly thought that homosexuality should be avoided, and he interpreted desire only within a heterosexual binary framework of sex.

At Hopkins, Money argued that the set of psychological tests conducted on Geraldine had confirmed that she was female. But how did the different medical teams test for Geraldine's gender role and other norms? At first, two separate Stanford-Binet form L tests for intelligence, one conducted in July and one in January, determined that Geraldine was "feeble-minded." Her IQ of 53, the teams noted, made the assessment of her judgment and evaluation difficult.[15] Money also used the thematic apperception test (TAT), designed to reveal a person's social drives or needs by studying how that individual interpreted a set of pictures of emotionally ambiguous situations, to determine Geraldine's orientation as female or male. Mostly, however, Money and Joan Hampson had relied on "oblique" observations of play and behavior and their interviews with Geraldine. Money commented that "despite the difficulty of obtaining extensive information about dreams, fantasies, and peripheral thoughts from a mentally defective child, the girl gave clear evidence in the TAT stories of a feminine orientation toward men" (782).

But what counted as "a feminine orientation toward men"? For one thing, according to Money, it was a rather socially determined notion of female endangerment. He noted that "she unthinkingly regarded females as constantly in peril of being suddenly scared or assaulted by men." This reaction, he acknowledged, was without a doubt connected to the specificities of the girl's family life. Her father was serving a prison term for an "incestuous relationship" with her sister, and Geraldine's experience with "a drunken, bad-tempered, incestuous father" was certainly enough reason to be scared of men. Money added, however, that it was significant "that the child automatically placed herself in the female role while narrating the stories." That is, Geraldine had already learned that in her family, to be female meant to live in fear. Most important, she regarded herself as a girl and, when prompted, chose to remain one. When Money asked her, "If some blind person came to you and said: 'Are you a boy or a girl?' What would you say?" Geraldine replied that she knew that she "was part boy," but that she wouldn't tell him. Instead, "she would tell him she was a girl" (782).

Despite the firm conclusions of the Hopkins team, Geraldine's statements were open to conflicting interpretations. In defense of the gonads, at the University of Pennsylvania György called on Dr. Rashkind, then a resident at Children's Hospital of Philadelphia, to repeat to the panel the kind of present Geraldine had wanted for Christmas. The girl, Rashkind said, had wished for "a holster . . . two guns, a guitar, and a tie." To add more evidence of her masculinity, "her favorite television program [was] Gene Autry with a close second being Hopalong Cassidy." Gender was in the eye of the beholder, however. Joan Hampson read the same wish as a sign of Geraldine's femininity. After all, she had not just asked for "two guns and a holster," she also wanted "a cowgirl suit to wear it on!" (788) Clearly, as this exchange about the gender of toys shows, the terrain between masculinity and femininity was highly contested and its meanings needed contextualization. That is, the repertoire of masculinity and femininity that these medical experts drew from was much more complex and messier than it might have seemed on the surface. At the very same time that doctors were debating Geraldine's gender role in light of her preferred toys, another Western TV series (1954–57) fictionalized the life of the sharpshooter Annie Oakley, depicting her wearing a fringed cowgirl suit and wielding guns. Half a year after the debate over which gender had been indicated by the child's interest in guns, the film poster for *Johnny Guitar* prominently featured a gun- (and holster-) carrying Joan Crawford. Ideas about the proper roles of men and women in the 1950s were not only up for negotiation but also more nuanced and contradictory than the standard historical account allows.[16]

Despite the Hopkins team's insistence on prioritizing gendered expression over biological sex, it was not that the body did not matter for them. Genitals, for example, mattered a great deal; they influenced what sex would be assigned at birth. It was important that a person's genitals were a convincing signifier of the assigned sex, both in form and in function. The minimum criterion was that they could be shaped surgically to meet these requirements. Hormones mattered too; they fashioned the kind of puberty the child would experience, though it was next to impossible to make a prediction. In all cases, early diagnosis was recommended, because it allowed the doctors to differentiate between cases of CAH, where the hormonal outcome was known and endocrine treatment available, and other cases of intersex, where prognosis was not always as clear-cut.

In the end, the doctors at the roundtable agreed that Geraldine should remain a girl—though they clearly disagreed about why. For Money and Hampson, it was the accumulation of experiences that shaped the child's psychosexuality; gonads and sex chromosomes did not matter when it came to the psychosexuality of children like Geraldine. Rather, these children's psychosexuality belonged "to the sex which was assigned to them on their birth certificate, the sex for which their hair was cut and their clothing bought."[17] Furthermore, Money postulated, "a child's psychologic outlook, sexually speaking—his psychosexual orientation—is a product of or is determined by the kind of life experiences that this child encounters and the kind of life experiences that he transacts" (780). This formulation—"experiences encountered and transacted"—would become a consistent formulation in future publications.

The Penn psychiatrist Kenneth Appel described Geraldine's case as one of bisexuality—"embryologically and anatomically and psychologically and sociologically." Rather than being shaped regardless of the gonads, the child's "libidinal direction" took shape "in spite of the gonads and personality development." He continued, "Behavior is determined, as we see here certainly in large part, by parental and social selection or guidance, by the experience the personality has lived through; so that we have to think both of biology and psychology and sociology when we are thinking of personality function." The anatomic potential of the child's genitals and the parents' wishes also mattered. In this case, the true sex was not the best sex for Geraldine. Adhering to the gonadal dogma would actually produce a socially problematic outcome, Appel maintained, since "if this boy were raised as a boy, he would be psychologically homosexual." He continued, "It seems to me that he would have more difficulties in that way than he would have in the decision that has been made" (789). This formulation is yet another indication of what was at stake here, namely the future life of Geraldine. It also depicts doctors as ostensible protectors of the welfare of their patients, a feature common to medical culture in the mid-twentieth century.

It was certainly not new for doctors to favor the sex that matched the behavior and characteristics of the child in question, especially when the individual was already a bit older. Hugh Hampton Young, urological surgeon and Hopkins's main expert on hermaphroditism before Wilkins, had done so in the 1930s, reasoning that behavior and character were shaped by hormones.[18] His clinical work was informed by two factors: one was his relationship with each individual patient and his observation of that person's character and wishes; the other was the maintenance of social norms such as marriage and heterosexuality. Young assessed the individual patient and prescribed the treatment he thought would be in his or her best interest, thus reinscribing social categories.[19]

At this roundtable discussion, the debate was a different one. The Hopkins team's question implied a radical clinical rethinking of sex: was the child's femininity or masculinity acquired regardless of gonads or hormones? Yet the participants' reaction revealed the pervasiveness of the idea that behavior and personality were structured by culture and environment rather than biology. Many of the practitioners at the table felt that the prevailing trend was favoring a cultural approach, and not all of them were happy about it. Frank Fremont-Smith, medical director of the Josiah Macy Jr. Foundation, which had funded this meeting (and the Hopkins research team), was pleased that "there has not been complete agreement, thank goodness. Thank goodness to you, Paul [György]."[20] His generation had been "brought up in a biological rather than a cultural tradition of learning" and thus assumed "boyness or girlness was biologically determined." "But relativity, which has been brought vigorously into physics," he continued, was "also a Johnny-come-lately in biology and medicine." In the end, it remained an open question to be discussed at "more seminars of this sort."[21]

Ultimately, the decision of which sex to choose for Geraldine was also a question of pragmatism. As it turns out, the participants were dealing with a fait accompli. Geraldine's undescended testes had already been removed in the course of examinations—a fact mentioned only in passing (788). During the surgical examination at Hopkins, her "testicle, epididymis, glans of the clitoris, and appendix were excised," while only biopsies were taken from her ovaries (778). This was a clear indication that the team at Hopkins had already decided on which sex was better for Geraldine at the time of the operation. They were "going to keep this child as a girl," and they could not predict whether her testes would at puberty secrete predominantly androgenic or estrogenic hormones. It would have been disastrous, Wilkins noted, if in a few years she might begin "to develop hair all over her chest and whiskers and various other masculine attributes" (783). He had no doubt that their decision was the ethically right one. None of the participants at the roundtable objected to these drastic surgical interventions.

It is an odd moment in the transcript of the roundtable discussion that reveals that much of the debate was moot in light of her testes having already been removed. But we don't learn how involved Geraldine's mother might have been in the decision, given that she wanted her to remain in the female sex. Shocking as the ad hoc decision in the operating room might seem to us today, it was not uncommon. From the early twentieth century to the 1960s, medicine was "a model profession" and physicians were held in high esteem, contrary to earlier periods in US history. Medical and surgical innovation in the wake of bacteriology and anesthesia; reforms and standardization of medical education after the 1910 *Flexner Report*; the subsequent professionalization and specialization as well as expansion of hospital care; and the general trust in science and expertism since the Progressive Era were all factors influencing why the medical profession was viewed highly favorably and regarded as trustworthy in public opinion polls. This trust was well reflected in parents' engagement with physicians and their at times unquestioned adherence to medical advice and recommendations. It was present as well in discussions among physicians regarding the extent and kind of health information that could be given to patients and their families.[22] Over the following two decades, this confidence in the medical profession would be chipped away through internal criticism of unethical behavior and a patients' rights movement initiated by women's health activism.[23]

"What We as Pediatricians Can Do or Should Do"

In early November 1954, John Money and Joan Hampson's theory of human gender role made its first public appearance—at of all places a conference about the adrenal glands. There Money and Hampson once more postulated that a child's outlook as boy or man, girl or woman, was not automatically determined by chromosomes, gonads, or hormones. This time, the decline of gonadal dominance was hardly debated. The audience at the symposium "Adrenal Function in Infants and Children" in Syracuse, New York, consisted of pediatricians from the United States and Canada; the discussion focused on the decisions they faced in their daily clinical practice—what to do, how to do it, and who should decide.[24] At this point, Money and Hampson had studied "fifty-five infants, children and adults, representing seven varieties of hermaphroditism and including 36 hyperadrenocortical females." At the meeting, they presented their psychological findings on patients with congenital adrenal hyperplasia (CAH), and in their conference abstract from 1954, Money introduced his new term *gender role* as signifying "all those things a person says or does to disclose himself or herself as having the status of boy or man, girl or woman respectively."[25]

Hampson's talk focused on the role of hermaphroditic genital appearance in sex assignment and gender role. Just like Money, she stressed that in the majority of the cases that they had examined, gender role was consistent with the sex in which the child was reared. If a child was reared as a girl, she would behave and express herself in a feminine manner, even if she had testes or XY chromosomes. Yet while chromosomal, gonadal, and hormonal sex played little role in the development of a child's gender role, genitals mattered. The inspection of genitals at birth determined sex assignment in most cases, and in children with CAH "early surgical feminization of the hyperplastic phallus was psychologically beneficial and in no way harmful."[26] It was harmful, however, to change sex after the age of two and a half years, she added, because by that time gender role was indelibly established.

The subsequent 1956 publication of the conference proceedings includes a transcript of the discussion that followed Money and Hampson's presentations.[27] Lawson Wilkins was the first to comment in support of his team; he felt that he "should present this from the standpoint of a pediatrician or a doctor faced with one of these babies, and state how we go about diagnosing and proceeding with the case."[28] The most important step was correct diagnosis right at birth. In cases of CAH, now easily confirmed by chemical analysis of the patients' urine for the 17-ketosteroids level, the trajectory based on clinical experiences of the projector and prognosis of the condition was clear. Cortisone treatment would prevent not only death in severe cases but also the gradual but inevitable virilization of girls through excess androgens. In such cases as girls with CAH, "the females should invariably be raised as females and treated with cortisone" (130). Only a few years earlier, and before cortisone was available, Wilkins had recommended raising these girls as boys.

But what should they do with the other cases, where such easy prognosis was not available? Wilkins continued. Here he expressed what can only be described as genital pragmatism—that is, to focus on whether genitals could be surgically shaped to fit the assigned sex. Based on clinical data acquired in Wilkins's clinic, Money and Hampson had claimed in their papers that genitals were an important factor in sex assignment. It was no surprise, then, that Wilkins in his introductory comment confirmed that the anatomy of the genitals should determine choice of sex of rearing. "We make the selection of sex on the basis of their external anatomy," he said. "If there isn't a phallus, you can't make a man. . . . So the decision should be based on the size of the phallus and/ or the presence of a vaginal pouch, and not on the type of gonad or on the chromosomal pattern as determined by the type of nuclear structure" (130).[29] As in Geraldine's case, the phallus was more important than the testis for male assignment. These assessments were shaped by a specific phallic standard in which a phallus that did not fit social criteria of sex and sexuality (large enough to urinate standing up and to penetrate a vagina) was deemed invalid and refigured as female genitalia.[30] This "sizeism" had another side—clitorises judged as too big or too phallic were quickly excised or shortened to ensure proper gender role development.

The symposium audience seemed pleased by the usefulness of the Hopkins studies.[31] Convinced that some kind of intervention was warranted, they worried about making the right decisions at the right time. For instance, Henry L. Barnett, an assistant professor at Cornell University Medical College who would join the pediatrics department at the Albert Einstein College of Medicine in the Bronx the following year, wondered what would be the right age to operate on genitals to make them fit the assigned sex. After cortisone became available, he had postponed clitoridectomies to see if cortisone would reverse the virilizing effects on the child's genitals. He had realized that "cortisone will not cause sufficient regression in the size of the clitoris to obviate the necessity for clitoridectomy" and was planning to do this operation in the future at an early age.[32] Hampson, the only woman on the Hopkins team, provided data in her talk that "early genital reconstruction" was beneficial (129). There was no objection to "amputat[ing] an enlarged phallus" in girls with hyperadrenocorticism, she said (125). Vaginoplasty, on the other hand, could be done when the patient was older or demanded it herself. The absence of a vagina was, Hampson stressed, not as problematic for girls as the presence of a "large phallus." The group she interviewed consisted of mostly grown women; one was 14, the others 22, 26, 30, 35, and 49 years old, respectively. Only the two youngest women endured clitoridectomies at or before the age of 8. The rest had the procedure at age 15, 20, 34, and 46.[33] Based on the experiences of these older women, some of whom had elected to have their clitoris amputated only a few years before the study, Hampson recommended that the procedure be done in early childhood, preferably before preschool age to avoid "psychological difficulties."[34] In the following discussion, she showed some consideration for the patients' capacities for pleasure. She responded to a question about the extent of surgical interventions on a particular case that "where surgical feminization would be totally destructive of all areas of erotic sensation" (133) the team would—at least—debate their surgical decisions in more detail. As discussed later in this chapter, Hampson had published her specific findings on the effect of clitoridectomies in 1955 in a single-author article. In it, she discussed the consequences for women's "eroticism" in more detail.

Another recommendation of the Hopkins team was that information and communication were key to successful adjustment and gender role development. Remember that Money had already complained in his dissertation that too many of the patients he interviewed were ignorant of the medical specificities of their condition and that this combined with a lack of knowledge about sexuality and sexual anatomy caused much pain and confusion. If delay of operations was "surgically indicated," the team recommended talking openly with children and informing them about their diagnosis and further steps. It was, after all, "the mystery of ignorance which seems to cause all the trouble," Money said. The children carried "themselves through quite a number of years, up to early teen-age, with remarkable aplomb, as long as they know what to expect" (135). Even more so for Money and Hampson, the Hopkins approach "medicalized" hermaphroditism in a positive way. They saw themselves as allies against outdated medical and popular prejudices. Geraldine's mother, for example, had been very upset that at birth the doctor "told her that her child was a freak," and she felt that she needed to protect her.[35] Their study, Money and Hampson thought, promised to bring the clear language of science to these cases and to reframe them not as abnormal but as unfinished development that could be helped by medical expertise.

Information and communication also included the parents and families of these children. Sexual ambiguity and unresolved sex diagnosis deeply upset some parents, and the pediatricians found themselves in situations for which they felt ill equipped and untrained. Again and again, physicians talked about their difficulties in not only making the "correct" decision but also in communicating with parents about their children's condition. These shared stories highlight the urgency some felt in such medical encounters and their readiness to embrace clear-cut recommendations and standardizations. Barnett related a story of one such case from his hospital in great detail. "I had hoped," he said, "that the speakers who have had this much experience with the psychological aspects of this disease would be able to tell us more about what we as pediatricians can do or should do in our relationship with the parents of these children."[36] The child in question had been thought to be a boy at birth, but after the baby showed signs of adrenal insufficiency, the parents were informed that "their baby was not a boy, but a little girl." The situation escalated over the next twenty-four hours. The father's first reaction was to declare, "We will not have this child a girl; we want this child to be a boy, and this is the way he will stay." "I discussed this with them at length," Barnett continued, "and suggested that they go home and think about it and come to see me the next morning. When they came in the next morning they said, 'We have made our decision.' I said, 'There is really no decision to make at this stage.' They said, 'No, it is not whether the infant is a boy or girl; we have decided that we don't want this baby'" (131). The parents were consequently sent to talk to a psychiatrist to help them accept their child—alas, to no avail. Over the next couple of days, Barnett kept communication open with the parents until he felt they were ready to accept the child. "I finally said to them in effect, 'Well, I think we know one another well enough now that I can tell you, in my judgment, it is wrong for you not to take this baby.' By this time it was clear that they were wanting someone to tell them, 'Look, you have to take this baby.' As soon as I said this, they said, 'Why, of course, this is our baby'" (132).

Barnett's story and how the conference audience related to it show the pressure under which pediatricians felt themselves to be operating in cases of intersex children. Granted, not every case was so dramatic, but the vulnerability of the parents and the burden pediatricians felt to make the right decision—Barnett was even scolded by his resident staff for being too passive—explain why the Hopkins recommendations were quite well received in this setting. The audience asked about how parents' general psychological needs were amplified in these cases; whether to let the surgeon decide the right age for "plastic reconstruction" of the vagina; how to preserve erotic sensation after clitoridectomies; the psychological problems of infertility encountered by some male pseudo-hermaphrodites assigned as girls; "active homosexual problems" in boys with CAH; feelings of guilt in parents; and possible neurosis in siblings of pseudohermaphroditic children. This is not to say that these concerns were warranted, but they exemplify how the cases were experienced as medical emergencies necessitating medical interventions and how practitioners were highly doubtful about how best to proceed. The research at Hopkins promised concrete solutions and guidelines based on a relatively large amount of empirical data transmitted under the support of an authority figure such as Lawson Wilkins.

Workers in Sex

Not even two weeks later, on November 16, 1954, thirty men and one woman gathered for three days at the Lord Jeffrey Inn in Amherst, Massachusetts, with one thing on their minds: sex. The group included some of the most distinguished scientists of the day in the fields of endocrinology, reproductive biology, psychology, psychiatry, and medicine; they had come together to attend a conference, "Genetic, Psychological and Hormonal Factors in the Establishment and Maintenance of Patterns of Sexual Behavior in Mammals." Among the attendees were John Money and Joan Hampson, who had traveled without Wilkins this time to present their findings in this prestigious setting. They had initially titled their paper "Psychosexual Development and Behavior Problems in Human Hermaphrodites," but at the last minute they revised it to "Human Hermaphroditism: Establishment of Gender Role and Erotic Practices," thus granting exposure to Money's new term, *gender role*.[37]

After the presentation of an array of papers on the sexual behavior of guinea pigs, rats, pigeons, cats, rabbits, and primates, the conference focus finally turned to the human species on the last day, and Joan Hampson, the only female attendee, presented the findings of the Hopkins group.[38] Hampson stressed the significance of their contribution for learning about human sexual behavior: hermaphroditism was a naturally occurring experiment that allowed practitioners to study the relationship between the sex of the body and that of the mind. As had Money two weeks earlier, Hampson introduced their new term, *gender role*, and claimed that the sex in which hermaphrodites were raised became their gender role, seemingly regardless of any contradictions with biological sex determinants. Genitals and hormones were the only biological categories that mattered.

After Hampson's presentation, Money claimed his place as first discussant and stressed again the importance of thinking about experiences as "encountered and transacted . . . in order to avoid the simplemindedness of the theory of environmental determinism." In front of this audience of prominent sex researchers, he was cautious to emphasize that he balanced the nature and nurture aspects of sex carefully. While experiences were important in shaping an individual's sense of sexed self, there was no "line-for-line correlation with how these experiences [would] be interpreted and what sort of conclusion the individual [would] come up with." Now it was the researchers' task to try to correlate gonads and chromosomes, hormones, and external genital morphology to assigned sex and to the experiences of the individual. The underlying mechanisms remained hidden to the observer—Money here referred to a "black box"—but one could nevertheless study the outcome. "And then our job is to observe how the individual himself added all this up together," Money explained, "and what sort of interpretation he came out with."[39] The discussion that followed went back and forth between questions about biological sex markers and the significance of the individual cases Money and Hampson presented. The team stated that they did not worry about their small and preselected sample. Their selection was based on the clinical condition. First, CAH was a rare condition, as was "hermaphroditism" in general (311). Second, the clinical setting demanded—in their eyes—being able to make quick decisions about sex assignment and treatment.

The team was, after all, providing what they considered to be much-needed advice to practitioners in the clinical setting. That had been clear already at the two conferences in Philadelphia and Syracuse, and even in this venue the embryologist George Corner, who was chairing the section, brought up the "surgeon's dilemma." "In defense of the surgeons," he said, "I remember being called on just as a casual amateur in an operating room once. The parents had not been able to make a decision. The case was one on the borderline that could be swung more or less satisfactorily from the surgeon's standpoint either way, and the patient was under anesthesia and was very young, so somebody had to decide, and the decision was made by council at the operating table. I hope we judged right." Hampson replied that she hoped that studies such as theirs would "help a surgeon who is under such admittedly extraordinarily difficult decisions." Money, on the other hand, thought that they would not "mind in the least making mistakes, because they are still very interesting to science." To which Hampson added, "but . . . if once you have made a mistake, for God's sake don't change your mind again. [Laughter]" (310).

This exchange and the note "[Laughter]" in the transcript highlight the inconsistencies and tensions of Money and Hampson's new model of gender as clinical yet experimental. Since the late nineteenth century, such so-called mistakes in sex assignments had provided "interesting" research material for generations of physicians and were utilized to provide unique insights into the study of human sexuality. Remember that many of the studies we discussed so far have referred to hermaphrodites as experiments in nature. Endocrinologists, who had performed hormonal experimentation on animals such as guinea pigs or rabbits, had felt, for example, that they could learn from such experiments how hormones affected sexual development in humans. Yet at the same time, physicians also felt an obligation of care for these patients, however misguided this care might seem in hindsight. They expressed an increasing clinical concern about how such mistakes in sex assignment affected the lives of patients under their medical care. With significant shifts in birth practices such as an increase in hospital births or births under a physician's supervision rather than a midwife's, physicians could intervene at an earlier age but were unsure of the right path forward in each case. Money and Hampson's findings made gender open to manipulation, rendering moot the concern over making mistakes. They provided a shortcut in which such mistakes and the consistent uncertainties physicians complained about did not matter, because it could guarantee the outcome of the establishment of one of two gender roles.

From Practice to Theory and Back

John Money and Joan Hampson returned to Hopkins, and together with Joan's husband, John, they started to write up and publish the results of their study of ninety-four patients between 1951 and 1955. These appeared as six articles in consecutive issues of the *Bulletin of the Johns Hopkins Hospital* in 1955 and 1956.[40] The articles were organized by the logic of their clinical setting. The first two single-author papers, sent to the *Bulletin* on March 2, 1955, and published in the June issue, focused on the main patient group in Wilkins's clinic, children with hyperadrenocorticism (or CAH), and presented the basic findings of the team's research. Money introduced his new term *gender role* and the conceptual framework of the study, and Hampson presented findings on the psychological effect of genital appearance and change of sex in girls with congenital adrenal hyperplasia (CAH).[41] The other four papers were all coauthored by Money and the Hampsons. Topics covered by these included evidence provided by another group of hermaphroditic patients;[42] recommendations on the management of hermaphroditism; an extrapolation on what their findings meant for human psychosexuality in general;[43]

and an evaluation of the psychological health of their hermaphroditic patients, which provided further support for their recommendations.[44]

In order to compare measurements among patients, the team had to establish what to measure. In Amherst, Money and Hampson had complained about "the age old problem of there being no standardized measuring rods or scales to employ" for an individual's sexual orientation (i.e., masculinity and femininity).[45] To resolve this dilemma, they decided to develop their own mélange of psychological appraisals, consisting of interviews, observations of behavior, and psychological tests.[46] Over the course of their study, Money and the Hampsons collected a large amount of data on each patient. They developed a case history, which included first impressions, a series of interviews, the social/family background, a thumbnail self-sketch, a description of day-to-day routines, an intelligence test, an appraisal of somatic growth and appearance, and finally questions concerning the patient's sexuality.[47] The psychological data they amassed was used to assess Money's newly introduced category of gender role.

Hopkins's Gender

As discussed in detail in chapter 7, Money and the rest of the Hopkins team used *gender* and *gender role* to convey a meaning quite different from the associations these terms have accrued since the 1970s. In his single-author paper published in June 1955, Money set out to define the new term: "The term gender role is used to signify all those things that a person says or does to disclose himself or herself as having the status of boy or man, girl or woman, respectively. It includes, but is not restricted to sexuality in the sense of eroticism."[48] His choice of *role* was a nod to the already circulating term *sex role*, but it was also shaped by Talcott Parsons's work on social roles. Parsons, who had chaired Harvard's Department of Social Relations, where Money received his PhD, thought that society was a structure with interrelated parts such as norms, customs, traditions, and institutions.[49] Individuals had expectations of other peoples' actions and experienced peoples' reactions to their own behavior. These expectations were not random but the result of accepted norms and values of the individual's society. As behaviors were repeated in multiple interactions and expectations became ingrained over time and an accepted part of a social structure, a "role" was created. "The system of social relationships in which the actor is involved is not merely of situational significance, but is directly constitutive of the personality itself," Parsons wrote in 1951, providing a framework that went on to shape Money's conceptualization of "gender role."[50]

During the Hopkins study, the team had subdivided sex into several variables. Five biological variables accounted for the different expressions of sex in the body: external genital morphology, internal accessory reproductive structures, hormonal sex and secondary sexual characteristics, gonadal sex, and chromosomal sex. Since Theodor Klebs's nineteenth-century classification of pseudohermaphrodites according to their true gonadal sex, testes and ovaries had been considered important signifiers of sex. With the newly introduced Barr body test, clinicians hoped to determine true sex via sex chromosomes. However, in practice neither gonads nor sex chromosomes were the fixed determinants of sex that scientists and doctors had hoped for. Additional biological variables accounted for the many aspects in which sex could be contradictory; these variables included hormonal sex, genital sex, and internal accessory reproductive structures. Money and the Hampsons added another essential category to this pool of sex markers: the sex assigned to the child at birth and in which the child was raised. They set out to systematically evaluate which of these factors would determine a seventh variable—namely, a child's gender role and his or her femininity or masculinity.

Sex assigned at birth/sex of rearing was the only truly social variable of sex in the mix. Though sex was often assigned based on a biological category, for example genital appearance at birth, Money argued that sex assignment was the main category that determined a child's role as man or woman in society, and it could well be in contradiction to gonadal and chromosomal sex.[51] In their analysis of these sexual contradictions, the team was building on experiences from Lawson Wilkins's clinical practice. Wilkins had often complained about the difficulty of assigning the "right" sex in cases of CAH. Thus, Money was working with a pool of patients who had all grown up with some inconsistencies between the sex they lived in and their anatomy. Girls with CAH who grew up as girls often lived for many years with male-appearing genitalia, masculinized appearance, and an unusually high level of androgens. A significant number of girls with CAH had been raised as males. Before the introduction of cortisone, Wilkins had recommended assigning the male sex to female CAH patients. These patients lived as boys despite having ovaries and female reproductive organs. In both scenarios, children's gender roles correlated with the sex in which they were living despite biological contradictions. Gonads and sex chromosomes did not matter as much as consistency in sex assignment.

Another group of patients served as a test case for contrasting gender role with chromosomal and hormonal sex: girls, formerly diagnosed as females with ovarian agenesis, who were tested with the new Barr test for chromosomal sex and reclassified as "simulant females with feminizing testes." In 1948, Murray Llewellyn Barr had found a dark-staining body in the cell nuclei that, he hypothesized, indicated the presence of the female's two X chromosomes.[52] By January 1954, the Barr body test was being used on patients in Wilkins's clinic to diagnose sex, under the assumption that females usually have one Barr body, while males usually have none.[53] The test, consisting of a buccal smear where cells were taken from the cheek, soon became a useful medical tool to differentiate between male and female as well as a means to explore the chromosomal setup of intersex, transsexuality, and homosexuality. Much to the surprise of the Hopkins team, the Barr tests showed that chromosomally, these patients were predominantly male. They had been uniformly reared as girls, and they had genitals that looked female (though infantile) and a "normal" female production of adrenal hormones. The team reported that they were struck by the "unequivocal femininity" of the eleven patients they evaluated: "In all respects, these individuals fulfilled the cultural and psychological expectations of femininity so completely that it was, in each instance, impossible to envisage the person as a boy or man."[54] Despite possessing male sex chromosomes, the patients all had female gender roles, Money and the Hampsons argued, and provided more evidence that gender role corresponded to the sex in which a child was raised rather than with biological sex variables.

The team utilized the comparison of gender role with the six other variables of sex as convincing empirical evidence that the most significant indicator of somebody's gender role was the sex in which the person had been raised. The tabulation of the data allowed them to argue that in most cases where a contradiction existed between sex of rearing and one of the five biovariables of sex, gender role was in close conformity with the sex of assignment and rearing. Factors such as gonads or chromosomes, which had been regarded as the essential signifiers of sex, proved to be a "most unreliable prognosticator" and gave "no reason to suspect a correlation."[55] In conclusion, they postulated what they had already been practicing at the clinic. "Evidently," they maintained, "there is a very close connection between, on the one hand, the sex to which an individual is assigned, and thenceforth reassigned in a myriad subtle ways in the course of being reared day by day, and on the other hand the establishment of gender role and orientation as male and female."[56] In short, the sex of assignment and the consequent experiences of living in this sex were more important than any anatomical, physiological, or even chromosomal factors in determining a patient's sex.

Transforming Sex

The implications of the study went beyond the management and treatment of hermaphroditic patients. Its aim was to transform sex, and hermaphroditism was an opportune model, an experiment in nature that would allow the team to make grander claims. At the beginning of the first publication, "Hermaphroditism, Gender and Precocity in Hyperadrenocorticism," Money made clear that "the psychologic pertinence of hermaphroditism in human beings is that it provides illuminating evidence concerning the determinants and concomitants of sexual outlook and orientation," and he followed through on his promise.[57] He had a clear advantage in making such claims; his clinical access provided him with enough "data" to argue for a new "psychologic theory of sexuality" obtained "from the study of hermaphroditism"; he skillfully applied a set of accessible metaphors to reveal the actual process of gender role development. In addition, he could rely on the scientific authority of the Johns Hopkins Hospital and his mentor Lawson Wilkins to be taken seriously. As a result, and without hesitation, he claimed "that sexual behavior and orientation as male or female does not have an innate, instinctive basis."[58] This did not mean, however, that gender role was a purely socially produced/determined category.

Money's claims need to be understood in the context of both clinical pragmatism (what works for our patients?) and the group's grander claims to be solving persistent problems in psychology. That is, the team at Hopkins were solving a clinical conundrum based on existing practices, *and* Money was extrapolating from his clinical data to address what he called the age-old problem of mind-body dualism, providing what would become his trademark solution to a common conundrum. As he had already noted in his dissertation, hermaphroditism in general was an ideal natural experiment to test his theories on body and mind. Psychobiology and psychosomatic psychology, he argued, were still caught up in the cause-effect relationship of body and mind. His goal was to transcend such dualities. "These double-barred terms do not resolve the mind-body dilemma," he noted in his 1957 textbook, *The Psychological Study of Man*, which was based on several of his term papers and early published articles in *Psychiatry* and the *British Journal of Medical Psychology*.[59] On the contrary, "whenever men speak of two things, then they will surely, sooner or later, allow one to be cause, the other effect; and so arises the controversy of whether somatic happenings are caused by the psyche, or vice-versa, or both."[60] He argued that by the observation of signs and signals, by the deciphering of messages, with the "mind as the information and communication function of the human organism," one would gain insights into the mind-body unit.[61] How did the psychic and the somatic form the individual without forcing the two components into a causal relationship?

The Mind-Body Unit

For John Money, gender role was neither purely a social nor an environmental variable. It existed, rather, at the level where the biological and the social intersected. Nor could one tease out biological or social "components" of gender role. His was not "a theory of environmental and social determinism." Gender role was determined at birth but built up "cumulatively through experiences encountered and transacted," yet this process did not follow a "simple, point-for-point correlation." "Spontaneously putting two and two together" sometimes made four and "sometimes, erroneously, five." These experience-driven transactions, Money argued, were "frequently highly unpredictable, individualistic and eccentric, for reasons as yet not fully ascertained."[62] The process was best understood through analogies.

He provided two metaphors for thinking about gender role. The first related to language.[63] When a child acquired its native language, Money reasoned, an inherent biological capacity for language acquisition was directed by the language to which it was exposed.[64] Every human being was capable of learning any language that it encountered in its infant stage. This language skill became a part of the individual, so that it seemed nearly innate. Everyone had the capacity for language, but which language they would speak depended on the environment and culture in which they were raised as a child. Similarly, Money believed, everyone had a physical capacity for sexuality, but how it was expressed was shaped by early impressions.

The second metaphor Money used was imprinting, which he borrowed from ethology. Imprinting, translated from the German word *Prägung*, describes the process of how some species of birds attach to the first moving object they see after hatching.[65] In 1935, the Austrian animal behaviorist Konrad Lorenz, working primarily on geese and ducks, had observed that his birds would accept a foster mother in the place of its biological mother, even if she was of a different species (e.g., Lorenz himself).[66] For Lorenz, this kind of behavior was restricted to a critical period, an age at which a behavior had to be developed or never would be. After this fixed time, a change was impossible; the imprint had become irreversible. As the historian of science Marga Vicedo puts it in her description of Lorenz's research, "Afterward the brain, like hardened wax, cannot be molded."[67]

In a 1936 collaboration with Nikolaas Tinbergen, who studied stimulus-response behaviors in gulls, fish, and insects, Lorenz formulated the notion of the fixed-action pattern: a distinct and completely stereotyped set of complex behaviors that was innate in origin but triggered by an event in the animal's environment. For example, as Tinbergen showed, hungry gull babies would peck at a decoy with a red spot on its bill—a characteristic of the gull. Lorenz, Tinbergen, and Karl von Frisch, who decoded the "waggle dance" that honeybees use to direct their hive-mates to a nectar source, pioneered the study of instinctive complex behaviors. The three scientists shared the 1973 Nobel Prize in Physiology or Medicine for this work. Of the three, Lorenz was the most successful at bringing his ideas to popular audiences. As part of a postwar popularization of science, his widely read studies of animal behavior included *King Solomon's Ring* (1949/1952), *Man Meets Dog* (1950/1954), and *On Aggression* (1963/1966).[68] In the mid-1950s, the findings of Lorenz, Tinbergen, and von Frisch were already firmly integrated into psychology textbooks.[69]

In one of his articles with the Hampsons, "An Examination of Some Basic Sexual Concepts," Money wrote that gender role became "not only established, but also indelibly imprinted," yet there was no reference to Lorenz. He must have read Lorenz at that time, since he also invoked a "critical period," Lorenz's signature phrase.[70] Only in 1957, in a paper summarizing the findings of the team and in his textbook published that year, did Money finally explicitly mention Lorenz.[71] In these instances, he chose an example highlighting that imprinting had a directionality. Lorenz had shown, Money wrote, that wild mallard ducklings, immediately upon being hatched, could be made to treat him as if he were their mother. Contrary to graylag goslings, who react to the first living being they see as if it were their mother, the ducklings followed Lorenz around only after he started making quacking noises and waddling. "Lorenz became established for them as their mother," Money noted. "The truly amazing sequel, however, is that the ducklings responded to Lorenz as if he were their mother from that day onward."[72]

Money never cited Lorenz's scientific papers, only his popular book *King Solomon's Ring*. He was not interested in building his new theory on Lorenz's reformulation of instinct; rather, imprinting and Lorenz's birds provided a striking image of how gender role worked. This might account for the discrepancy between Lorenz's definition of *imprinting* and Money's use of the word. For Lorenz, imprinting in its original conceptualization had little to do with learning. Instead, it was caused by a bird's "innate urge to acquire the imprint of its species." "Imprinting," he explained, "is a process with a very limited scope, representing an acquiring process occurring only in birds and determining but one object of certain social reactions."[73] A bird would undergo this attachment process, as Vicedo puts it, "through a single impression, without conditioning, trial and error, or any period of learning."[74] This process was irreversible.

Lorenz's imprinted birds were a useful metaphor for Money, not a comparable example in a greater theoretical scheme. Using imprinting as a metaphor helped Money explain gender role as a behavior learned in a manner so fundamental that it became as innate as an instinct, yet was environmental and social as well as biological and elemental. He argued that there was no separation of body and mind, just as there was no distinction between maturation and learning. Concerning the process of growth, he wrote, "the contrast usually drawn between maturation and learning is not simply a contrast between ineradicable and eradicable. It is also tacitly conceded that maturation takes place mechanically and automatically, whereas learning must be activated by some drive or some promise of reward."[75] Money's intention was to transcend the binary opposition of biology and environment. He argued that these boundaries were not as closely drawn, that genes could be changed by environmental conditions, and that learned behavior could become ineradicable. Maturation and learning "belong together in the unitary process of growing up."[76]

The metaphor of imprinting suggested, at least in Money's interpretation, a certain fluidity of a gender role, the direction of which was not predetermined. A gosling could "choose" Lorenz as mother goose, if that was the option present at hatching, and a child could develop a male or female gender role, contingent on whether this child was raised as a boy or a girl. Yet gender fluidity had limits in Money's gender concept. Again he borrowed from ethology to introduce the notion of a critical period, which was crucial for the sense of "medical and social emergency" that the protocols invoked.[77] "Birds, of course, are not human beings," Money admitted, but the examples showed "that for the different phases and manifestations of growing there are critical periods during which development takes place and thenceforth cannot be undone." In "critical periods" certain influences, biological or social, had to occur, or else there would be a loss that could not be recovered. "At a year of age," he argued, "a child has no native language, but by the age of two establishment of native language is well on the way." In regard to hermaphrodites, this meant that "children born with genital anomalies so that their sex looks ambiguous . . . may be assigned to the sex contradictory of their chromosomal sex, of their gonadal sex and, at puberty, of their hormonal sex."[78] Based on data provided by Joan Hampson, he was convinced that with rare exceptions, children established the gender role of the sex they were assigned to and—if reassigned to the other sex—they were "unable to grow up in the new sex without some signs of personality 'nonhealthiness'" after the age of about eighteen months.[79]

Flexibility and Rigidity

Based on their theory of a learned gender role that would become indelibly imprinted in a child's mind, the Hopkins team proposed concrete treatment and management recommendations. A child would adjust to either gender role regardless of biological characteristics if the assignment of the sex of rearing was firm and consistent. It was essential that neither the parents nor the child have any doubts as to whether the child was a boy or a girl. As in their previous talks and presentation, the team stressed that clear communication with the child concerning his or her status was essential. The parents and physicians were called to speak openly and scientifically; for example, it was important to impress on children that they were not "physically half boy, half girl," as many still believed. Anatomical and embryological knowledge "that the child is, in fact, a girl or a boy who did not get finished, genitally," would help to bring "enlightenment to parents and children alike."[80] For Money, scientific language and clear, science-based explanations served as a bulwark against outdated prejudices against hermaphroditic children as freaks of nature.

Openness had its limits, though, and those limits were chromosomal. "Girls with gonadal agenesis and male chromosomes," the authors maintained, "are benefited if they remain uninformed of their chromosomal status. Should they obtain this information, they may be . . . unnecessarily confused and influenced by present day misconceptions that the entirety of one's sexuality is genetically determined."[81] In this reasoning, objective scientific and medical explanations and focused, carefully preselected information were the key to solving social problems. This approach also put increasing emphasis on the parents; with the medicalization of child-birth, "hermaphroditic" conditions had been diagnosed early and long before children could have a say in or consent to their treatment. The parents thus needed to be educated and brought in as allies to ensure the children's social adjustment and psychological health.

Building on Lawson Wilkins's existing practice and their theory of gender role, the Hopkins group recommended basing the sex of rearing on the child's external genitals as a visual signifier of sex—something that most parents and doctors were already doing anyway, they argued. Genitals that did not match the sex the child was living in only raised doubts in the minds of parents and confused children, who were prone to compare genitals. "Genital appearance is an important factor," Joan Hampson wrote, and "in assigning a sex to a newborn hermaphrodite, regardless of the etiology of the condition, primary consideration should be given not to the chromosomes, gonads, or hormones, but to external genital morphology."[82] Thus, the team recommended that "all further surgical and hormonal endeavor should be directed toward maintaining the person in that sex."[83]

Not only was it important that surgery to adapt genitals to the assigned sex be performed at an early age, but it was also inadvisable to change the sex a child was raised in after early infancy. "Though gender imprinting begins by the first birthday," the Hopkins team maintained, "the critical period is reached by about the age of eighteen months."[84] "By the age of 2½ years," Hampson claimed, based on a sample of ten patients, "gender role was indelibly established and thus change of sex should in general be avoided."[85] During the critical period, a change was possible; afterward, it would only lead to psychological "unhealthiness."[86]

The commitment to clear assignment and unambiguous rearing in one sex necessitated a clear-cut gender role division. Gender role had to be "clearly defined and consistently maintained," Money and the Hampsons wrote. Genitals had to be "corrected" so that these patients could eventually fulfill their social roles as men and women. Take this instance, in which Money and the Hampsons addressed criticism that keeping a CAH girl in her assigned sex as a boy would interfere with her fertility and render her sterile. In response, they argued that parenthood and marriage, too, were social categories. "The answer to this objection," they wrote "is that actual child bearing as distinguished from potential biological fertility is not determined by chromosomal, hormonal, and gonadal sex alone. It is also determined by the social encounters and cultural transactions of mating and marrying, which are inextricably bound up with gender role and erotic orientation."[87]

If this child could not fulfill her social role because her gender role was male, as was her assigned sex, then fertility did not matter. "The greater medical wisdom," they continued, "lay in planning for a sterile man to be physically and mentally healthy, and efficient as a human being, than for a fertile woman to be physically well but psychologically a misfit and a failure as a woman, a wife, or a mother. Thus a boy, changed to wear dresses once ovaries were discovered, may continue to think, act and dream as the boy he was brought up to be, eventually falling in love as a boy, only to be considered homosexual and maladjusted to society."[88] In the psychiatric model of maladjustment, homosexuality was linked to psychological "unhealthiness." A person's social role, even if only as a prediction for the future, trumped biological sex and reproductive capacities as determinants of gender. Health was folded into a broader notion of being able to fulfill one's social role.

Homosexuality plays a peculiar role in this reasoning. During the post–World War II era, an extraordinary moral panic arose—a surge of fear and social concerns about homosexuals in what is often referred to as the Lavender Scare. Homosexuals had become more visible during World War II and formed new communities in port cities afterward. Yet with the rise of Cold War anxieties about containment and political deviance, politicians and the public alike increasingly viewed homosexuality as sexual deviance that was not only corruptive and potentially contagious but also a first stop on the road to treason. After all, the reasoning went, homosexuals were susceptible to blackmail by foreign agents and thus should be prevented from taking government employment.[89] At the same time, scientists such as Alfred C. Kinsey normalized same-sex practices by showing how common they were in modern America and across populations. In his new quantitative notion of sexual norms that he first postulated in *Sexual Behavior in the Human Male,* one of the so-called Kinsey Reports, homosexuality became one of six possible sexual outlets and one reference point on a scale of human sexual orientation. Some read Kinsey's data as inspirational for thinking about homosexuals as an oppressed minority. For others, the data just confirmed their worst fear that a fifth column of homosexuals had infiltrated American society at every level.[90]

At the Hopkins clinic too, homosexuality was regarded as far from a desired outcome. To a degree, this anxiety about homosexuality was multiplied in cases where sex was considered ambiguous, contested, or undecided. If a person's sex needed to be contained within the categories of male and female to avoid accidental homosexual pairings, gender role complicated these assessments, because it might not match biological sex. Since for Money gender role was intrinsically heterosexual in its orientation, changing the sex of a child with an already established sex role would condemn that child to homosexual behavior. Homosexuality was yet another argument against changing sex after gender role was established.

The Lavender Scare of the 1950s left its mark on Money and the Hampsons' publications. Most important, they were worried that their research would be connected to the stigma of homosexuality and the sensationalism of transsexuality, which would run counter to their attempt to "medicalize" hermaphroditism as a legitimate health concern. "Most parents need to be told," they wrote, "that their child is not destined to grow up with abnormal and perverse sexual desires, for they get hermaphroditism and homosexuality hopelessly confused."[91] In another article, Hampson felt it important to stress that a "hermaphrodite's request for a change of sex" was not the same as requests "for mutilatory surgery or hormonal treatment from anatomically normal people, homosexual transvestites, for instance." Rather, the team was concerned with "only voluntary requests in older individuals with ambiguous genital appearance."[92] These anxieties about homosexuality were shared by their patients in their case studies, who took pains to describe themselves as heterosexual and reject any suspicion of homosexuality or association with "some of the queer flabs around."[93]

In the end, the team at Hopkins formulated a set of clear-cut recommendations for "treating" all variations of sexual development which addressed the practitioners' concerns and uncertainties: assign any sex as early as possible (though preferably the sex that would fit the external genitalia best); stick with this assignment firmly and consistently; do not change a child's sex after the age of two and a half; and use surgery before the child becomes a toddler to "reconstruct" the genitalia to fit the assigned sex of rearing and thus the child's gender role. These recommendations were firmly based, they claimed, on the empirical data of the clinic and underwritten by the theory that a child's gender role was learned through experiences and became ineradicably imprinted in the child's mind in the first years of life. Finally, the Hopkins team provided a standardized and manageable treatment protocol for doctors who felt uncertain about how to treat these patients.

––––––––

The formulation of gender role emerged from a range of different factors. First, there was an urgent clinical need for a practical and general solution to what was perceived as a medical, social, and psychological problem. Second, psychiatrists, psychoanalysts, and psychologists increasingly claimed that patients' psychological sex had to be considered to evaluate their sex. At Hopkins, an interdisciplinary team attempted to balance this complex endeavor across disciplinary boundaries, trying to provide all medical practitioners with a pragmatic and standardized solution. This clinical sense of emergency was underwritten by a set of ideas that had shaped US social thought over the last decades and seeped into the clinic. Among them were the ideas that behavior was learned and that personality was shaped by the culture and environment in which a child was raised. Hormonal experiments in the 1920s and 1930s had shown the body (and sex) to be malleable, plastic, and open to manipulation. Social sciences had shown that the same was true for the human mind and behavior by way of culture. These seemingly contradictory ideas of human plasticity allowed the team at Hopkins to propose that gender role was learned and that the body could be surgically and hormonally adjusted to fit the gender role of the child.

The findings and recommendations of the Hopkins team were shaped by perceived medical needs, the availability of medical technology, and John Money's mélange of theories and metaphors which postulated that gender was open to manipulation. Rather than positioning a purely social or environmental category of gender (mind) in opposition to a biological notion of sex (body), Money created the idea of an interactive mind-body unit that allowed the Hopkins group to study sex in a more complex way. His gender concept seemed to promise an astonishing fluidity of sex, and it deconstructed the naturalness of masculinity and femininity. In the clinic, though, gender role created a treatment regime that saw that role as fixed and rigid after a critical period, and regarded the body as the flexible unit that could be shaped to fit somebody's gender.

The team at Hopkins was caught within this paradox; the idea that any sex could be assigned was transformed into the recommendation that one sex must be assigned. Their goal to humanize a group of patients through science—that is, to speak freely, openly, and without prejudice about their anatomy, sexuality, and treatment goals—was undermined by their assumptions about humanity and their unquestioning acceptance of cultural scripts and norms of masculinity and femininity. Their ultimate inflexibility was shaped by cultural anxieties about sexuality and gender, some of which the patients and their families shared. As social determinism and social engineering replaced biological determinism, the Hopkins team inscribed these norms onto the body—and though not fixed to any biological root, they were strictly enforced in the name of psychological health, proper adjustment, and personal happiness. More than this specific contribution, Money and Hampson had reframed the question of true—or correct—sex from biological truth to social functionality and personal happiness. An exchange at the 1954 conference in Amherst aptly summarizes this shift from sex to gender. In the discussion following Hampson's presentation, the psychologist Calvin Stone asked her how sex could be assigned "correctly in every case." "Well, correct with regard to what?" Hampson replied. "I assume you mean so that the individual can grow up happily?"[94]

FIVE

Gender in the Clinic: The Process of Normalization

In January 1951, Mr. and Mrs. Smith took their ailing new-born son, Andy, to Baltimore to have him treated at the Johns Hopkins Hospital's Harriet Lane Home for Invalid Children. They were deeply worried, because they had already lost their first son to "severe dehydration + vomiting." The admittance record listed the referring physician's observations: "Could not tell if boy or girl, urinates often, drinks much, vomits occasionally."[1] When the Smiths left the clinic six months later, Andy's life-threatening symptoms were under control, thanks to the new drug cortisone. In addition, the infant had been reassigned as a girl. In the hospital record, on the line for name, "Andy" had been crossed out and replaced by "Ann."

Andy/Ann's diagnosis was congenital adrenal hyperplasia (CAH), and when the infant first entered the Pediatric Endocrinology Clinic in January 1951, its director, Lawson Wilkins, and his colleagues had just introduced cortisone as a treatment for the condition.[2] In November, when Ann was readmitted "for study and reevaluation of her congenital adrenal hyperplasia," John Money and Joan Hampson had just begun their psychological evaluation of the cortisone treatment and their formulation of the concept of gender role and standardized treatment guidelines. Over the next two decades, Ann's life, and that of her parents, was structured by the medical logic of the clinic as she returned for examination, assessment, and consultation at least once a year up until 1960. At face value, Wilkins and his team's goal was straightforward: to make Ann "healthy."

Yet health is a historically specific concept, articulated through a set of bodily practices, cultural meanings, and social norms. As the French philosopher and physician Georges Canguilhem has observed, medical treatment is always, in a sense, about normalizing the body.[3] Vital norms, according to Canguilhem, stem from the normativity of life, the capacity of an organism to adapt to its environment. In this context, health is a dynamic category denoting the ability to function in the world. Social norms, on the other hand, represent a particular order of society, and it is the incorporation of the social into the vital that this chapter explores. Normalization, as described by Foucault, becomes a process in which vital and social norms coalesce and overlap, and are integrated into a historically contingent notion of health. In this context, treating adrenal hyperplasia with cortisone to lower a patient's 17-ketosteroids (17-KS) level, which Canguilhem would label a vital normative procedure, and carrying out surgical and psychological procedures to make the same patient appear and act more feminine, thereby satisfying social norms, both become medical attempts to "heal."

In theory, the team at Hopkins developed standardized and one-for-all protocols for treating children with intersex traits. These protocols would allow them to achieve their treatment goals by manipulating gender role to ensure that these children became clearly gendered boys and girls, men and women. As psychiatry and psychology emerged during the two world wars as important fields for evaluating and treating individuals, the idea of a psychological sex that could be more authentic than biological sex had already found some degree of acceptance in medical circles. The Hopkins protocols and recommendations were developed in the context of a general understanding that much of what had been previously perceived as biological was indeed culturally specific and environmentally shaped human behavior. Even reluctant culturalists had to at least partly accept the new dominance of culture. By the end of World War II, the idea of culture shaping behavior and personality had shifted toward an idea of manipulating this process to produce a welcome social outcome—that is, to ensure well-adjusted and productive citizens.

In practice, this process of normalization was not a straightforward, universal, standardized route. The messiness of medical practice, in which doctors made sense of a condition that encompassed the biological and the social, was quite distinct from the polished logic of published case studies and stories. We often think of modern biomedicine as a precise science and imagine the process of diagnosis and prognosis as standardized and exact. Yet the messiness of diagnosing and managing chronic conditions, of encounters between physicians, patients, and their families, and of experiences inside and outside the clinic tells a different story. It reveals medicine as a social practice and discloses how understandings of health and disease are shaped by the world in which they are arrived at. The historian of medicine Charles Rosenberg, for example, used the metaphor of framing to refer to the process through which disease is defined and the consequences these definitions have on the lives of individuals or groups.[4] Factors such as the availability of intellectual definitions and diagnosis of disease, concepts of the body, and medical technologies as well as cultural and social meanings attached to disease shape the perceptions of physicians and patients as well as the broader public and public health officials. Historians of medicine have also pointed out the sometimes uneven relationship between theory and practice and the disparate ways in which medical knowledge and theories of the body are dispersed. For example, when bacteriology and germ theory revolutionized medical theory in the last decades of the nineteenth century, the practical application of germ theory still built on older theories of dirt and diseases to some extent, and its adaptation to medical therapeutics differed widely.[5]

Medical cases often tell a story that is different from published reports. They reveal *how* those involved in the clinical encounter know something rather than *what* they know. For example, instead of weighing medical definitions of sex against patients' conception of their sexual identity, one might ask how sex is given shape in clinical practice. Publications from the Hopkins clinic might state that chromosomal sex was determined by a Barr body test, yet patient records reveal a complicated process of contesting information, weighing diagnosis and test results, probing and examining the body, and considering seemingly nonmedical factors such as the sex noted on the birth certificate and the sex that parents preferred.[6] In a similar manner, patient records reveal how particular meanings of health and disease were negotiated in and through daily practices and routines. Accordingly, the stories about diagnosis, treatment, and maintenance depicted in this chapter probe the tensions and inconsistencies in these clinical encounters.

In the clinic, three types of practices structured the medical encounters among CAH patients, their parents, and medical experts: diagnosis, treatment, and maintenance. Parents took their children to the clinic to be diagnosed, and physicians there situated a child's symptoms within the framework of a condition they were in the process of defining. Part of the diagnostic process involved the determination of the patient's sex—a crucial element for deciding on a course of treatment—and one that was much more difficult and messier on the ground than depicted in published case studies. Although the diagnostic process was similar in boys and girls, treatment was specific to the assigned sex of the child.

Physicians determined their patient's sex to design a treatment program that was explicitly sex specific. For this reason, the Hopkins treatment protocols and "gender role assessment" were not just about determining sex but also a crucial part of the treatment regimen. As social norms were integrated into the medical norms of health, correct gender role was folded into the treatment process as one of many markers to check. Finally, the third practice concerned what I call management/ maintenance. Treatment consisted not only of immediate interventions to counter the life-threatening effects and symptoms of CAH that were perceived to be problematic. CAH is a chronic condition—and cortisone was not a cure but an intervention for management of the chronic condition: it had to be taken throughout a patient's life. The practice of maintenance set in after patients were "controlled on cortisone." It included yearly checkups for adequate cortisone dosage, somatic development, social adjustment, and gender role development.

Diagnosing CAH

Andy's parents arrived at the clinic worried because their infant was unwell. He did not feed well, he vomited, and consequently he became increasingly dehydrated despite drinking adequate fluids. What brought them to the clinic was alarm over their child's health and hope that physicians there could improve his condition. Although Andy's obvious dehydration was his parents' most urgent concern, it was not their only concern. Uncertainty about Andy's sex had arisen at birth, and his parents were hoping for medical answers. These two concerns—one life-threatening, the other upsetting for the child's parents—were the reasons most commonly listed for why parents sought the advice of medical experts. More and more, that expert was Lawson Wilkins.

How did Wilkins and his team diagnose CAH? And how was that diagnosis related to sex and sexual development? Diagnosis started with the parent. First, doctors collected a patient history of the child from the parents. This included a narrative of the child's development, appetite, diet, and any similar cases in the family. The child was then examined, measured, assessed, and tested. The thorough general examination assessed genitalia and sexual appearance, skin pigmentation, and hair growth. Doctors measured height and weight and compared the results to average measures for age to determine advanced bone growth. X-rays were made for further assessment of bone development. Some tests, such as a tuberculosis test and a test for syphilis, were performed on all children who came to the Harriet Lane Home.[7] Others, such as the urine test for 17-KS, were specific to diagnosing CAH.[8] In practice, collecting a complete urine sample over a twenty-four-hour period was quite invasive, and babies and infants had to be strapped to a special metabolic bed for the entire period.[9]

These diagnostic procedures were the same for girls and boys. Physicians were concerned primarily about the child's metabolism and checked for any salt-losing tendencies. They constantly monitored his or her development, including bone growth, height, and physique, to identify precocity. They repeated urine tests to determine the child's 17-KS level and checked for obvious effects of increased androgen levels such as skin pigmentation, depth of voice, acne, hairiness, and muscular development. Reading the child's genitals for signs of adrenal overexposure was contingent on diagnostic expectations and prognosis of sex. In boys, precocious enlargement of the child's penis was read as an indicator of CAH. In girls, such as Ann, "virilization" of the genitals was interpreted as a sign of CAH. However, this was not the only possible reading of genitals that appeared male. Without the CAH diagnosis, Ann's genitals (and her sex) had simply been considered as male at birth.

In practice, diagnosis was a messy process that was often contingent on the physician's experience with the condition, the cooperation of parents and patients, and the success of tests. Tests could fail or offer inconclusive results, and in some instances, parents had decided to leave before a diagnosis was finalized. When James was born in 1945, his parents and his doctor—Wilkins—examined him for signs of the condition. They had every reason to be concerned: two of his three siblings had already been diagnosed as having CAH.[10] At the time of his birth, Wilkins had thought that James "was strong and vigorous. The penis was perhaps a little large for a newborn, but was normally formed and could not be considered beyond normal limits of size. The testes, though small, were not abnormal." Wilkins expected "another occurrence of congenital adrenal hyperplasia in the family," and when one-week-old James started losing weight rapidly "in spite of the fact that he was taking ample feeding," the physician considered his assessment confirmed. In light of this family's medical history, he interpreted weight loss, a common childhood problem, as evidence of CAH.

At first, the chemical confirmation of his diagnosis failed; Wilkins could not get sufficient blood or urine samples from the baby to conduct a urinalysis. When James's condition improved, his mother had brought him home before more tests could be performed. She "had no further feeding difficulties with him" and returned a year later with her baby. At this admission, Wilkins finally confirmed his initial diagnosis through an examination, measurements, and tests: "there was definite growth in the size of his penis" and "a little short blond fuzz" on the genitals, and the child showed advanced growth and "rather strong, well developed musculature." X-rays confirmed advanced bone development, and blood and urine tests confirmed that this was "unquestionably a case of congenital androgenic hyperplasia of the adrenal causing macrogenitosomia precox." During the next two years, James was seen at regular intervals to confirm his diagnosis and to monitor his development.

Diagnosing Sex

Sex had to be diagnosed as well. Although in most cases the local physician and the parents had chosen a sex at birth, this assignment was reevaluated when a child was diagnosed as having CAH. In most instances, a child's sex had been debated at birth or doubted shortly thereafter, and parents expected doctors to diagnose the "true sex" or to confirm the assigned sex. Consequently, the diagnosis of sex and hormonal pathology went hand in hand—they were mutually constitutive. In their quest to determine sex, clinicians faced two basic questions and problems. First was the tension between diagnosing a child's true sex—an enterprise that was surprisingly complex and protracted in mid-twentieth-century America—and determining the right sex for a child, which did not always correspond to their diagnosis. Second, and specific to CAH, was the realization that the determination of the better sex, the sex that the child could live in successfully, shaped the direction of treatment and management.

Patient records from the clinic reveal that diagnosing a child's sex was far from easy and was contingent on a set of factors including experience, technique, test results, the age of the child, and parental wishes. Despite significant medical advances, diagnosis of true sex in the mid-twentieth century still relied on the physicians' experience and the medical and surgical techniques and technologies available.[11] A child's appearance could be deceiving, and diagnostic procedures could be inconclusive. Physicians used palpating techniques, such as feeling for testes or ovaries or penetrating the urethra and anus with instruments and fingers to feel for a vagina or a womb. Feeling the inside of the body was often misleading, however, and techniques to make that visible, including X-rays and the insertion of liquids into bodily orifices, were sometimes inconclusive. A laparotomy was sometimes the only way to know a child's sex for certain. Because prenatal androgen exposure mainly affected external genitals and appearance, the presence of a uterus, ovaries, and fallopian tubes indicated female sex for the physicians.

In the 1940s and 1950s, the practices of sex determination were lengthy and contentious. Take Carol's case, for example (discussed at greater length in chapter 2). At her birth in the fall of 1941, "an abnormality of external genitalia"—that is, an "enlarged clitoris"—had been noted.[12] Her "parents were told that the baby was a girl." Wilkins "saw the baby at the Women's Hospital when she was 12 days old" and diagnosed her as "female pseudohermaphrodite" caused by "hyperplasia of the androgenic zone of the adrenal occurring in very early embryonic life." Carol's mother concealed this diagnosis from her husband, worried that he might not be "emotionally stable" enough to bear that something was wrong with his daughter.

Diagnosis of sex was made by the examination of external and internal reproductive organs and in conjunction with the diagnosis of CAH. At first, Wilkins based his assessment on the inspection of Carol after birth and on her symptoms, which indicated CAH. Hopkins gynecologist Dr. Richard Wesley TeLinde, who examined Carol two years later in 1943, was not convinced by Wilkins's diagnosis of sex at birth.[13] To be certain, he recommended a laparotomy to determine the child's internal organs and gonads. If the "internal pelvic organs [were] found to be definitely female the clitoris should be amputated," he wrote, and "should any testicular tissue be found intra-abdominally it should be removed." Wilkins, though convinced that Carol was a girl based on his experience with her condition, accommodated his colleague's wishes. "Following this examination," he wrote, "I felt quite satisfied that the child had the usual anatomical abnormality which is regularly present in cases of female pseudohermaphroditism due to androgenic hypertrophy of the adrenal in early embryonic life. Dr. TeLinde, however, felt that to settle absolutely the question of the sex of this child once and for all it would be advisable to perform an exploratory laparotomy and demonstrate the presence of ovaries." Carol was admitted to the

Harriet Lane Home clinic "for exploratory laparotomy and amputation," indicating that there was already an expected outcome. During the procedure, doctors confirmed that Carol had a uterus, fallopian tubes, and ovaries, and upon the diagnosis of female sex, her "enlarged" clitoris was amputated. The diagnosis—that is, the determination of sex "once and for all"—triggered a follow-up procedure that adjusted Carol's body to the diagnosed sex. In Carol's case, the diagnosis of true sex correlated with what was determined to be the better sex for her. In other cases, decisions were not as clear-cut.

Chromosomes, often thought to be the definitive marker of sex, did not solve the puzzle of sex as the practitioners had hoped.[14] As we saw in chapter 4, in 1948 Murray Llewellyn Barr had discovered a dark-staining body in the cell nuclei—the "Barr body"—that he hypothesized indicated the presence of the female's two X chromosomes.[15] Today, the Barr body is understood as one of the X chromosomes that has been inactivated. Humans, who have two X chromosomes per cell, inactivate one or the other to prevent a "double dose" of the X chromosome genes. As Fiona Alice Miller has pointed out, this discovery allowed scientists and clinicians to "see" something that was otherwise invisible, and for a decade it was, as Miller shows, "good enough" science to be used to determine the sex of intersexuals, transsexuals, and homosexuals.[16] The Barr body test came to constitute only one step in a complex process. Throughout the 1950s, researchers supported an emerging three-stage model of sexual differentiation consisting of sex chromosomes as a first stage, sex hormones as a second, and environment—introduced by John Money—as a third.[17]

The Barr test was introduced into clinical practice at Wilkins's clinic in 1954 and increasingly used on patients to determine their sex. Even sex chromosomes, however, could be ambiguous. Take Richard's case. He was born in January 1949 and first came to Hopkins in the summer of 1954 at the age of five.[18] He had been diagnosed at the local hospital as a precocious boy with metabolic problems due to adrenal hyperplasia. He also had a history of convulsions. Richard's parents took him to Johns Hopkins's cardiac clinic to find out the cause of his convulsions and for evaluation of his cortisone therapy. When they arrived at the hospital, they did not doubt the sex of their son. In the general examination, a physician confirmed the child's sex as he examined and measured his penis and stated that the "right testicle was palpable and of the size of a small olive. Left testes [sic] could not be felt." During his stay at Hopkins, Richard's diagnosis was confirmed as "salt-losing type of adrenal hyperplasia." Dr. Judson Van Wyk, the treating physician in

Wilkins's absence, was mainly concerned with controlling the acceler-ated growth caused by the boy's excess androgen level and thought that "with adequate suppression he could probably attain a socially accept-able stature." It was recommended that Richard come back in the fall or spring for further evaluation by Wilkins himself and for dosage adjust-ment of his cortisone treatment.

In 1955, Richard returned, and this time the testis, which had been felt at the boy's last visit, was nowhere to be found. Wilkins, who examined the boy, wondered whether he might not be a female pseudohermaphro-dite with congenital adrenal hyperplasia after all. Last year's testis might in fact have been an "inguinal lymph node"; Wilkins also noted that "this boy's phallus does not seem to be as hypertrophied as most males with macrogenitosomia precox due to adrenal hyperplasia." He thought it wise "to exclude" this possibility "by means of a study of the sex chro-matin pattern in skin biopsy and by urethroscopic examination to deter-mine whether there might be a communicating vagina." Richard's Barr test, however, revealed an "apparently male pattern."[19] Dr. Scott did a urethroscopic examination and found no evidence of a vaginal pouch.

Despite the chromosomal and anatomical proof of sex, Wilkins re-mained doubtful. At Richard's next admission in the summer of 1956, he ordered an exploratory laparotomy and another chromosomal sex test. The result was surprising. This time, the pattern was female; Richard "had buccal mucosa smear this AM which revealed female sex chromosome pattern, so on [2 days later] at 10AM will have laparotomy to remove female gonads." It had taken two years for Wilkins and his colleagues to pinpoint Richard's sex, and in the end, genetic sex and the presence of a small uterus and ovaries—which could now suddenly be felt via rectal exam—indicated female.

Trusting his experience with the physical examination of CAH pa-tients over gonadal and chromosomal evidence, Wilkins had remained skeptical about Richard's sex. Although genetically female, the child had been raised as a boy, and upon finding gonadal and chromosomal proof of his female sex, Wilkins and his team stuck to the initial diagnosis of Richard as male. The file shows no discussion of the implications of this decision. In Richard's record, the operating surgeon, Dr. Howard Jones, simply stated, "A routine total abdominal hysterectomy was then per-formed with excision of both tubes and ovaries. The vaginal vault was closed . . . in the usual manner."[20] For the physicians, psychological sex, or gender role, and Richard's having already lived as a boy for seven years supported their decision to keep him in the male sex. Accordingly, the postoperative diagnosis read: "congenital adrenal hyperplasia in a genetic female with psychological sex of male." Once the decision was made, biological traces of femininity were surgically removed.

Contrary to the published reports, patient records reveal the imprecision of the new Barr body test and the questions it raised rather than answered. In cases of CAH, the test was applied at a time when recommendations concerning the diagnosis of sex had shifted with the introduction of cortisone. Wilkins thought that with the new therapy, newborn girls should be raised as girls. He was uncertain, however, about whether to change sex in cases where girls had already been living as boys. Sex chromosomes were added to the diagnostic process to confirm female sex, but they did not automatically determine the right sex for a child. In the end, the diagnosis of sex in CAH children was structured by available medical technologies, the skill and experience of the physicians in performing the Barr test, the presenting symptoms of the endocrinological condition, the families' wishes, and the sex already assigned at birth.

Sex chromosomes did not matter if the results of the Barr test contradicted the parents' understanding of or personal preference for their child's sex. Parents did not always yield to physicians' authority in this regard. For example, as we saw in the introduction, when Charles was born in the fall of 1955, he was "said to be a normal male infant at birth."[21] When he started growing pubic hair at the age of two, his parents took him to the local physician, where a Barr test revealed a female pattern. When he was admitted to the clinic in 1958, the emotional turmoil this announcement had caused resonated in the patient history the attending physician recorded: "The parents were told the findings, the diagnosis of congenital adrenal hyperplasia was made, and it was recommended that the patient undergo plastic repair and be raised as a female. Some family members objected to this approach and the pt [patient] was referred here for further evaluation and Rx [prescription]."

At Wilkins's clinic, Charles was diagnosed as having "congenital adrenal hyperplasia, female pseudohermaphrodite, salt losing type." The gynecological examination revealed female reproductive organs, and another Barr test confirmed the female pattern. To resolve the issue, the mother met with John Money, who was "of the opinion that this entire family is strongly oriented in the direction of masculine gender for this patient." Charles was only two and a half years old, and with the advent of cortisone treatment the recommendation would generally have been to reassign him as a girl.[22] However, as I have pointed out in the introduction, "the parents seem to feel rather strongly about raising this child as a boy [emphasis in original, with pen]." A few days later, Jones removed the fallopian tubes, ovaries, and uterus. Charles's genitalia were consistently referred to in terms of penis, phallus, and scrotum from the first day, though the anesthesia record reads "Diagnosis and operation: Female pseudo-hermaphroditism due to congenital adrenal hyperplasia." At the top of the page, where the patient's sex was noted, F for Female was circled, then crossed out, and M for male was circled.

As the case records show, knowing a patient's sex for certain was a contentious negotiation, which depended on the available medical technology and techniques as much as on the physician's experience with the specific condition, along with the manifold ways "sex" presented itself to the observer. Even in the face of gonadal and chromosomal "evidence" of a child's sex, Lawson Wilkins, who by the mid-1950s had observed 80 cases of CAH—60 female and 20 male—relied on his experience.[23] However, even if sex had finally been pinned down to a specific category—increasingly a genetic one—this category often did not make sense to the parents and the physicians in the face of contradictory somatic, psychological, and social variables.

Treatment

Andy's arrival at the Pediatric Endocrinology Clinic in 1951 was a medical emergency. "Obviously," Dr. John Crigler wrote in a summary, "control of her electrolyte abnormality was the most important and primary object."[24] Diagnosis was translated into immediate medical interventions. The physicians instantly placed Andy on a special diet with extra salt and started treating the infant with cortisone. The dosage of the new therapeutic had to be adjusted individually to each patient, monitored, and evaluated.[25] Andy's diagnosis as female also triggered another set of medical interventions. One was surgical. In 1954, her clitoris was "excised," and in 1959 Hopkins surgeons performed a "reconstruction of the external genitalia" and her vagina. The other intervention concerned her "adjustment." After her sex (and name) was changed to female, Ann was psychologically evaluated and tested to assess her development and evaluate her happiness. Often, these assessments were worded like this one from 1957: "She is an attractive, intelligent and cooperative little girl who is extremely well poised. The body build is somewhat stocky with square shoulders and well developed muscles although definitely feminine." CAH created a medical emergency on two levels. One was the life-threatening effect of the adrenal hyperplasia. The other was the diagnosis of sex and girls with a phallus or a large clitoris. In this section, I address how the first "emergency" was reconciled with the second.

Cortisone restructured the medical approach to CAH and to sex. It transformed CAH from an acute condition into a chronic one. It also reframed the question of finding the better sex for CAH patients. Before cortisone, some children had died. Boys raised as boys faced sexual precocity and the prognosis of stunted growth. Girls raised as girls faced an increasingly masculine appearance. Girls raised as boys, a path recommended by Wilkins, appeared male despite their chromosomal sex. With the introduction of cortisone, Wilkins's treatment recommendations shifted. Cortisone worked beyond the usual surgical intervention targeting the underlying condition. It reduced the androgen levels in girls with CAH, which "feminized" their overall appearance and promoted breast growth and menstruation. It also arrested and reversed the problematic premature growth and disturbances in salt metabolism in both CAH girls and boys.

To be sure, excessive "virilization" in CAH children was never regarded as a good thing. However, to Wilkins the degree of intervention depended on the prescribed sex. In CAH girls raised as girls, the prescribed goal of the physicians was to completely check all effects of excessive androgen through cortisone therapy and surgery. In CAH girls raised as boys, cortisone therapy was often reduced or supplemented with testosterone to achieve "adequate" virilization, though carefully balanced so as not to arrest growth prematurely. In CAH boys, who looked sexually mature far beyond their age, cortisone therapy was aimed at arresting precocious virilization and sexual development.

Salt loss and its threat to the infant's life made CAH a medical emergency and cortisone a lifesaver. But what about the surgical interventions that surgeons performed routinely on children in Wilkins's clinic? What kind of emergency was a large clitoris? These procedures were regularly performed and taken for granted; in not one of the patients' records or published case studies were these amputations questioned by physicians, surgeons, or parents. The voices of the children who underwent these procedures are mostly absent from these records; the majority had been too young to object.[26] In all but one of the sixteen cases in my sample where "enlarged clitoris" was listed as one of the "complaints," surgeons performed a clitoridectomy at the earliest possible time after admission.

Clitoridectomies were far from new—we find them in Hugh Hampton Young's cases as much as in Wilkins's precortisone recommendations.[27] Hopkins seems to have had an unusually strong surgical tradition, but as the historian Sarah B. Rodriguez has shown, clitoral surgeries (including clitoridectomies) were routine medical treatments for different "ailments" in the United States from the mid-nineteenth century far into the twentieth century.[28] Physicians were well aware of the clitoris as a sexual organ, but female pleasure was read through a prism of social norms and health.[29] Physicians removed all or parts of a clitoris if it was deemed "unhealthy." In the late nineteenth century, many of these cases revolved around fears about masturbation; the size of a clitoris was considered both cause and sign of masturbation and, increasingly, homosexuality. In this context, clitoridectomies were conceptualized as treatment to restore a patient's health.

In the patient records, frequent erections and masturbation in boys and girls are flagged as major concerns for the children's adjustment. These observations were made by doctors and parents alike. Physicians regularly inquired after such behavior, and parents, upset by their daughters' large clitorises, addressed these issues in conversation with clinicians.[30] Take Linda's case. At birth, she had been "considered a normal female and even at several examinations by a pediatrician during subsequent months." Her parents had noted very early, however, that her "clitoris was enlarged." Linda did not have a severe life-threatening form of CAH, but she showed signs of precocity (growth and pubic hair). In 1944 when she was three years old, her parents, upset by her large clitoris, underwent the long journey from the Midwest to be seen by Hugh Hampton Young at Hopkins's James Buchanan Brady Urological Institute.[31] At the age of five, Linda was referred to the Clinic of Pediatric Endocrinology for "treatment with newer steroids which may suppress the secretion of adrenal androgens." During this admission in 1946, her parents discussed their concerns about their daughter's genitals: "When she was a very young baby the parents noticed a little fullness about the genitalia but did not realize there was something abnormal. . . . When she was 2 years old and the younger sister was born, [the] parents realized that this child's clitoris was definitely enlarged." Normality had a reference point: Linda's clitoris enlargement became noticeable once her parents compared it with her little sister's.

Observation of Linda's "enlarged clitoris" was integrated into her therapeutic plan. "Although she plays with her genitalia some, masturbating has not become a problem," the clinician wrote, adding, "she's always hungry." When Linda returned to the clinic half a year later, Wilkins summarized, "The child has been well all summer. Has continued to grow rapidly and pubic hair has increased. Parents hope to enter her in kindergarten or school this fall. I advised before this was done the clitoris be removed as this is the source of sex excitation and curiosity and would probably be a cause of trouble with the other children in school." The parents agreed—they were planning to have Linda start school ahead of time, "because her school career will be interrupted by surgery necessary for her congenital anomaly." Shortly thereafter, her clitoris was "completely dissected out."

In Linda's case, clinicians and parents agreed that her large clitoris had to go. Why this insistence? Her patient records suggest that for her parents, the large clitoris raised doubts about her sex and heightened existing anxieties about her sexuality. What about Wilkins and his medical team? On the one hand, they saw the increased size of her clitoris as caused by the underlying pathology, her adrenal hyperplasia and excess androgen output, and thus something that could be corrected. On the other hand, they worried about masturbation and, increasingly, the danger of psychological maladjustments. Difference in appearance that triggered her neighbors' curiosity and doubts about her sex could cause such maladjustment—a conviction already deeply ingrained in Wilkins's reasoning in the mid-1940s.

A year after her clitoridectomy, Wilkins evaluated Linda's social development alongside an assessment of her growth (rapid), health (she had the measles), skin (acne on face and seborrhea on scalp), development (pubic hair had increased considerably), and behavior (very active and energetic, not unruly or hard to manage): "There have been no new problems in contact with other children. No undue sex curiosity. Asks only the usual questions in regard to sex and does not realize that she is different from other children." In his report on her genitalia, he remarked, "Since the removal of the clitoris the external genitalia superficially simulate those of an adult woman except that labia minora are lacking and the only orifice is the narrow urogenital sinus." In a psychological follow-up from 1950, a report by Linda's mother grants the only glimpse at how Linda might have felt: "She said to me once that she thought there was a difference. She said it looked different (after we took her home). She didn't seem to be very curious about her operation. I think when the clitoris was there it bothered her. She used to put her hands down there. I used to say 'Don't do that, you might hurt yourself.' I didn't have to say it very often." This exchange between mother and daughter shines a different light on parents' perceptions of masturbation than we find in the prescriptive literature of the time. In post-Freud America, the ideas that children had an innate sexuality and that sexual questions should be addressed in a "frank, friendly fashion" were prevalent at least in manuals promoting sex education at home and in schools, and could be found as well as in some psychology textbooks.[32] These authors cautioned parents that if they found "that their child masturbated, he [was] not marked out thereby as a potential 'pervert,' nor has any sin been committed."[33] On the contrary, there were "very, very few children" who never masturbated, and the "sporadic practice" was not to be "held in abhorrence although it is not to be encouraged."[34] If anything, "habitual performance of the act continued into adult life" would be a problem.[35]

In practice, the reasoning behind the amputation of "enlarged clitorises" was multifold. Masturbation and anxieties about children's sexuality played a role in the decision-making of the older generation of practitioners. In cases of congenital adrenal hyperplasia (CAH), the reasoning was also medical. Clinicians saw a clear correlation between the underlying pathology of the adrenals and the growth of the clitoris, which justified drastic surgical interventions such as clitoridectomy. Increasingly, the incentive to act was a psychological one as well. Wilkins, who stressed the importance of variation in growth and development and who cautioned other practitioners and parents to avoid medical interventions in children who were simply developing in their own manner, nonetheless recommended surgery in cases where difference in appearance would cause "maladjustment."[36] Based on this rationale, he paid close attention to creating a sex-specific convincing appearance. It was deemed important to appear believably as one's sex, the sex that had been assigned to one at birth or sometime afterward. Therefore, it sufficed if the girls' operated genitals simply "simulate those of an adult woman." The impetus to desexualize a girl by shaping her into a "woman" is representative of an approach to sex where "passing" and appearance were prioritized.

Appearance trumped function—in order for the patient to function convincingly in the world as a girl, the erotic function of her clitoris had to be neglected. In some cases, surgeons would construct a cosmetic clitoris after amputation—devoid of pleasurable sensation but giving the appearance of convincing female genitals.[37] Two-year-old Betty was operated on in 1954, and the surgeon noted in her report, "The clitoris was then excised, leaving a flap of the ventral mucous membrane for a cosmetic clitoris."[38] Surgeons also constructed an artificial clitoris for nine-year-old Dorothy after her subtotal clitoridectomy in 1955.[39]

Although clitoridectomies were performed in the 1930s and 1940s— Linda's operation dates from 1946—their raison d'être was reformulated and psychologized in the early 1950s. Lawson Wilkins's psychological team set out to address two questions: One, how did clitoral amputation or reduction affect the sexuality of adult women with CAH? Two, should the Pediatric Endocrinology Clinic continue performing clitoridectomies on girls who had received early treatment with cortisone? Joan Hampson found only six adult women to interview, but her results were unanimous.[40] The interviews revealed that "adult untreated women with hyperadrenocorticism . . . have been driven more often than not to frequent masturbation, sometimes with desperate urgency, despite personal taboos." In these patients, the "feminine role had become so thoroughly ingrained" that possessing an "erectile phallus" caused "immense distress, morally if not physically" (270).

Based on this evidence of psychological suffering and potential maladjustment, Hampson developed a rationale for clitoral amputation. She was well aware that "many surgeons have hesitated to deprive a patient of what some authorities have declared the most significant erotic zone in the female." Her data showed otherwise, she wrote: "The evidence demonstrates that clitoral amputation in childhood or later proved detrimental neither to subsequent erotic responsiveness, nor to capacity for orgasm" (270). Leaving a large clitoris in place was, however, detrimental to a girl's psychological adjustment and could lead to problems with her gender role. Weighing the pros and cons, Hampson cautioned that one should not underestimate "psychologic difficulties consequent on growing up with a large phallus" (271). "To make normal-looking female external genitals," she stated, "it is often conspicuously advisable to extirpate or amputate an enlarged phallus in addition to plastic remodeling of the urogenital sinus" (270).

Cortisone promised a long-term chemical solution to all these issues. If applied at an early age, it would arrest any further virilization, save the lives of children with severe salt loss, and halt precocious development in children with CAH. Its promise was circulated via medical and popular channels. Wilkins trained a generation of pediatric endocrinologists who would open their own clinics and refer their patients to him. Others heard about Wilkins and cortisone in the media. Donna's mother said she took her daughter to Hopkins in 1953 because she had read about "the use of cortisone in treatment of adrenal hyperplasia in a popular magazine."[41] Cortisone treatment was biomedicine's promise of a better future for these children, but as so often happens, the story was more complicated.

Management

Kathleen's mother saved for a whole year to raise the money to take her sick three-year-old daughter to Hopkins in 1952.[42] Her doctor suspected a "glandular problem or a tumor" and convinced her that the doctors at the Pediatric Endocrinology Clinic would be able to help her child. In examining Kathleen, Wilkins and his team noted pubic hair, an enlarged clitoris, advanced bone age, and elevated 17-KS, and they diagnosed her as "female pseudohermaphrodite due to adrenal hyperplasia." They also proclaimed her to be a "severely mentally defective child."

Kathleen's experience seems typical at first. She became part of Wilkins's studies and stayed in the hospital for the next three months until she was "well controlled on cortisone." She was treated with cortisone because "it was felt that this patient was particularly suitable for the various studies, in as much as she was so mentally impaired that the restraint was no particular hardship or handicap and that she had no electrolyte defect which might jeopardize her and that she was the only untreated case of adrenal hyperplasia available." The physicians explained "the scientific impact of the studies" to Kathleen's mother and charged the "costs of hospitalization for most of the period of investigation" to a fund. Doctors also noted that "the mother was quite willing and probably relieved to have her [daughter] stay in the hospital," an assessment that did not consider the hopes she placed on the clinic's medical care.

Cortisone was not a cure but part of a lifelong management strategy for a chronic condition. A process of normalization combined biological and social interventions to shape a child into a functioning, well-adjusted, clearly gendered citizen. What makes Kathleen's case exceptional are the ensuing debates among members of her medical team about whether to even continue her long-term treatment with cortisone. Her mother had come to Hopkins filled with hope that she would find a way to improve her child's condition. Cortisone had restored some aspects of Kathleen's health but would not change the diagnosis of "mental deficiency." Wilkins and his colleagues consequently discussed whether they should continue treatment, given that she could not be normalized. "It seems debatable," they wrote, "whether to continue with prolonged cortisone therapy because of her severe mental defect." Cortisone was expensive, the girl did not suffer from a severe and potentially life-threatening form of CAH, and gender role and sex assignment did not matter in a girl who would never live independently. They explained to her mother "that no improvement of her cerebral condition could be expected. The only advantage of treatment would be to prevent progressive virilization and to attempt to regulate somatic growth and osseous development at normal rate."

In the end, Wilkins and his team decided to continue treatment for two reasons. One was to make the parents' lives easier. "The mother insists on keeping the child at home for her full life-time, so the cortisone therapy is considered justified to make it less of an ordeal for the family. The size of the clitoris will not diminish—surgery would be necessary if considered aesthetically necessary." The other reason was that "scientifically," Kathleen's was an interesting case to follow. "Since we have comparatively few cases of this age group in our series," they noted, "it was of interest to us to continue treatment for a number of years to see how successful it might be particularly in regulating somatic growth and development and delaying premature puberty. We therefore arranged to supply oral cortisone free for her further treatment [emphasis in original, with pen]." Kathleen was discharged in late winter 1952, and her parents were given cortisone for her treatment. Her record ends with a follow-up note in 1954 that her mother had a baby boy "who seems to be normal."

Kathleen's case underscores the fact that in the long run, medical management of CAH patients aimed at making the patient into a fully functional social being; gender/sex was only one aspect of this ongoing and tenuous project. With Kathleen, who in the eyes of the treating physicians had no chance of one day living independently due to her mental deficiency, masculinization and its implications for proper gender orientation became less of an issue. There was no incentive for the complicated—and no doubt costly—cortisone treatment, as it did not matter in this case. Nor are there references in Kathleen's record to suggest that doctors performed a clitoridectomy on her during her 1952 stay. There is only the assessment among the handwritten progress notes from 1952 that "surgery would be necessary if considered aesthetically necessary." If normalization was not an attainable treatment goal, genital appearance was negligible. Ultimately, the reasons that Kathleen's treatment was continued reveal both sides of this medical encounter: the (sometimes futile) goals of care and restoring a notion of health that encompassed the social, and scientific interest in a case that would provide insights into the workings of a specific rare condition.

The goal of management encompassed both vital and social adjustment. Its goal was to restore metabolic health through cortisone treatment, to control for psychological health by assessing happiness and adjustment, and to ensure the development of the proper gender role through surgery and the ability to pass as the assigned sex. Gender role was folded into the management of CAH as one aspect of successful treatment. Health was never a purely biological goal in these interventions. The clinic's management goal was to make these patients into what Wilkins and his team perceived as psychologically well-adjusted and functional, clearly gendered men and women who could "live a normal life." How did this goal translate into markers of success? It meant to fit in socially, to be accepted as boy or girl, as man or woman, to succeed in a chosen education or profession, and to be happy and cooperative. After the introduction of cortisone, it also entailed dating and getting married. Gender role was measured through an assessment of the child's behavior during examination and through psychological interviews and tests. In this context, deviation from gender role was entered in the records in the same manner as elevated 17-KS levels.

For Wilkins and his team, gender role was on a long list of physical and psychological markers to be checked in the process of normalization. Richard, who despite his female chromosomal sex remained a boy, returned to the clinic four more times until 1964, and his body and behavior were observed for signs of maleness and femaleness.[43] A physician described him as a "large, somewhat clumsy male child appearing well," whose "well proportioned hips have contours somewhat female in type with no deformity." Dutifully reporting Richard's progress in letters to the physicians, his mother wrote in 1960 that "he is all boy now, well adjusted with his playmates and will be in the 6th grade when he passes this June." The treating physician commented, "This patient is actually a female who has been ovariectomized," and he wondered how best to balance the continuation of the cortisone treatment for avoiding precocious growth and the administration of testosterone for masculinization. Four years later, the mother again confirmed her assessment of Richard's gender by writing to the physicians, "With exception of his height, he is an average boy of 15 years."

Management was contingent on desired outcome. In Richard's case, masculinity had been the goal. In Carol's case, virilization was a matter of concern. Carol's behavior over the years was noted and closely followed during each admission as Wilkins and his colleagues assessed her appearance and her performance. In 1944, before cortisone, they had written, "She is a very bright, active, precocious child. Appears quite intelligent. Her appearance and actions seem to be quite feminine." The following year, Wilkins thought she had a "very feminine appearance." In 1946, he was worried that the "child continues to grow and virilize at a rapid rate," but in his opinion, "the patient is not abnormal in her sexual interests and curiosity." The question of sexual normality had come up because of "the neighborhood problem"—Carol's condition had put her at the center of "much sexual attention" by little boys. "One of the neighbors has called on the mother to get more detailed information about [Carol]'s condition," Wilkins wrote, and he advised the parents to move. He continued to assess Carol's gender at every visit, noting in 1948 that she was a "tomboy," was hyperactive, and had a deep voice. She was not only "rough" in her play but also played "as easily with boys' toys as with girls', which causes her mother some concern."

In 1950, nine-year-old Carol was started on cortisone treatment, and physicians measured the improvement of her condition and the decrease of virilization in tandem. While it was easy to measure her decreasing 17-KS values, her behavior and appearance were often in the eyes of the beholder. While Wilkins was of the opinion that "there were no changes on physical examination," her mother "thought she was much less boisterous and more feminine in her actions." This change, Wilkins cautioned, "could be reasonably ascribed to her long hospitalization and its attendant benefits in the way of good discipline and mental hygiene." In any case, the apparent behavioral change was only of short duration; her mother reported that after her first round of treatment, Carol "was more feminine in behavior for a while but later became boyish again." Gendered behavior was often evaluated according to cultural tropes of gender and heterosexuality. In 1954, Carol had "a boyfriend, who took her to a ball last night," Wilkins noted. Two years later, she came to the examination "wearing high heels and acting quite grown up"—all markers of a "normal" female gender role in the 1950s.

Restoring and managing health proved quite complex in the treatment of CAH. On the one hand, new medical problems emerged. Cortisone caused side effects such as obesity and Cushing's syndrome–like symptoms, described as "Cushing's moon face."[44] On the other hand, cortisone, sex assignment, and gender role had to be managed together. Girls growing up female faced new complications with the onset of cortisone treatment. Before, CAH girls had rarely menstruated; but with cortisone, initiating a regular menses became one of the main markers of control over the disease. This in turn created new incentives for surgical intervention, as Wilkins's colleague, the gynecologist Howard W. Jones, would attest. As he wrote in an article he coauthored with his wife, the reproductive endocrinologist Georgeanna E. S. Jones, in 1954, "It has only been since the beneficial effects of cortisone have been known that the gynaecological surgeon has played an important part in the therapy of individuals with severe hyperplasia." Now that these girls menstruated, the surgeon was called on to provide "a suitable passage for the menstrual blood." Menstruation was, however, only the beginning; its presence implied "the possibility of pregnancy and the desirability of a functioning vagina," the Joneses pointed out.[45] They were convinced that operating in early childhood was of "psychological advantage"[46]—a recommendation that resonated soundly with the guidelines John Money and Joan Hampson were developing at the same time.

Management and maintenance of health make visible the conflation of social and vital norms. The "desirability of a functioning vagina," for example, became a more central treatment goal with cortisone. It was a process that entailed multiple operations, with a long-term maintenance process that included dilation of the constructed vaginal opening. If the girls were followed right from birth, the first operation was performed as early as age two. Others came to the clinic later and were operated on shortly after first admission at age four, six, nine, and ten.[47] Practitioners generally thought it was safe to delay the procedure for a few years, contrary to clitoridectomies, which were mostly performed early after first diagnosis to ensure proper gender role development and consistent sex assignment.

Vaginoplasty was seen as both a corrective procedure aimed at reconstructing the "right" genitals for the assigned sex and a benchmark of treatment success. More clearly, the "desirability of a functioning vagina" was part of measuring treatment success and long-term management. Wanting a vagina signified successful gender role and adjustment. Carol, for example, after twenty years as Wilkins's patient, demanded a vaginoplasty at the age of twenty. In 1961, she visited Hopkins's gynecology clinic to discuss what could be done about her vagina and expressed concern about "her chances for leading a normal married life and for having children." She was quite frank about her reasons for wanting the operation: she was afraid, she said, to get carried away on a date. She also brought up her concern about her small breast size and extensive hair growth on her face and legs. In her preoperative visit in 1962, she talked again about why she wanted to go ahead with the vaginoplasty. She was planning to get married, and her fiancé and she wanted "to try sexual intercourse to be sure everything was all right." When the engagement was broken before the operation, she still wanted to go ahead with the procedure.

Much work was invested in these surgical constructions of normativity. They were never isolated but always part of CAH management. Gender roles and their appropriate bodily representation were part of a continuous long-term process of normalization that went hand in hand with daily dosages of cortisone. After vaginoplasty, girls and women were supposed to dilate their reconstructed vaginal canal to successively widen it—another form of maintenance that many patients experienced as uncomfortable, painful, and embarrassing. The dilation could take place in the doctor's office, but it was also performed at home by the parents, and it eventually became the responsibility of the adolescent and adult patients.[48] Functionality meant not only a womanly appearance—to convincingly pass—but also physiological processes such as menstruation and intercourse, with the latter, not surprisingly, defined by heterosexual standards such as penetration. Reproduction was trumped by social role, because being well adjusted was deemed more important than being fertile. But with the introduction of cortisone, pregnancy became a possibility and an option for CAH girls.

Carolyn's case shows the simultaneous triviality and severity of the struggle to become a woman both biologically and socially.[49] Born in 1954, she had been under medical supervision almost from birth. She was diagnosed as suffering from salt-losing virilizing congenital adrenal hyperplasia and put on cortisone.[50] Surgeons performed a clitoridectomy when she was two years old in 1956, and four years later her external genitalia were "reconstructed." In 1966, the doctors worried about whether the previous surgery had been enough. "I think the vaginal orifice is going to be alright," Jones wrote, "but I would be very anxious to see her when the menstrual periods begin to be sure there is no obstruction here." Carolyn was "just beginning to understand her problem" at the age of thirteen in 1967. In 1968, Jones was wary about another possible complication. He feared that she might, like other girls with CAH, suffer from enuresis— the inability to control the flow of urine and involuntary urination. "We discussed her condition in general, the pros and cons of Medic Alert and Tampax. She seems to be a well-adjusted girl to whom athletic participation is very important."

Occasionally, however, Carolyn would not take her cortisone—a common complaint with adolescents and young adults who were starting to monitor their own treatment—and her period was very irregular. As the children grew up, responsibility for the management and evaluation of their conditions shifted from their parents to the children themselves—a peculiar disciplining of the self that included monitoring body and mind constantly. These young adults did not always comply with the clinic's instructions. They forgot to take their cortisone dosage, often on the weekends; they did not send the required urine sample, often because their living situation in dorms or shared apartments was not conducive to collecting urine; sometimes they simply refused because they resented the medical mementos of their condition.

The prescribed practice of dilation, too, was structured by the lives these young women lived outside the clinic. In 1971, Carolyn's mother called to inform her physicians that her daughter "would probably have vaginal reconstruction this summer." In 1972, a year after the operation, Jones examined Carolyn and thought that while the "vagina has exteriorized alright, . . . the orifice is quite small." It would have to be dilated if Carolyn wanted to wear a tampon, though it seemed to Jones that "this was too much of a deal" just for being able to use one. The teenager would discuss it with her mother. A year later, in 1973, Carolyn returned to the clinic with the same problem. Jones tried out dilators with her and expected her to continue using them to widen her vagina after she returned to school. A few months later, he wrote, "Because of the lack of privacy at school, patient really has not been able to work with the dilators very well." He reasoned that "it seems to me there is no point in urging [Carolyn] to work with the dilators when she is not motivated to have a functioning vagina at this moment." Also, she was going to summer camp, where she would have no privacy to dilate.

In winter, Carolyn dropped in on Jones without any appointment. "She is concerned about her vagina, but as it turned out she does not do a thing about [it]," he noted. In 1973, she had said she was not using the dilators, as she had "no opportunity for privacy at school." Anatomically, Jones saw no problem. "On examination, the vaginal outlet is quite satisfactory. . . . There is no mechanical obstruction here, there is no real problem. She says it hurts terribly and it probably does." The dilemma, Jones thought, was that she was not motivated enough to endure the discomfort of dilation. "I tell her to stop worrying bout [sic] the vagina and leave it along [sic] if it is giving her a fit," he wrote, "and if when [sic] the time comes for her to want a functional vagina I think she will be motivated enough to put up with the discomfort of the dilation." The problem, however, did not go away.

In 1975, Carolyn returned and complained, according to the record, "that she is unable to use even tampax due to pain. She has not used the dilators at all as they are too large. She has not been able to have sexual relations, and feels that this problem interferes with her life." Carolyn was very upset and "cried when talking about her small vaginal opening." Jones was now convinced that the problem was psychological and advised her to see Dr. Money's group. In 1977, the treating doctor wrote in the admission record, "When last evaluated, in December 1975, it seemed that she desired additional vaginal reconstructive surgery. Dr. Howard Jones thought, however, that her main problem was psychological in that she could not dilate herself and disapproved of further surgery at that time." The medical dismissal of Carolyn's pain shows a strange disjunction between anatomical norms and bodily experience. Her pain and the doctor's conceptualization of her body suggest an incommensurability that is hardly ever acknowledged in these medical encounters.

Management of the multiple components of CAH was intertwined with all aspects of patients' lives. Physicians and parents alike were concerned about the psychological adjustment of CAH children. While this concern was connected to the perceived "problematic" sexual status of these children, it was also an effect of problems caused by patients living with a chronic condition. Again, the treatment goal was concerned with but not limited to sex. It also addressed social problems arising from CAH children looking "different" in ways that were not only sexual. Children with CAH looked much older than their chronological age, thus raising a set of social and intellectual expectations they could not fulfill. For these patients and their parents, being healthy often meant eliminating signs of visible difference, including height, axillary hair, acne, male baldness, masculine features in girls, excess weight—cortisone often led to obesity—and skin pigmentation. In complicated ways, some of these signs were connected to sex. But being healthy was always also about being able to function in the world.

The administration of cortisone and the assignment of gender role made the goal of a "normal" life possible, an idea structured by the physicians', the parents', and often the patients' belief in the existence of only two sexes, male and female. Cortisone therapy, correct gender role, and matching (genital) appearance only mattered if this goal was attainable, as the singular case of Kathleen, discussed earlier in this chapter, shows. Kathleen's mother had saved for a year to take her daughter to Hopkins, where she was diagnosed as having CAH and mental deficiencies. In her case, physicians discussed whether the child should even be treated with cortisone, at the time a rare and expensive drug, because she would never live an independent life. In addition, they did not perform a clitoridectomy despite noting that Kathleen's clitoris was "enlarged." Restoring biological norms only mattered in conjunction with the constitution of social norms. Once social functionality was deemed unfeasible, the process of normalization was halted.

―――――――

Diagnosing and assigning sex at the Pediatric Endocrinology Clinic in the 1950s was sometimes a long and contentious enterprise as Lawson Wilkins and his team struggled to pinpoint sex. Furthermore, in one of two cases of CAH girls being raised as boys, it was the parents who insisted that their child was a boy and kept her, with the psychological sanction of John Money, in the male sex.[51] Treatment and management of CAH at the clinic was an enduring process that included quick medical interventions in the case of severe salt-wasting CAH and a lifelong management of what was perceived as a chronic adrenal disorder. Physical development and hormonal levels, psychological adjustment and healthiness, and sexual appearance and gender role were checked and controlled in yearly evaluations. In this manner, finding and adjusting to the optimal gender role was folded into the management of CAH as one aspect of its successful treatment.

Clearly, CAH's sexual symptoms, such as "virilized" genitals in girls and precocious genitals in boys, caused anxieties in parents and physicians. Medical/surgical intervention provided a solution to a social problem of ambiguous or precocious sex. It seemed easier to fix ambiguous bodies than rigid gender roles, which would become imprinted during the child's early years. Nevertheless, Wilkins and his team defined CAH as a complex endocrinological disorder caused by adrenal hyperplasia, affecting the whole development of children of both sexes. They considered its sexual symptoms in conjunction with other somatic effects of adrenal hyperplasia. The physicians' and parents' main treatment goal was for their children to lead a "normal" life—that is, a life unhindered by what was defined as a chronic endocrinological condition. This goal was structured by the highly normative sexual roles of the 1950s as much as by the actual underlying adrenal pathology. Normalization was a process in which treating somatic effects and assuring psychological healthiness were deeply enmeshed in the conviction that a normal life was only possible as a clearly gendered and sexed person.

SIX

The Circulations of Gender, Cortisone, and Intersex Case Management

Things Fall Apart

In 1958, just three years after John Money, Joan Hampson, and John Hampson had formulated the optimum gender of rearing model of intersex case management, their partnership dissolved rather dramatically. On April 6, Money sat down to pen an angry entry in his diary. "Wednesday, March 19th, was the day of the big snow," he wrote. "Baltimoreans remember it as a day of destruction when every drooping thing collapsed under the clinging weight of watery snow."[1] A storm had dumped up to two feet of snow on the state, the Baltimore *Sun* reported, leaving many homes without electricity and at least five people dead.[2] Money, however, had been preoccupied with a different crisis in the aftermath of the storm: "I remember Wednesday was the Day of Jacob and Esau, the day my birthright was wheedled away; the day my strong branches strained under the Jacob-weight of an advantage unfairly taken." This rather strong wording marked the end of his collaboration and friendship with Joan and John Hampson.

Money was feeling bitter and betrayed. The team, he wrote, had worked as "a research brotherhood," and John Hampson was not just his "colleague in research" but his "academic brother." Or so he believed. This "brotherhood" had actually begun as his collaboration with a woman,

Joan Hampson, in 1951, with her husband, John, joining them later. As Money was scribbling away angrily, crossing out lines and switching pseudonyms chosen for the people involved, it occurred to him that their collaboration had been ill fated from the beginning. John Hampson was ambitious and "clambered for prestige." "It was in him an obsession, you might say, to maintain, in everything, the appearance of success." Money ruminated that he had needed the Hampsons' cooperation to handle the workload and as "a safeguard against . . . going off half-cocked." Yet, he complained, he had done most of the hard work, with John Hampson shunning long work hours. He felt that he had had to compensate for his colleague's "infertility of ideas" by making his ideas seem like Hampson's. This was a narrative Money would uphold for the rest of his life. The concept of a gender role and all other conceptual ideas had been his, and only in the spirit of teamwork (and to add medical authority) had he agreed to coauthorship.[3]

Working with Joan Hampson was not easy either, he added. "She had disabling bouts of myxedematous depression," Money diagnosed. Moreover, she struggled with being John Hampson's "professional competitor" and his wife at the same time. Of course, Money admitted in retrospect that he himself must have been difficult to work with. His "marriage [to Grace] was on the rocks," and he knew that "it would be perilously easy for any woman, Joan included, to become the target of [his] distress." "Divorce and depression," he mused, "they were disturbing intrusions."[4]

In 1954, the trio had still presented a united front. They had gone to John Whitehorn, chief psychiatrist of the Henry Phipps Psychiatric Clinic at the Johns Hopkins Hospital, demanding a promotion above instructor for all three of them. All or none had been their demand, and all three had been made assistant professors as a result. Four years later, "on the day of the big snow," John Hampson had asked for another promotion but this time without telling Money, who was busy in his office. Unbeknownst to him, the wheels were set in motion at an extraordinary pace. "In two hours John had his application papers ready. Joan submitted them for him," and in another half hour, Money fumed, "his request had been approved." The next day, John Hampson told Money what he had done, but the big snow kept Whitehorn away from the office until Monday. By then, he had announced that he would not make any more appointments or promotions for the year. "This is how my birthright was stolen from me," Money wrote less than two weeks later in his anger and resentment.[5]

What Money described with a flair for the melodramatic and a great deal of negative emotion was the end of the team. After 1958, they were no longer on speaking terms and effectively stopped collaborating. By 1959, the Hampsons had departed to Washington, where John Hampson took a job as full professor and proceeded to head the Gender Identity Research and Treatment Clinic at the University of Washington in Seattle.[6] He and Money were to meet again only once, briefly, in 1967. Money never saw Joan Hampson again.[7] What had been planned as a triumphant collaboration for William C. Young's third edition of *Sex and Internal Secretions* was divided into two chapters, one authored by Money and one by the Hampsons.[8]

Like John Money and the Hampsons, the legacy of the Hopkins study took different paths over the next two decades. What connected these circulations, transmissions, and adaptations of the team's findings was the weight lent to the clinical data acquired by the Hopkins group. In each of these applications of gender, the evidence gained from the Hopkins patients (and others whose case histories were added later) was significant for each new—and at times even conflicting—reformulation of gender. The circulation of cortisone treatment for children with congenital adrenal hyperplasia (CAH) and the set of recommendations developed by the team and underwritten by the concept of a learned gender role came to be known as the optimum gender of rearing model of intersex case management (ICM).

The Hopkins Protocols are often depicted as a hegemonic treatment regimen that was formulated in a discrete moment and subsequently followed both nationally and internationally. Yet tracing the circulation of medical knowledge and practices in the case of ICM demonstrates that the optimum gender model was not a monolithic regime but a multifaceted practice. Here I use the image of a knowledge/practice package to stress that this exchange of knowledge and practices consisted of several components that, in the process of exchange, acquired differential and shifting importance. One component of this package was the substance cortisone itself and, more specifically, the intimate relationship between the cost and the scarcity of the substance and the development and execution of specific therapeutic practices. A second part of the knowledge package was a set of ICM recommendations (often referred to retrospectively as the Hopkins Protocols) developed by a team of psychologists and psychiatrists and based on existing clinical practice at Lawson Wilkins's Pediatric Endocrinology Clinic. These recommendations, in turn, were grounded in a newly formulated theory of human psychosexuality that proposed a learned gender role. This concept of gender role formed a third key component of the knowledge package. Following these multiple aspects and actors reveals dynamic concepts that changed over time and acquired different meanings in different settings. Which parts of the Hopkins Protocols traveled well and which did not? What kinds of networks enabled their circulation, and how were the Hopkins recommendations and concepts adapted to other sites of clinical practice?

CAH, Cortisone, and the Hopkins Recommendations

Shifts in medical knowledge and practice do not happen in isolation but within national, and often global, networks and communities. In the late 1940s and early 1950s, researchers in the emerging subspecialty of pediatric endocrinology often had overlapping research agendas. Many within this community had been trained or at least shaped in clinical style and research trajectory by Lawson Wilkins in his clinic at the Johns Hopkins Hospital's Harriet Lane Home for Invalid Children. In the 1950s, as Wilkins's fellows and pediatric academic faculty with informal training backgrounds established new pediatric endocrinology clinics and pediatric endocrinology programs at other hospitals across North America and eventually in Europe, an independent research community and network developed.[9]

In other words, the Johns Hopkins group did not work in isolation. Wilkins's Pediatric Endocrinology Clinic had been the first of its kind in 1935. Nathan Talbot established a second successful pediatric endocrinology clinic at Boston's Massachusetts General Hospital in 1942.[10] The Wilkins group consequently had "a friendly but intensely competitive rivalry"[11] with Frederic C. Bartter and his colleagues at Massachusetts General, and the introduction of cortisone as a possible therapeutic for CAH happened nearly simultaneously at these two locations.[12] The textbooks of these two groups, published within two years of each other and right at the cusp of cortisone treatment, reveal similar concerns and a few subtle differences.[13] Talbot and colleagues' textbook, which came out of the research at Mass General, shared many of Wilkins's convictions about the treatment of intersex patients: the importance of early and "correct" diagnosis at birth "from both psychological and sociological points of view"; the attention to psychological health; and the belief that these cases were best handled by experienced and competent medical experts with the treatment goal "to help patients live comfortably in the sexual status which is psychologically most congenial to him."[14] While the clinician-researchers at Mass General agreed that it was best for proper sex assignment to attain a diagnosis as early as possible, they seemed—at least on paper—more cautious about irreversible genital surgery. Though the authors advocated the amputation of the clitoris "if the enlargement of the organ embarrasses the patient," they cautioned to "postpone this procedure until the patient is old enough to take part in the decision."[15] This was certainly a recommendation that the team at Hopkins would contest in their findings. Based on Wilkins's practice, they linked genital appearance to proper development of gender role and hence recommended early surgery.

How Knowledge Travels

One of the consistent claims in literature on ICM is that the version developed at Hopkins was quickly integrated into medical textbooks and clinical practice and became the dominant form of medical engagement with intersex patients. But how did this integration happen? What were the pathways ICM took, and how did it change through these adaptations? By considering in detail the circulation of knowledge and practices produced at Hopkins, a more complex picture emerges. Initially, Wilkins as a figure and cortisone as a new treatment certainly lent the Hopkins Protocols weight. Wilkins's authority as the leader of the field, and cortisone's as a newly availably "miracle" drug, comprised the means through which many of the early Hopkins recommendations had been circulated even before they were published. In the early 1950s, when Wilkins first published on treating CAH with cortisone and Money and the Hampsons were conducting their study at his clinic, knowledge and practices were exchanged through personal contacts, in discussion at conferences, on research visits, in consultations, and in letters.

One early site for the transmission of the Hopkins recommendations was the University Children's Hospital in Zurich, Switzerland. Looking at the Zurich case study[16] allows us to understand how personal contacts and the establishment of an international research network around CAH had enabled the circulation of many of the Hopkins recommendations before they were published, how cortisone and treatment plans enabled the spread of ICM and the notion of gender role, and finally, how local medical cultures shaped the uptake of some aspects of the protocols but not others.

In the summer of 1950, the first postwar international pediatric congress was held in Zurich, and Lawson Wilkins, who at the time was on a European tour with his family, was part of the program.[17] He presented his research on cortisone treatment for CAH. He had also prepared an exhibit of his new textbook of pediatric endocrinology.[18] Wilkins, however, did more than talk. At some point during the conference, he accompanied his Swiss colleagues, Dr. Guido Fanconi and Dr. Andrea Prader, to the University Children's Hospital in Zurich to examine one of their patients (B. M.). The ailing Baby M. of "undetermined sex" had previously suffered a metabolic crisis. Wilkins confirmed the diagnosis of "female pseudo-hermaphroditism with adrenal cortical insufficiency," and he advised the Swiss doctors to treat the child with cortisone.[19] This therapeutic intervention was successful, and Fanconi movingly acknowledged the triumph of Wilkins's recommendation: "The future of our patient remains unclear. What is certain is however that the child was saved from sure early death through the diagnosis of the metabolic disorder and through a purposeful treatment" (426).

This dramatic intervention was the beginning of a lasting relationship between Baltimore and Zurich and a process of circulation, transmission, and adaptation. From the beginning, practitioners at Zurich's University Children's Hospital selectively adapted the Hopkins recommendations; some elements easily fell into place in a new environment, while others fit clumsily with the existing practices and theories. Taken by Wilkins's presentations and his clinical assessment that cortisone could be an effective treatment in CAH cases, Prader and Fanconi were inspired to pursue their own clinical trials (426n2). In contrast to the well-established Wilkins, thirty-year-old Prader was only just about to qualify as a pediatric specialist. In the fall of 1950, he departed for a year in North America, where he spent the majority of his time training at Bellevue Hospital in New York with L. E. Holt Jr. In the summer of 1951, however, he spent a few weeks in Baltimore with Wilkins. Prader became part of an emerging international network of pediatric endocrinologists and in coming years would regularly attend the same panels and colloquia on cortisone and CAH as Wilkins and his colleagues.[20]

Cortisone knowledge exchange was fairly straightforward, and in many ways the Swiss research replicated the framework and setup of Wilkins's cortisone studies. In 1953, Prader published the results of Zurich's own long-term cortisone treatment trials.[21] In his correspondence with referring physicians, he continuously stressed the expertise he had gained in the United States and supported his recommendations with reference to Wilkins's medical authority and apparent success with cortisone treatment. In December 1951, he corresponded with referring doctors about diagnosis and treatment recommendations.[22] In diagnosing a patient as having adrenogenital syndrome, he wrote, "The only available therapy at the time is long-term treatment with cortisone. I have only recently been in the USA with Dr. Wilkins and could witness his extraordinary success."[23] Yet while knowledge and data on cortisone therapy for CAH patients circulated freely, the substance itself did not. Cortisone's synthetization was still a complex and expensive process, and it was not until it was successfully produced from soybeans in 1954 that it became widely available.[24] In 1951, the substance's scarcity and its high price affected therapeutic possibilities for clinicians in Baltimore and Zurich alike.[25] Prader, for example, cautioned in 1953 that initial success triggered great hopes in patients: "Especially with girls, treatment should only be started if the possibility of cortisone provision is secured." The treating physician should keep in mind that "a short-term treatment followed by a relapse is actually futile and carries the danger of psychological problems."[26] Prader also provided samples of the substance to ensure further treatment.[27]

While Prader therefore followed many of the Hopkins team's recommendations regarding cortisone, patient records and published notes reveal a complex adaptation of other aspects of the Hopkins recommendations at the Zurich Children's Hospital. Take, for example, the warning by John Money and the Hampsons that sex changes after a certain age (eighteen months to two years) should be avoided because they caused psychological "unhealthiness." In December 1955, Prader discussed whether to change the sex of his patient Anna, who had been declared a boy at birth by Prader and his colleagues.[28] When Anna was two years and three months old, he wrote that they had diagnosed her as a "true hermaphrodite." Since the external genitals were predominantly female and could be made completely female through surgical "correction," the doctors argued it would be best to declare the child a girl "for once and forever." After the removal of the testes, they thought, hormonal intervention during puberty would ensure Anna's female character. Prader supported this change, stressing that the child was "barely above the critical [age] limit." However, he did not refer to Money and the Hampsons but to his fellow pediatric endocrinologist Wilkins, writing, "The main reason against [choosing the female sex for this child] is Wilkins' recommendation that sex should not be changed after the second year without adverse psychological damage."[29] In another case, colleagues contemplated changing the sex in a girl he had diagnosed as having "testikuläre Feminisierung" (testicular feminization), a condition in which the "outer body development is entirely female" while the chromosomal sex is male (XY).[30] Prader, who disagreed, wrote to the physicians that "last year Wilkins in the USA (*Pediatrics* 16:287, 1955)—based on his unique great experience—has shown in an expressive example that after the second year any change of sex—independent of diagnosis—has a psychologically disastrous effect," yet again referring to Wilkin's authority in the field.[31]

Prader fully embraced the recommendation not to change the sex of "hermaphroditic" children after they reached a certain age. Yet despite appearing on a conference panel with Money and the Hampsons (as well as Wilkins) in Copenhagen in 1956, he did not refer to their research in his letter or in patient records.[32] Rather, he consistently referred to an article in which Wilkins summed up the results of his own work on CAH and the results of the accompanying psychological study. In this article, published in September 1955 in *Pediatrics*, Wilkins described the classification, diagnosis, and selection of sex and summarized treatment recommendations for "hermaphroditic" patients based on his research; he included the results of the Hopkins team.[33] In addition, he summed up Money and the Hampsons' gender theory in detail, stating that gender role was established through the cumulative experiences of years of living as a boy or a girl.

Pediatric endocrinology and cortisone treatment comprised the framework through which these treatment recommendations were exchanged. In Prader's practice, reference to Money and the Hampsons was omitted, while Wilkins was identified as the main, even the sole, expert in the matter. It is clear that Prader moved most comfortably within his own subspecialty and that Wilkins, as the "father of pediatric endocrinology," carried more authority in his eyes than the young psychological/psychiatric team. Notes and comments in Wilkins's papers also hint at frequent personal exchanges of CAH case histories among physicians to strengthen studies of this rare condition and allow for comparison.[34] By following Wilkins rather than Money and the Hampsons, Prader not only relied on Wilkins's particular authority but also adopted his simplified version of the gender concept: a concept that relied on Money and the Hampsons' gender role theory without postulating a general theory about human psychosexuality.

The crucial difference, however, resided in Prader's psychosexual theory and, consequently, his rationale for this treatment regime. Here he relied on the findings of two Swiss psychiatrists, Manfred Bleuler and Walter Züblin. In the early 1950s, Bleuler, son of the famous psychiatrist Eugen Bleuler (who coined the term *schizophrenia*) and head of the psychiatric hospital at the University of Zurich (Burghölzli), was working on his book *Endokrinologische Psychiatrie* (Endocrinological Psychiatry) supported by a generous five-year grant of USD 16,800 from the Rockefeller Foundation.[35] Also financed by this grant, Bleuler's colleague

Züblin was given access to Fanconi and Prader's CAH patients to pursue a psychiatric study of the "adrenogenital syndrome in congenital adrenocortical hyperplasia," which he subsequently published in 1953.[36]

Züblin's study, published two years before the publications of Money and the Hampsons, reveals a subtle difference in approach to the team at Hopkins. Züblin considered the American approach driven by a focus on the environment rather than on hormones or other biological factors.[37] In his evaluation of the psychological sex of his sample group of twelve CAH patients—nine females and three males—he concluded that in most cases, the psychological sex matched genetic sex. Most important, he noted that all patients were slightly depressed, anxious, and withdrawn. He concluded that their "social and psychological sex patterns" did not follow "arbitrary environmental sex." Rather, psychological sex in these patients was somewhat childish, immature, and aimless. Their sexual drive direction was not fixed by a deep urge of sex/gender (*Geschlechtsempfinden*), he argued, but by "the wish to be a normal human being or at least to appear as such." These patients were considered much more malleable in terms of their behavior than patients deemed to be in possession of "normal psycho sexuality."[38] In other words, while Money and the Hampsons argued that all children learned their gender role, Bleuler and Züblin argued that these patients—due to their specific hormonal constitution and the effects of their appearance on their social lives—had a lower psychosexual drive and, as a result, were more adaptable than other children.

In his 1957 habilitation thesis on intersexuality, Prader relied on Züblin's study to argue that social ostracism affected the psyche of girls with CAH. "This explains why female patients previously preferred to live as men," he wrote, "and why before cortisone therapy it was advised to raise such girls as boys, since they would attract less negative attention and better fit in socially this way." Prader conceded that some of these physical attributes might be specific to the adrenogenital syndrome, yet he stressed that they had to be considered symptoms of what Bleuler called the "endocrine psychosyndrome."[39]

Prader's conclusions in his thesis differed in two fundamental respects from those of Wilkins and his team. The first difference lay in the relationship between the specific and the general in the two doctors' proposals. At Wilkins's clinic, the psychological team started by observing patients with CAH but soon extended their study to all "hermaphroditic" cases. In the Hopkins optimum gender of rearing model, the specifics of the condition mattered less than questions of timing: the age at which gender roles become indelibly imprinted in a child's behavior and psychology. The universality and simplicity of the model—just pick a sex early and preferably one that matches the genitals—was part of its attraction. Prader, by contrast, warned against generalizations and argued that some patient groups consistently adjusted well to particular sex assignments. "It would be dangerous," he continued, "to generalize that psychosexuality in healthy individuals is determined only by external factors such as upbringing and environment."[40]

A second departure from Wilkins was in how the two interpreted the results of their studies. Prader argued (following Bleuler) that other researchers had simply drawn the wrong conclusions from the "evidence" of intersex studies, maintaining that the exceptional state of intersex psychosexuality made CAH patients more adaptable. This contrasted sharply with Money's claims that his theory was universally applicable and that CAH patients (and all other intersex people) were psychologically within the norm if their bodies were adapted to the chosen sex early enough. Bleuler, who used CAH as an example of endocrine psychosyndrome, positioned them outside the norm—in other words, as extraordinary.[41] Those who debated whether the sexual orientation of intersex patients was male or female, Prader argued, were simply asking the wrong question. Sexual orientation should be considered not in terms of its *direction* but in terms of its *quantity*. Intersex patients adjusted to their assigned sex and believed in it, even in the face of chromosomal and gonadal contradictions, not because they were psychosocially male or female, but because their psychosexuality was weak and only slightly differentiated. If this "natural process of adjustment" was suddenly disturbed by an externally imposed change of sex, harmonious psychological development would no longer be possible, and these patients would develop mental disorders that were otherwise seldom found in intersex patients.[42]

Andrea Prader's ICM recommendations can be summarized as follows: choose a sex of rearing early, based on genitals; do surgery at an early age; and don't change a child's sex after the age of three. At first sight and in terms of implementation, these recommendations seem strikingly similar to those from Hopkins: a focus on genitals, a strong impetus to "surgically correct" genitals and to operate early, and an urge for consistency and consensus in sex assignment. Money and the Hampsons based their recommendations on their findings that children could learn any gender role and that this gender role would become indelibly imprinted on their minds. Prader based his similar treatment recommendations on a different framework—it was the weak psychosexuality of intersex patients that allowed them to adapt easily to any role.

Though Prader cited Money and the Hampsons in his thesis, he warned against generalizing the gender theory to suggest that "normal" human psychosexuality was also dependent merely on exogenous factors such as education and environment.[43] He had adapted the Hopkins guidelines on sex assignment, sex change, and surgery to the Zurich context.

Follow the Textbooks

As the Zurich case shows, the Hopkins model was widely circulated (and adapted) not merely through publications in journals but through personal contacts, clinician-researcher networks, personal correspondence, and professional conferences and meetings. The next important step for new research to become standard medical knowledge was its integration into textbooks. These volumes, often consisting of several hundred pages, typically go through new editions every five to ten years to integrate and adapt to new research findings. As sources that summarize and cite new research, they disclose medical networks and collaborations as well as reveal the extent and speed with which knowledge becomes codified. As was the case with clinical exchanges, not all aspects of the Hopkins study were considered equally important; omissions and exclusions of certain elements of the Hopkins recommendations and gender role formulation allow us to understand what might have been considered controversial and how theories became facts. Like stones skipped over water, the Hopkins Protocols created a ripple effect—initially, and most prominently, in textbooks on pediatric endocrinology and genital surgery written by various members of the Hopkins group.[44] Starting in the late 1950s, the Hopkins findings were also integrated into major pediatric textbooks, such as the 1953 revisions of Luther Emmett Holt's classic treatise on the diseases of infancy and childhood and Waldo E. Nelson's 1959 *Textbook of Pediatrics*;[45] and by the 1960s and 1970s, the next generation of pediatric endocrinology textbooks was published and integrated some aspects of the Hopkins findings.

Networks and References

Between the early 1950s and the early 1970s, the Hopkins findings were widely circulated and adapted as standard medical knowledge. Not surprisingly, clinician-researcher networks played an important role in this process through integrating the findings into textbooks. Lawson Wilkins and his close colleagues not only authored a set of textbooks themselves but also contributed sections in other related textbooks. Wilkins's textbook had first been published in 1950, the year he presented its content at the pediatric congress in Zurich. As its publication coincided with his first cortisone study, he included only a short note on the prospect of cortisone treatment for patients with CAH. By the 1957 edition, the findings of the team at Hopkins had been fully integrated. Money and the Hampsons' "studies and management of the psychologic problems of adjustment . . . have been of the greatest benefit to us and our patients," Wilkins gushed. "Some of their findings have had a profound influence on fundamental concepts of psychosexual development."[46] The new edition also included a thorough discussion of the success of cortisone therapy and the recommendation to assign the female sex to female pseudohermaphrodites with CAH, "since one can be sure that with proper cortisone therapy the patient will grow and develop as a normal female, maturing sexually at puberty with ovulatory menstrual cycles."[47] Money and the Hampsons' recommendations were integrated into the section on abnormal sex differentiation; it was advised not to change sex after the age of eighteenth months to two years (except if an adolescent patient strongly requested a change), and the section included a discussion of the psychological management of parents and patients. In five pages, Wilkins discussed how the sex of rearing should be chosen and whether sex should ever be altered after early childhood.

The third edition published in 1965, two years after Wilkins's untimely death from a heart attack, was "carried through to final publication by his colleagues, Drs. Robert Blizzard and Claude Migeon."[48] That it was John Money who commemorated Wilkins's life and achievements in the text's first pages shows how well established he had become by that time. A few changes had found their way into the new edition, mostly because of the findings in human genetics in the previous decade.[49] Language-wise, gender had also become firmly integrated into the text, and in the section on psychosexual orientation, we find titles such as *Selection of the Gender of Rearing and Treatment* and *Change of Gender Role after Infancy*. Although the recommendations remained the same, the switch from *sex of rearing* to *gender of rearing* and the use of the term *gender role* instead of *sex* was remarkable.

In 1958, two Hopkins surgeons—the gynecologist Howard W. Jones and the urologist William W. Scott—published another "internal" textbook, which focused on "hermaphroditic" anatomy and surgical techniques developed to "repair" genital anomalies.[50] Both Jones and Scott had performed genital surgeries on intersex patients in Wilkins's clinic;

and in a celebratory foreword to the first edition, Wilkins himself drew a line from Franz von Neugebauer's 1908 treatise, a compilation of clinical descriptions of over a thousand cases, to Hugh H. Young's 1937 classic *Hermaphroditism* monograph. In their first edition from 1958, the authors replicated the findings of the Hopkins team and summarized their conclusion that "gender role more nearly followed assigned sex than any other factor" (50). "To put the matter more simply," they wrote, "it seems that sex orientation is much more dependent upon hair style and clothes than upon the morphologic criteria of sex. It follows that the sex of rearing is a most evident consideration in describing sex and should be a weighty factor in the therapeutic orientation of the physician" (49–50). This was quite different from the recommendations that their surgical predecessor Young had made in 1937. He had still insisted on "a sex of rearing consistent with the gonadal sex," though at times he had been "persuaded that the social and psychologic implications of such a change were such that he permitted a continuation in the contradictory sex somewhat against his real feeling in the matter" (55).

In a volume focused on surgical techniques and skills, it is not surprising that in the discussion of preserving the sex of rearing, Jones and Scott's emphasis was a surgical one. Gender role was contingent on proper rearing in the assigned sex, and it was essential that children's genital appearance matched the sex they were raised in. The authors had developed "unique and in some incidences unorthodox surgical procedures" needed by this new emphasis on genital form. Their assessment included a discussion of the consequences of clitoridectomy. Remember that it had been Joan Hampson, the only woman on the Hopkins team, who had argued that removal of the clitoris had not affected the orgasmic abilities of her admittedly small study group, and that this procedure did less harm than the psychological pain of living as a woman with a phallus. Jones and Scott eagerly used this finding to argue that Hampson's work had shown that "removal of the phallus including the glans at an early age is entirely consistent with later normal feminine sexual manifestations including orgasm." They concluded that "the older idea that the clitoris was entirely the site of erotic sensation in the woman must be modified" (57).

Jones and Scott thus acknowledged the centrality of the clitoris for female sexual pleasure, yet they stressed the importance of psychological health. This fits well with Sarah Rodriguez's claim that physicians had been well aware of the important role of the clitoris in female sexuality throughout the long nineteenth century and well before the sex researchers William H. Masters and Virginia E. Johnson in their study of sexual responses insisted on the importance of the clitoris in the 1960s—though each generation of doctors (and feminists) seemed "almost to rediscover the clitoris as a sexually important organ."[51] There was a long tradition, she shows, of surgically altering the organ to redirect female sexual pleasure, not necessarily to get rid of it, but to contain it and force it into the right channels—that is, within marriage.[52] We have seen that Wilkins and his team focused on genital appearance—a focus that often neglected genital functions such as pleasure. Accordingly, Jones and Scott argued that "every effort should be made to provide, by surgical means, external genitalia which are as normal as possible in appearance, for it has long been recognized that genital deformities are a source of embarrassment to the patient and the cause of a serious psychologic handicap."[53] In this reasoning, pleasure was contingent not just on anatomy but psychological healthiness and social functioning.

Expanding the Circle

When it came to textbooks published by groups not affiliated with Hopkins, the inclusion of gender-related content was contingent on whether the editors were part of the broader Hopkins networks and research affiliations. Where this was the case, Hopkins authors often contributed several sections to the volume. For example, Lytt I. Gardner was an associate at Wilkins's clinic from 1950 to 1952. When he published his own pediatric endocrinology textbook in 1969, he not only used the term *gender role* but also asked Money to contribute about five pages on the role of psychological counseling in cases of hermaphroditism. Money's contribution was taken from an article he published in *Pediatrics* in 1965 and expanded for the textbook.[54]

By the 1960s, the optimum gender of rearing model of ICM was also integrated into the new editions of the classic textbooks of pediatric medicine. A comparison of two significant pediatrics volumes shows the importance of networks for the integration and adaptation of the Hopkins model. In 1896, L. Emmett Holt, professor of diseases of children at Columbia University, wrote the first edition of *Diseases of Infancy and Childhood*, which quickly became the definitive book on pediatrics and went through several revisions until 1926. From 1927 until 1962, L. Emmet Holt Jr. and Rustin MacIntosh were responsible for its revision, and in 1962 they shared this responsibility with Henry L. Barnett, who became the main editor after 1968.[55] In the new editions of 1962 and 1968, a new section, "Abnormalities of Sex Differentiation (Hermaphroditism, Intersexuality)," was included. It fell to Melvin M. Grumbach, who had been an associate of Wilkins's from 1953 to 1955, to integrate the findings of the Hopkins team into the section on management.[56] In referring to Money and the Hampsons, he stressed the main features of the Hopkins model: the significance of "early diagnosis and skillful management"; the importance of assigning patients to "the sex which conforms to the genital morphology"; the claim that psychosexual orientation was "a result of growing up and of all the experiences which this implies"; and the age range for the establishment of gender role (1½ to 2½ years). In all of this, Grumbach wrote, the role of physicians was of utmost importance. Their task was to relieve "parental apprehension and misconception" and provide "the parents with practical guidance."[57] Appropriating the language of the Hopkins Team, who had insisted on the importance of explaining the science of embryonic development to families of intersex children, he suggested that physicians "reassure the parents that their child is not 'half boy and half girl.'"[58]

Other pediatric textbook authors were farther removed from the Hopkins network and more selective in their integration of the Hopkins model. Waldo E. Nelson's *Textbook of Pediatrics*, first published in 1933, was one of the leading pediatric textbooks, and it went through multiple editions. Nelson was a longtime editor of the *Journal of Pediatrics* and head of the pediatrics department at Temple University School of Medicine. The seventh edition of the textbook in 1959 included "Hermaphroditism (Intersexuality)," a short section in which the recommendations for treatment and sex assignment in children with CAH were replicated, including plastic procedures "between eighteen months and four years of age" and the centrality of genitals and their potential for surgical reconstruction as the determining factors for sex assignment, even if they were "contradictory to the gonadal or chromosomal sex."[59] In 1959, the authors of the seventh edition referred to "psychosexual orientation" rather than *gender role*, even though they referenced Wilkins's and Jones's textbooks as well as one of Money and the Hampsons' 1955 articles.[60] *Gender role* eventually entered the textbook in the revised editions of 1964 and 1969, though with a slight adaptation in usage. The authors advised that "the diagnosis of the adrenogenital syndrome should be unequivocally established or negated and the appropriate gender role should be assigned"—replacing *assigned sex of rearing* with *the assignment of a gender role*.[61] In the updated text in the section about hermaphroditism, the term of choice remained *psychosexual orientation*.

"Useless Findings and Erroneous Claims"

Some physician-researchers expressed doubt early on that the sex of rearing would always dominate in patients with intersex, but they found that those who criticized the Hopkins findings faced an immediate admonition. In 1959, a team of Canadian researchers from the University of Toronto published an article titled "Psychosexual Identification (Psychogender) in the Intersexed" in the *Canadian Psychiatric Association Journal*, which had been established only five years earlier. Daniel Cappon, who was leading the Psychodynamics and Psychopathology section in the Department of Psychiatry at Toronto General Hospital, and Calvin Ezrin and Patrick Lynes, both of whom were working out of its Department of Medicine, claimed that their study of seventeen hermaphrodites contradicted the findings of Money and the Hampsons that gender role was determined by the sex the child had been assigned at birth and raised in. They criticized the methods of comparison used in the Hopkins study because these "failed to relate the physical and psychological wholes of the person and only compared component parts without submitting these comparisons to mathematical validation."[62] Even more so, the Hopkins study was problematic because it mainly focused on the "congenital hyperadrenocortical female" and lacked studies of male pseudohermaphrodites. According to their own research, Cappon, Ezrin, and Lynes maintained that most of the patients examined had a "psychogender" that fit their somatic body. Even though they acknowledged that the environment had "a strong influence on gender role"—citing Konrad Lorenz among others regarding the crucial influence of imprinting in early infancy—they were nevertheless convinced that "in humans deciding their psychogender the most important factor is the body with both its internal image and its concomitant physiology."[63] In their opinion, individuals with intersex who were assigned a social sex contrary to their somatic sex presented simply "a mask-like face of acceptance of the imposed gender role," causing them "the greatest intra-psychic conflict." Cappon, Ezrin, and Lynes were especially concerned about male pseudohermaphrodites with a small or no penis who were assigned to the female sex. Remember that the Hopkins team believed that for the development of a consistent (learned) gender role, the child's genitals had to fit assigned sex; therefore, one could not develop a proper male gender role without a penis. The authors accordingly strongly objected to Money and the Hampsons' recommendations and advocated "correcting" any contradictions in upbringing and anatomy in "the direction of preponderant somatic sexuality"

(99). Yet many of those individuals were hindered in their quest to change their sex, they lamented, "because the current medical opinion, sponsored by the John Hopkins Hospital group of Money, Hampson and Hampson, was that it was too late to reverse the sex now and to go along with the originally assigned gender" (97).

Cappon and his colleagues' reference to "the current medical opinion" was certainly an indication of the perceived dominance of the Hopkins Protocols, yet the article also shows how differently they applied and adapted Money's nomenclature. When the Toronto team criticized Money and the Hampsons for recommending that gender role never be changed after infancy, they revealed an intriguing misunderstanding of Money's terminology. What he and the Hampsons had actually suggested was to avoid changing the assigned sex a person was living in after infancy because by then a gender role would have been firmly established. In their understanding, it was gender role that could not be changed once it was imprinted; thus, a person's assigned sex could not easily be altered. Even more so, as Money and the Hampsons would point out in their response to the article, they had always stressed that "in the exceptional instance of an hermaphroditic child who has privately construed that an error of sex assignment has been made, and who has secretly half-resolved on a change of sex, successful negotiation of a change may prove possible." These requests usually came from teenagers, and though they were rare, "they deserve serious evaluation."[64]

The Canadians' misinterpretation of the Hopkins findings not only reveals their perception that the Hopkins recommendations were dominant but also displays the subtle ways in which the gender concept and its recommendations were adapted, reformulated, and politicized. It is less remarkable that they tried to develop their own nomenclature, in which they described the combination of "the person's gender identification, hence role" and "the orientation towards a sex object, hence sexual behavior" as "psychogender."[65] After all, the ambitious article was clearly set up to counter what they called "the only other comprehensive psychological study . . . carried out by the John Hopkins Hospital group of John Money, Joan Hampson and John Hampson" and to present an alternative study in which the data supported the claim that in humans the body was the most important factor in deciding their "psychogender" (98–99).

What stands out is how clearly some understood the potential social and political implications of the Hopkins findings. In the last paragraph of the article, Cappon (one assumes, since the "we" of the article switches to "I") makes the connection between sex differences and equal rights much more explicitly than Money would have done at the time:

I will not sum up except to say that when one thinks of the pelvic tilt of the coquettish 5-year old girl which distinguishes her so boldly from behind from her male playmate who simply could not swing a kilt in such delightful rhythm; when one remembers that from skin and buccal mucosa to nerve cells and even the healing granulation tissue, man is different from woman; when one surveys the social delinination [sic] of gender role, the distribution of gender labour, and finally when one takes account of this study showing the vast array and depth of psychological differences between the sexes one cannot help but be amused by this anachronism: that science has uncovered at last the profound differences between man and woman just when the suffragette cry for equality is so perversely vindicated and fused with the findings of science as to inspire the pun "one can no longer tell the sex of a person by what is in the genes." (103)

As I discuss in chapter 7, the new "suffragettes" of the women's liberation movement eventually adapted Money's gender concept to reinforce their "cry for equality."

From today's perspective, the paper ultimately had little impact, but Money and the Hampsons' response to it was swift and harsh. In their reply, published in 1960, they did not mince words when they wrote that the "paper needs examination as both a scientific and medical document" and that they hoped that responsible physicians and scientists would "disregard the useless findings and erroneous claims of Cappon, Ezrin, and Lynes."[66] They rejected the findings of the Canadian researchers based on their selection of patients. Of the seventeen cases they had presented, only four were genuine cases; the others had been born looking like "normal" females or males and raised as such, so it was "no surprise that they turned out to be psychologically female and male, respectively." In short, the authors' conclusion and contradictory finding to the Hopkins study were due to the fact that they did not look at cases where there was "no preponderant somatic sexuality."(131) Four, moreover, was "too small a sample from which to prove any point" (132), implicitly referring to the large number of patients with intersex examined at the Hopkins clinic. Further, the Hopkins team wrote, the authors were not up to date on science, and despite stressing the importance of sex chromosomes and the Barr body test, they had missed that some of their patients had previously been genetically misclassified, and they had based their results on these misclassifications.[67] Hopkins had the data, the numbers, and the access to the newest scientific discoveries.

Ten years later, in 1970, another controversy around the publication of a critique of the Hopkins study occurred. The New York pediatrician and child psychiatrist Bernard Zuger submitted a paper to *Psychosomatic Medicine*. Zuger, who worked in the Department of Psychiatry and Neurology at New York University School of Medicine in New York City, was interested in gender—he was studying effeminate behavior in boys, linking it to adult male homosexuality—and he set out to critically examine Money and the Hampsons' 1955 findings and recommendations on gender role formation and sex assignment. Specifically, in this paper he argued that "the evidence for the claim that individuals with ambiguous sex at birth will accept the sex role of rearing over that indicated by chromosomes, gonads, hormones, internal or external genitalia was wanting on methodologic and clinical grounds." "The conclusions drawn from it," Zuger wrote, were unacceptable.[68]

Money, who reviewed Zuger's paper before publication, was extremely upset and angry, to say the least. "It is difficult for the seeing to give art instruction to the blind," he wrote, but of course he tried anyway and in much detail.[69] Money insisted that the paper should only be published in the journal if Zuger subjected his manuscript "to a very radical, total revision." If he did not "feel capable of meeting this demand," the editor should "perhaps publish his manuscript as it is, and follow it with this memorandum." Money kindly included "a carbon copy of it" to be forwarded to the author.[70] Zuger was not amused and rebutted all of Money's claims in an equally hostile manner.[71] A complete revision of the paper according to Money's demands was impossible and would only stall the paper forever, he wrote. "I would like to avail myself, therefore, of your second alternative. . . . I will await your reply on this. As for including Dr. Money's memorandum, I agree to that. I am sure that you will consider it only fair also to include my rebuttal to it."[72] The paper was subsequently published with Money's critical review and Zuger's reply to it.

What was at stake in this controversy was not the quibbling about methodology, clinical data, and the proper diagnosis of patients with intersex traits. This was a deeper debate about the implications of the Hopkins findings and recommendations and their power to shape the subsequent debates on this matter. It was the beginning of a debate about the return of biological sex as the main determinant of behaviors and personality. Zuger cited Cappon, Ezrin, and Lynes's paper and two of Milton Diamond's articles as the only criticism of Money and his collaborators.[73] Diamond rejected the basic conclusion that there existed "a state of sexual neutrality at birth"—meaning that any gender role could be imprinted on the neutral sexual state of a child. In 1965, he had argued that "in sexuality, as in so many other areas, the human being is extremely flexible and his behavior is a composite of prenatal and postnatal influences with the postnatal factors superimposed on a definite inherent sexuality."[74] In contrast, Money and the Hampsons' findings actually allowed for the subtle influence of hormones (and genitalia) on the development of gender role. By 1965, Money had already started conversations with biologists who postulated that prenatal exposure to hormones organized neural pathways toward masculinity or femininity in the brain.[75]

Money, on the other hand, saw no contradictions, just an utter misrepresentation of and failure to understand his work. For him, "interactionism" was the key concept. "It is not a case of constitutional versus acquired," he replied to Zuger, whom he accused of carrying researchers "back in futility to the nineteenth century by setting up, once again, that fake dichotomy." "A more productive schema," he continued, was to see "gender identity as the end product of a sequence of events that begins with the sex chromosomes and ends with social learning." Yet he insisted that the period of social exposure in the early years of life was essential for the differentiation of gender identify to the extent that it could "override antecedent events in the sequence, including chromosomal sex, in certain circumstances."[76] What really concerned him, however, was not Zuger's false claims but the consequences for patients with intersex traits.

Both Zuger and Money framed their debate in terms of causing suffering to versus helping patients with intersex traits. Zuger feared that the Hopkins recommendations, which were based on faulty methodology and simply inaccurate findings, caused other physicians to unnecessarily hesitate "in deciding on change of sex where indicated and practical"[77]—even though he found that in fifteen of eighteen published cases in his analysis, the assigned sex did not take completely. Not only did the group of female or male pseudohermaphrodites all change their sex as teenagers or young adults to their "biological" sex, their adjustment after a sex change was described as good or excellent, they were "happily married, with full sexual adjustment," they were "cheerful and optimistic," and their sex lives were "extremely satisfactory."[78] In his critique, Money, too, addressed the happiness of patients that was at stake: "What really worries me, even terrifies me, about Dr. Zuger's paper . . . is more than a matter of theory alone." He feared that it would be used "by inexperienced and/or dogmatic physicians and surgeons as a justification to impose an erroneous sex reassignment on a child or

adolescent, omitting a psychologic evaluation as irrelevant—to the ultimate ruination of the patient's life." He had in his twenty years of experience in hermaphroditism "witnessed the tragedy of young persons'
lives ruined, in this respect." He had also seen "the tragedy of refusal
of a sex reassignment in selected cases of youthful hermaphroditism
whose gender identity demands it." In the original 1955 publications,
Money had already stated that in exceptional cases and when desired
by patients themselves, sex could be changed after infancy and "never
backtracked on that recommendation."[79] Both he and Zuger claimed
they only had the best interests of their patients at heart, best being in
the eye of the beholder.

———

The implementation of the Hopkins recommendations was swift and far
reaching. Recommendations to diagnose early, to assign one of two sexes
firmly, to choose a sex that fit the child's genitalia (or to which the genitals could be surgically adjusted), to reformulate intersex as unfinished
embryonic development, and not change a child's sex after the age of
eighteen months to two and half years (unless the child desired it) were
incorporated into medical literature as well as medical school curricula
and teaching hospitals all over the United States. Hopkins's position as
the primary center of intersex diagnosis and treatment and a network
of affiliated practitioners contributed to this extensive implementation,
and in turn reinforced Hopkins's position of authority in these matters. The success of cortisone treatment and Lawson Wilkins's authority
as the father of the field of pediatric endocrinology likewise contributed
to the success of intersex case management circulation. As interventions
became more routine, intersex case management was standardized and
further disseminated. Not everything was taken up in the same way,
though. The experiences of intersex patients over the following decades
reveal that John Money's recommendation to speak openly in scientific
terms with parents and patients about the condition and the options
was not followed universally. Many intersex patients only learned as
adults about the procedures that had been performed on their bodies
when they were children.[80] Most of all, these recommendations did not
take into account that gender itself underwent many transformations in
the decades after it was first formulated in the Hopkins clinic.

Despair

The human being is a recording instrument of uncertain and variable powers.

Throughout this book, I have tried to resurrect the voices of patients as they experienced clinical encounters at the time. In so doing I have relied on patient records, but these are difficult sources through which to understand a patient's experience. They consist of standardized forms and graphs, and the logic of modern patient records clearly privileges the physician's voice. We learn little about patients such as Janet. Her voice can be found only on the margins of the record in moments when a disjunction occurs between her narrative and the medical storytelling. Here I present a snapshot of her life that is discernable in the records.

In 1981, Janet came to the Johns Hopkins Hospital for carpal tunnel surgery and treatment for hypertension.[1] The admitting intern noted a "30 year old white female with congenital adrenal Hyperplasia (partial 21-hydroxylase) with poor compliance to her steroids, particularly during adolescence." The intern also noted that Janet was very obese, and that despite having had several genitourinary reconstructions, her vagina was still "tiny" and her urethra in the wrong anatomical place. Seemingly a little perplexed, the intern added that the patient "would not let me examine her genitalia." As it turned out, Janet was not a newcomer to the clinic at Hopkins: she was returning after she had temporarily removed herself from clinical encounters there. Her admission records before 1974 and clinical records before 1962 were missing. Therefore, the admitting intern felt it necessary to take a very detailed medical history.

A careful reading of this narrative reveals the tension between Janet's account of her health, her body, and her identity, on the one hand, and what was thought to be medical fact, on the other. Although her story was mediated by the format of the medical record, the handwritten notes made upon her admission tell her story with surprising immediacy. In the admission record, words like *apparently* and *supposedly* are frequent, and the physicians who wrote them stress the impossibility of verifying Janet's narration through prior patient records. This concern is far from unusual. Physicians routinely seek to access a patient's prior record in order to check for preexisting conditions and previous treatment protocols. Furthermore, as Arthur Kleinman suggests, "the doctor is expected to decode the untrustworthy story of *illness as an experience* for the evidence of that which is considered authentic, *disease as biological pathology*. In the process, the doctor is taught to read experience—at least the experience of the sick person—as fugitive, fungible, and therefore invalid."[2] Such an encounter devalues the patient's experience and delegitimates her suffering. However, I want to suggest another reading of this encounter: the fact that the doctors needed to cast doubt on the authenticity of Janet's own assessment of her life and medical past highlights the disjunction between medical history and biography. I take the occurrence of words such as *apparently* and *presumably* in the narrative as moments in which Janet's voice inserts itself in the record—emphasized by the doctor's suspicion.

Janet told the admitting intern that she had been one of Wilkins's patients in 1950, "originally thought to be a boy when she was born and christened [with a male name]—however about 5 days after birth, Lawson Wilkins diagnosed her with congenital virilizing hyperplasia. She *apparently* [my emphasis] spent much of her first two years in the hospital on a metabolic bed with little normal human contact." Long hospitalization had indeed been a defining feature of the early treatment of children with congenital adrenal hyperplasia (CAH), and small children were strapped to a metabolic bed to facilitate collecting their urine for analysis.[3] That the doctor taking the notes felt it necessary to add an "apparently" to her story reveals that physician's unfamiliarity with the condition. It also highlights a moment of intensity, when Janet insists on her own description of the past, "with little normal human contact," that constituted her experience of being a patient.

Janet's refusal to be a good patient, or at times to be a patient at all, might have made her narrative even more suspicious to the intern. She had been put on cortisone, the story continued, and "supposedly" very high doses were necessary to suppress her 17-ketosteroids values, which were checked regularly after she left the hospital. Janet returned to the clinic when she was four years old, and "a clitorectomy and plastic reconstruction of the genitalia was performed." The medical reason cited was "because of severe masculinization." The doctors also performed a laparotomy, which showed "normal female uteral organs." At this point, "a small vaginal pouch was found off her urethra; at age 11 an attempt was made to exteriorize and enlarge this but this was unsuccessful and that patient has refused further cosmetic surgery. She had frequent adrenal crises during childhood." That refusal—Janet's insistence on deciding which part of her would be subjected to treatment and which would not—suggests both her increasing agency and her growing despair over time, as she found herself increasingly confined to a space where her pain and the relief offered were incommensurable.

Refusing most medical interventions from the age of eleven onward, Janet slowly retreated from the world. At age thirteen, she "apparently" quit school. As "details of schooling [were] missing because of no chart available before 1967," the intern taking the admission notes had to take her word for it. After she left school, Janet "lived at home almost exclusively during her adolescence." She left the house only to go to the store, "but that was all." She "developed quite severe psychological disturbances and had difficulty in co-operating with her sibs [sic] and mother." Assuming that Janet did not use the phrase "psychological disturbances" to describe her emotional state during her adolescence, the doctor was translating her story into medical terms. Her trouble, he thought, was rooted in her gender role. He noted that Janet "had a very poor body image as a teenager and apparently rejected her femenity [sic] almost completely." Janet told him that she "apparently" had had a "very masculine appearance with phallus, during childhood." She emphasized this point by showing him pictures of herself as a girl, but the intern was skeptical and noted at the margin: "Pictures show a cute little girl."

We can only speculate as to whether Janet's masculine appearance was shaped by her self-perception, or whether the intern applied measurements of masculinity and femininity in the 1980s that were different from those applied in the 1960s. Her suffering, however, was real and intense. She told the intern that "at age 11, she tried to commit suicide by swallowing her cortisone pills." The same year, as I have noted above, her genitals were operated on for the last time and she refused any further cosmetic surgery. The doctor, it seems, did not make a connection between the operation and her refusal. Again, the disjunction between Janet's narrative and what the intern took to be a reliable account is quite telling. While meticulously scribbling down every detail of her account, the intern was safeguarding the realm of objective truth by marking Janet's story semantically with the injection of the word *apparently*. It was not only her self-assessment of her body's sexual appearance that the intern doubted; one also wonders how, with the progressive narrative of her medical history, her emotional despair was translated into the language of medicine.

As Janet grew older, she did not menstruate and continued to virilize. She also struggled with her weight. She tried dieting but "could not keep this up indefinitely and generally was overweight throughout this period." Her weight and control of her diet would become a prominent theme in the following hospitalizations. "Apparently," Janet's bone age also progressed "more rapidly than her height or chronological age," and then with some relief the intern noted that "data on her bone ages can be found in the chart noted c. 1968." Still a little skeptical, he wrote, "This androgen effect presumably also contributed to her obesity." This caution was not only a sign of reluctance to believe her story. Janet had come to the general hospital admission as an adult, rather than returning to the Pediatric Endocrinology Clinic, where she had been a patient as a child. The intern may well have been unfamiliar with the symptoms of CAH, in contrast to the physicians who had treated Janet at Wilkins's clinic.

Janet's psychological condition seemed to worsen throughout adolescence. She developed "extreme agoraphobia and she never left the house between ages 17 and 21." At home, isolated and anxious, she grew exceedingly distressed. She developed an eating disorder, which the intern described as follows: "During this time her eating habits become extremely bizarre—eating 1 lb spaghetti/day with hamburger and salt, along with much junk food." Janet could not sleep at night "because of fear." Again, the intern added an "apparently," indicating that this came directly from Janet, and that for him this was not verifiable. To deal with her anxiety, Janet ended up going to bed at dawn—we do not learn what she was afraid of. She "refused to take her prednisone and developed fairly severe hirsutism during the period."

In 1972, after eleven years of absence from the medical record, Janet resurfaced. She became a patient again, and her case was followed from this admission until the 1980s. At this point in the record, the intern who was taking her patient history started adding values as objective assessments of her condition. The tone of the account of Janet's patient history changes significantly as it switches from her narrated patient history to the subject of her prior patient records. The intern wrote that Janet's "first <u>documented</u> [emphasis original] medical admission was in 1974 for an episode of urinary tract infection"—the underlining of the word *documented* in the record a literal sigh of relief at finding a reliable and recognizable assessment of the patient's previous history. At this time, a female doctor had performed a vaginal exam on Janet, which "showed only a rudimentary clitoris [unreadable] to previous surgery." Her vaginal opening was so small that it "barely admitted a Q-tip." The doctors treated her with vaginal estrogens to "relieve the severe atrophy of this area."

Janet returned later the same year for another procedure. The goal of this operation was an "exteriorization of the vagina to relieve her symptoms of incontinence which were caused by urine backing up in her vagina and continually leaking." Surgery on genitals such as the procedure Janet endured served multiple purposes. One was clearly cosmetic and gendered to construct genitals that accorded with the doctors' standard for feminine; other interventions sought to achieve anatomical functionality—sometimes gendered to enable heterosexual intercourse, sometimes—as in Janet's case—to fix an anatomical problem. It is unclear how much of her problem with incontinence had been caused by previous operations.

After the 1974 operation, Janet again fell out of the medical gaze. She had been given a vaginal dilator, which she was supposed to use at home.[4] Janet refused to use the dilator, which is noted in the record. We do not know whether she talked about the pain and discomfort these devices caused, but in any case, her reasons were not included in the record. Nor did Janet go to her scheduled follow-ups in the Department of Gynecology, another act of refusal neither explained nor further investigated. All that is offered is a note stating that she "has remained essentially unchanged since that time."

From the admission pattern, it seems Janet only came to the hospital when it was absolutely necessary and never for gynecological examinations. She did come to Hopkins again the following year for another urinary tract infection, which had been "complicated by an Addison Crisis." This pattern continued as Janet returned in 1976 for an "evaluation of dizzy spells." She had difficulty breathing and would start feeling dizzy as her chest tightened. This was followed by numbness, tingling, and severe headaches; her heart would start beating rapidly, and she would start sweating excessively and experiencing "visual symptoms." Janet went to the neurology department to get help for these dizzy spells. Her primary care physician had been unable to explain them, and the intern at Hopkins also noted, "No definite etiology for the spells was discerned." Her symptoms were considered secondary to anxiety and hyperventilation. When she returned in 1978 complaining of carpal tunnel syndrome, the doctors had something more concrete to address. Pages upon pages are filled with diagnosis, prognosis, and treatment. Again, however, Janet's reluctance to engage with medical practitioners got in the way of what they perceived as successful treatment. The assessment ends with "however none of this has been followed up."

My reading of Janet's story in the record suggests that she was not feeling well, had not been feeling well for a long time, and had been upset both by her condition and by her encounters with medicine. As I noted earlier, medical records are structured by the logic of the clinical encounter and the format required by the record. It has been argued that they construct the patient and that the patient, already silenced by the shift from symptom to sign, becomes so heavily mediated that we have little or no access to the authentic patient's voice.[5] However, even if we cannot access the authentic voice of a patient—and I might add that authenticity is never a given, anyway—we may still be able to encounter *a* patient voice. It is in these moments, when the logic of the record does not work; in these instances of resistance, disruption, and refusal and in encounters with errors, mistakes, and misunderstandings, that we detect the glimmer of a patient's voice. This is the moment when medical personnel feel the need to comment, and often to interject with their own puzzlements, annoyances, and disbeliefs. It is through these interjections that the historian can catch a glimpse of what a patient did or did not want. Similarly, there are moments of disjunction when patient and doctor reach a particular terrain where the pain and the emotion cannot be measured or explained by medical means.

Janet's life in the record is full of such moments of incommensurability: her initial refusal to have any more surgery at the age of eleven; her refusal to take any cortisone as a teenager; her refusal to use a vaginal dilator; and her refusal to come to follow-ups at the gynecology clinic in the 1970s. These moments impress on us what it means to not want to be treated—to just want to be left alone. For the doctors, her body was speaking a language of neglect—she had bad dental hygiene, she was heavily virilized (despite the availability of treatment), she had never menstruated (a marker of therapeutic success for CAH patients), and she was obese. For the doctors, it was incomprehensible from a professional standpoint that she would refuse medical treatment.

During her last hospitalization, Janet only reluctantly and selectively accepted her physicians' treatment plan. Her hospital stay turned into a tug-of-war, a contest of suggestion and refusal, and finally, it seems, a decision was made to comply with her—to accommodate her and make her comfortable. This accommodation was born of necessity rather than being an achievement of commensurability. Janet remained firmly resistant to any medical intervention she did not want. The medical personnel noted again and again: "Patient poorly compliant." They also noted that she had "severe psych. problems (afraid of strangers, nights, P[atien]t poorly compliant)." There was a disjunction between the doctors' assessment of Janet's state of mind and how Janet said she was feeling. In the interview done upon her admission, the intern had referred to her as "unfortunate"—yet at the same time, he wrote that "pt states that she had been doing very well." He added that she was "fairly vague about these complaints however" and "pt. states that she has been taking her meds."

More than anything, I would suggest, these disjunctions were caused by different points of reference. The doctors' reading of Janet's symptoms came from the perspective of vital norms. Janet's assessment of herself was embedded in her life and experiences, her relations with other people, and her conception of herself. She may not have been doing well, despite her assurances (maybe these defiant remarks were meant to ward off the overwhelming medical attention that she found so oppressive)—but clearly there was a disparity in perception. What the doctor saw was this: "Morbidly obese, short ♀ [with] marked facial hirsutism, well developed musculature." What Janet was to herself emerged on the margins of the record, moments of denial within which she set her own priorities, or in which she refused to be objectified.

In the middle of Janet's progress notes, we find a page where both entries start with a direct quote from her. The first, "I want to go home," is simply followed by medical data. The second entry explains this wish: " 'I want to go home.' Pt. would like to be treated as outpatient. She feels that her hospitalization is not needed for her condition. She has no objections to the [*unreadable*] care or any member of the staff. She says she has not slept in the past 3 nights but has not requested any sleeping pills. Her suitcase is packed but she will not leave until she receives approval by [her doctor]. . . . Appease pt. to wait for [doctor's] reply." Janet wanted to go home, not only because she rejected the hospital routine, but also because she was caring for her ailing parents. Again, different priorities intersect. In the end, the medical personnel came up with two solutions for how to treat Janet. One was "to advise pt. on home care for her father." The other amounted to an acceptance of her wishes. The nurses were instructed to "create non-aggressive atmosphere. Try to encourage pt to discuss phobia and implement approp. therapy." The medical personnel had decided to accommodate her needs, even if those impinged on their own notion of what would constitute the best therapy.

This approach was followed until Janet's discharge. When her arms were found to be too large for a normal-size sphygmomanometer cuff to measure her blood pressure, an effort was made to find a larger cuff. Janet found daily life in the hospital immensely frustrating. She had "been stressed by her demented roommate. We have discussed this and she has also discussed it w[ith] Dr. Money. We will try to find a quiet roommate if the other bed in her room has to be filled." This the staff did, and Janet's mood improved: "She had a quiet roommate and had a much better night." The next day, the attending doctor wrote: "Pt was upset this AM because need for liquid diet was not explained to her. She also is worried because of the double dose of Mag[nesium] citrate + Dulcolax. I've given her permission to refuse any aspect of prep she wants." Janet's records—especially as her discharge date approached—are full of these moments of refusal, when she knew what was best for her. One day she insisted, "My stools are getting clear—I don't think I need the pills [Dulcolax]" and "refused Ducolax [sic] tabs." The same day, it was noted that she "appeared in good spirits" and that "patient refused IV." It was also noted in her own words in the record, "I don't want this IV now."

The record ends with yet another moment of defiance. Although further treatment had been suggested, "the patient feels this could be done as an outpatient and she isn't keen on staying." In her own words, again inserted into the record: "I feel good. I'd like to go home." The doctors were not convinced, but Janet was discharged, and this how the record of her clinical life ends.

SEVEN

The Life of Gender: Reformulations and Adaptations

Gender soon took on a life of its own. In the late 1960s, the notion of psychological sex and the idea of a learned gender role were reformulated in the field of psychology as gender identity; applied in the study of and clinical care for transgender individuals; consolidated with new theories about brain development; and eventually adapted by feminist activists and academic feminists to their own disparate ends. In all these transitions, gender was a dynamic concept shaped and informed by shifts in American culture and policies. Each adaptation largely relied on both well-known and new evidence drawn from patients with intersex traits. John Money's use of patient data represented a rare instance of studies of human rather than animal behavior, and many physicians found helpful the standardized recommendations on intersex case management developed at the Pediatric Endocrinology Clinic. Both the human data and the authority of the Johns Hopkins Hospital as a leading center for research carried significant weight for those who then used the concept of gender to make arguments about the relationship between nature and nurture. Gender took on multiple meanings as it was adapted to the needs of different disciplines, groups, and activists. Feminists and queer communities often used the word *gender* indiscriminately and inconsistently, while others engaged with its precise meaning in debates about transsexuality and sexual difference.

This chapter probes a number of questions: What happened to gender once it entered fields and contexts other than the clinic and pediatrics? What happened when it was applied in research on what some psychologists and physicians considered to be the new and intriguing phenomenon of "transsexuality" in the 1960s? How did feminists utilize the term in the 1970s for the politics of women's liberation? Were the intersex patients who served as Money's clinical evidence and their stories acknowledged in these projects, or were they rendered invisible?

Gender Identity

In the first two decades after the original publication of results of the study of children with intersex traits at the Johns Hopkins Hospital, psychologists and psychiatrists adapted and reconceptualized the concept of gender that had been developed within it. Robert J. Stoller was one of the first psychologists to take up the notion of gender and adapt it to his research priorities. Born in 1924 just north of New York City, Stoller spent his student and professional years on the West Coast. He received a BA and an MA in psychology from University of California at Berkeley and became a faculty member in the Department of Psychiatry at the UCLA Medical School in 1954. By 1958, he was working on questions of psychological sex, and in 1962 he and his colleagues opened UCLA's Gender Identity Research Clinic, the first of its kind.[1] Stoller reformulated Money's concept of gender role to encompass a person's innermost conception of self and called it gender identity. In the following years, he reshaped the concept of gender in strategic conference presentations, publishing his findings in articles in the *International Journal of Psycho-Analysis*. In 1968, he presented his research on gender identity in his book *Sex and Gender*.[2] By this time, his focus on gender identity had shifted from intersex patients to transgender individuals.

One of Stoller's contributions to scholarship was his differentiating between a person's conception of the self (gender identity) and the behavioral manifestations of gender (gender role). Gender identity described "the sense of knowing to which sex one belongs, that is, the awareness 'I am a male' or 'I am a female.'"[3] Stoller was clearly influenced by the work of John Money and Joan and John Hampson in his adaptation of what shaped a person's gender identity. He described three essential elements of gender formation, two of which were clear references to the Hopkins study. The first was anatomy and physiology of the external genital organs, and the second was the influence of parents, siblings, and peers.[4] Though he also acknowledged the influence of the environment, Stoller added another quite contradictory element. He thought that there must be a third element, a rather mysterious biological force which provided "some of the drive energy for gender identity."[5] That force, yet to be identified, could be strong enough, he argued, to overwrite the usual patterns of learning and anatomy.

Case studies of patients with intersex traits served as "natural experiments" to explore the formation of gender identity by comparing their sex characteristics with their psychological sex. Stoller wrote, "Intersexed persons—those who for genetic and/or constitutional reasons have defects in the appearance of their external genitalia or a strong shift in secondary sex characteristics toward those of the opposite sex— provide 'natural experiments' which permit us to study, in purer culture than is possible in the anatomically and endocrinologically normal, the variables responsible for this development." In principle, he agreed with Money's claim that most "intersexed patients" developed a gender identity according to the sex they were reared in and which had been assigned at birth. But what about cases of "rare individuals" in whom neither the external genitalia nor the gender role assignment and attitudes of the parents determined their gender identity, but for whom some other factor seemed to be of decisive importance, overriding both of these considerations? (220) These individuals were few in number but would offer new insights into the factors that contributed to gender identity formation more broadly.

Stoller based his claim of a mysterious third element—a yet-to-be-determined biological force at play in gender formation—on two of these rare case histories. The first case was presented as a simple sex assignment error in which one force (sex chromosomes) overrode all others, both biological and environmental. The young girl had been declared female at birth and raised as a girl for fourteen years. Her genitalia and appearance were entirely female. Much to her mother's dismay, however, the girl rejected the female gender role and seemed to take on a male role in all her behaviors and interactions. During her adolescence, tests showed that "she was in fact a chromosomally normal male," and it was during that time she was first seen at Stoller's clinic for psychiatric evaluation. The psychologist noted in his report on the case that "since she had such a tremendous desire to be considered a boy, and since the anatomical and laboratory tests indicated that she was unequivocally a male, it was decided to tell her she was a boy." The girl acted as if she had been told something she already knew, Stoller added, and she went home and "took off her girl's clothing and became a boy, immediately beginning to behave like other boys in the community" (222). The parents moved to a new neighborhood—in line with doctors' usual advice to parents, this was a common practice in sex reassignment. In the new community, there was no doubt about either his being a boy or his masculinity. Stoller described the child as a well-adjusted boy, stressing that only his genital status—that is, the lack of a penis—caused him concern.

For Stoller, this was a remarkable case in which a child had known his gender identity despite his appearance and sex of rearing. The only reason he had been maladjusted in the first fourteen years of his life, Stoller reasoned, was because he had been forced into a gender role that did not fit his gender identity. "Somehow, preconsciously, the child must always have known his true gender identity and has had no doubt about it," Stoller explained. Of course, Money himself had encountered errors in the development of a proper gender role, and he mostly blamed families' inconsistency in raising and their doubts about a child's sex. He also insisted that a boy without a penis could not live as a boy. Yet Stoller argued that none of this was true about the case he was describing. The child had "always felt (though not consciously) that he was a male" and never shifted "his identity." The patient did "not shift from female to male, but only had the rights of maleness confirmed by society," Stoller concluded (223). The source of this core gender identity therefore had to lie in nature.

Stoller interpreted the details of this case as evidence of a fundamental sense of maleness, which the child maintained despite anatomical structures and environmental pressures to the contrary. There was, Stoller explained, "an overpowering drive unalterably and continuously thrusting this child towards maleness" (223). This strong force was without a doubt biological in nature, and though at the time Stoller could not be more specific, he wrote that "someday, such a force may be found to be the algebraic sum of the activities of a number of neuroanatomical centers and hierarchies of neurophysiological functions" (224). Despite the vagueness of this prediction, he was convinced that "a sex-linked genetic biological tendency towards masculinity in males and femininity in females [worked] silently but effectively from fetal existence on, being overlaid after birth by the effects of environment, the biological and environmental working more or less in harmony to produce a preponderance of masculinity in men and of femininity in women. In some the biological is stronger and in others weaker" (225). That Stoller framed this claim as controversial was a clear indication of how pervasive the environmental stance had become in some disciplines (though not so much in others, as we will see).

In the same paper, Stoller cited the case of another patient whose gender formation did not sync with the sex of rearing or anatomy, shaping his research trajectory for years to come in unexpected ways. In October 1958, Agnes was referred to him and came to see him at the Department of Psychiatry at UCLA.[6] She was described as a nineteen-year-old single white girl who looked by all accounts convincingly female; she was "tall, slim, with a very female shape . . . dressed in a tight sweater, which marked her thin shoulders, ample breasts, and narrow waist."[7] Yet there was something different about her. Agnes had been declared a boy at birth, had male genitalia, and had been raised as a boy. By the age of seventeen, however, she had developed all the secondary sex characteristics of a girl. Also at seventeen, she changed "to a female" and "lived completely as a female undetected by either females or males." Testing at the clinic revealed large amounts of estrogen, presumably "produced since puberty," when her feminine transition began. After many hours of conversation, Stoller concluded that "from the beginnings of memory at age 3 [her] conscious fantasy life consisted completely of playing at being a female."[8] In March 1959, at the age of twenty and by her own wish, Agnes underwent surgical procedures to remove her penis and testes and to create an artificial vagina.[9] She continued coming to UCLA for weekly consultations until August 1959.

Stoller understood both cases as intersex individuals whose core gender identity did not follow their sex of raising. His diagnoses of these patients as intersex were essential for his theory of a biological force. According to the Hopkins study, these children should have formed a gender identity in conjunction with the sex in which they were raised. For Stoller, the fact that they did not was clear evidence of an element at work in gender identity formation besides environment, genitalia, and appearance. However, in 1964 Agnes revealed that her development of female secondary characteristics had not been spontaneous.[10] At the age of twelve, she had started taking her mother's stilbestrol, the synthetic estrogen prescribed for a wide range of indications, among them sometimes to feminize girls with congenital adrenal hyperplasia (CAH). Stoller and his colleagues had been using Agnes's diagnosis as intersex to argue that in some cases, gender identity did not follow sex of rearing. So in 1968, Stoller published an article that corrected his previous assumption, revealing that Agnes "was, instead, a male transsexual, a biologically normal male who nonetheless feels himself to be a female and who wishes to be transformed into a female."[11]

The rediagnosis of Agnes quickly became an important opportunity to test the hypothesis of what caused transsexuality in boys. Stoller argued that psychological problems in childhood and adolescence could cause a female core gender identity in a biological male. The guilty party here was a familiar character in America's repertoire of villains: mom. Stoller had already pursued this line of research into why some boys identified as girls, and Agnes's case would allow him to test his hypothesis that mothers were the main contributing factor in producing "dysfunction" in the core gender development of their young sons, making them into future male-to-female transsexuals. "I was most curious to know," he wrote, "if the findings in the little boys . . . were present in the histories of adult transsexuals." These included "the special bisexual personality of the mothers, the excessive body contact that the mothers indulged in with their infant sons, the mothers' great pleasure in promoting their sons' femininity, the fathers' almost complete absence from the family and lack of interference with the feminization of their sons" (364–65). Stoller's vocabulary is quite revealing in his assessment of the mothers of his transsexual patients. He interviewed four of the "empty women" in "joyless but unending marriages" who had raised such children, who "prevented their infant sons from separating from their bodies," sons who consequently developed a female gender identity. Stoller was convinced that this particular constellation would allow him to predict psychological development in boys resulting in males thinking they are female (367). As usual, mothers were at the center of debates about raising children properly.[12]

Despite the focus on mothers as the psychological cause of errors in development of a person's gender identity, Stoller insisted that biology still played an important role.[13] Even in light of Agnes's revelation, he contended that "this patient's case does not disprove such a theory; by now six biologically intersexed patients have been seen who, while they cannot be discussed now, seem to exemplify the presence of such a biological force."[14] It is revealing, however, that he thought that "this concept of a biological force [determining gender] would seem to be controversial."[15] The journal that published his 1968 article also included a comment by Marcel Heiman, clinical professor of psychiatry at the Mount Sinai School of Medicine and attending psychiatrist in the Department of Psychiatry at the Mount Sinai Hospital in New York City. Heiman noted that Stoller's contribution was groundbreaking, an "unexpected and dramatic denouement to the case of this baffling patient." He was, of course, referring to Agnes. Heiman argued that her case actually disproved Stoller's theory of a biological force. He was convinced that Stoller was so fixated on finding this biological force that he ne-glected taking human agency into account. "Stoller's firm belief in a bio-logical force," he wrote, "made him less perceptive to the accumulating evidence of his patient taking oestrogen, and interfered with a fully ob-jective assessment of the patient's personality and psychopathology."[16]

Stoller's book *Sex and Gender* seems to have been the first American book with the word *gender*, in its nonlinguistic usage, in its title.[17] Split-ting gender identity from gender role meant that one could have a "gen-dered identity without necessarily being locked into social expectations of how that identity should be expressed or indeed experienced."[18] "The advantage of the phrase 'gender identity' lies in the fact that it clearly refers to one's self-image as regards belonging to a specific sex," Stoller wrote. "Thus, of a patient who says: 'I am not a very masculine man,' it is possible to say that his gender identity is male although he recog-nizes his lack of so-called masculinity."[19] He also offered a term for the outcome of what Money and the Hampsons had described as the critical period of gender acquisition.[20] Stoller used the concept of a core gender identity to formulate a theory about the outcome of the "imprinting" process.[21] *Core gender identity* meant a person's unalterable sense of being either male or female. It could be in contradiction with gender role and biological sex, thus opening up a model of explanation for patients who were biologically male but had a female core gender identity.

Making the Transsexual Patient

Since the 1950s, public and medical interest in individuals who felt a strong desire to "change" their sex and live in a sex other than their biological one had been steadily increasing. Even though there are ear-lier sources of sensational press accounts, puzzling obituaries, memoirs, and medical cases, the publicity of Christine Jorgensen's "sex-change" surgery in Denmark in 1952 focused attention on what was referred to as "false gender role orientation."[22] At the time, physicians and psychia-trists applied a set of different terms, from *genuine transvestitism* to *eon-ism* to *transsexism* to *contrasexism*.[23] The English term *transsexual* was first used by the US psychologist David O. Cauldwell in 1949. In his journal article "Psychopathia Transexualis," he described the case of a woman who desired to live as a man. "Among both sexes are individuals who wish to be members of the sex to which they do not properly be-long," he wrote. "Their condition usually arises from a poor hereditary background and a highly unfavorable childhood environment," linking nature and nurture in his explanatory model. Cauldwell recommended "rehabilitation" and "preventive"[24] social education for the individuals whose "pathologic-morbid desire to be a full member of the opposite sex" was so powerful "that the individual insists on—often impossible—elaborate surgery that would turn him into a complete woman, or her into a biologically perfect male."[25]

It was a German-born and German-trained physician, however, who shaped the medical definition of transsexuality for years to come. Over time, the endocrinologist and sexologist Harry Benjamin became deeply committed to helping individuals obtain "sex reassignment surgery." He was one of the six founders of the oldest professional sexological organization in the United States, the Society for the Scientific Study of Sex, in 1957.[26] Benjamin had encountered ten such patients between 1938 and 1953, and he was among the few who published on trans-sexuality during that period.[27] As his clinical observations steadily increased, he became one of the few medical experts on the topic and was invited to report his clinical experiences at New York University School of Medicine in October 1963. Benjamin also gave a talk, "Clinical Aspects of Transsexualism in the Male and Female," at the Sixth Annual Conference of the Society for the Scientific Study of Sex in New York in November of that year and at Jacobi Hospital of the Albert Einstein College of Medicine in April 1964.[28] Part of a network of sexologists that included Robert Stoller and John Money, he described transsexualism as "a striking disturbance of gender role and gender orientation,"[29] and he proposed that "since, in the case of transsexualism, the mind cannot be adjusted to the body, the opposite seems to me not only permissible, but indicated in carefully selected cases."[30] Benjamin, who displayed a great deal of paternalistic empathy with trans individuals, concluded his talk with a passionate plea that "with an accumulation of more cases, studied from the psychiatric, the genetic, and the endocrine angles, a more objective attitude of society in general, and the medical profession in particular, may finally emerge—together with a happier future for some of these patients."[31] Happiness or the alleviation of suffering would continue to play an important role in the argumentation for the establishment of gender identity clinics in the years to come.

In 1966, Benjamin published *The Transsexual Phenomenon*, where he combined an older vision of universal bisexuality (everyone shared male and female characteristics) with the new concept of gender role. "Sex is a matter of anatomy and physiology," he wrote. "Gender, however, can be considered a mixture of inborn and acquired, that is, learned characteristics. 'Masculine' and 'feminine' are therefore expressions belonging to the gender concept."[32] In 1963, he had still exclusively referred to *gender role* and *orientation*, but by 1966 *gender identity* had entered his vocabulary. Benjamin also devised a Sex Orientation Scale, modeled on Alfred C. Kinsey's famous scale of sexual orientation, in which he used the terms *gender "feeling"* (masculine or feminine) and *gender discomfort*.[33] At the time, he was the strongest proponent of making medical and surgical procedures available to transsexuals who wanted to "change" their sex. He also worked closely with trans activists, including Reed Erickson, a trans man who in 1964 founded the Erickson Educational Foundation with the goal of funding medical research, symposia, publications, and conferences on transsexuality. Between 1964 and 1977, the foundation spent around $2.4 million on supporting the trans community and transsexuality studies.[34]

In the early 1960s, John Money also became increasingly interested in transsexuality—although, true to his nature, he tried to coin his own term: "contrasexism."[35] (It did not catch on.) He claimed that transsexual patients were referred or referred themselves to him "because of his prominence in the corrective surgery of hermaphroditism."[36] Money served on the Harry Benjamin Foundation's advisory board, and he arranged meetings between three of Benjamin's patients and several Hopkins surgeons to persuade the latter to perform "sex reassignment" surgery at their prestigious institution. By 1965, he had become involved in a project to install a gender identity clinic or research unit at the Johns Hopkins Hospital, which would include members from different specialties. "Such a clinic, integrated with both the inpatient and outpatient services in psychiatry, would provide a practicable base of operations for the handling of, among others, transvestite and transsexual cases," he wrote in a memorandum to Joel Elkes, psychiatrist-in-chief at Hopkins, on December 9, 1965.[37] John E. Hoopes, assistant professor of plastic surgery, became chairman of the Gender Identity Committee and served as spokesman for the group, which by 1966 had included psychiatrists, plastic surgeons, gynecologists, urologists, and endocrinologists.[38] The psychologist of the illustrious group was unsurprisingly none other than Money himself. By the early summer of 1966, the Gender Identity Committee had "finally worked out the mechanics of the Gender Identity Clinic."[39] It was to meet at 1:00 p.m. on the third Friday of each month at the Johns Hopkins Hospital's Moore Clinic, followed by a clinical conference. For the first meeting, on Friday, July 15, 1966, an individual was invited to travel to Baltimore from New York to be evaluated as the first official patient of the clinic. The Gender Identity Clinic at Hopkins differed from Stoller's Gender Identity Research Clinic established four years earlier in that Stoller and his colleagues were cautious about performing or even endorsing sex reassignment surgery and focused instead on the gender identity of children. One reason was that UCLA's staff were worried about the legal implications of reassignment surgery.[40]

In contrast, the Johns Hopkins Hospital had a history of intersex case management, a flair for heroic surgery, and a position as one of the leading medical institutions in the country. Its doctors made the surgical aspects of transsexualism prominent in setting up the clinic, although in practice they performed very few sex reassignment operations. The Gender Identity Committee's line of reasoning built on established practices to adjust patients' bodies to their minds. Their patients had "extreme adjustment difficulties" and felt "as if their mind [was] in the wrong body," explained group chairman Hoopes.[41] Psychiatrists had tried in vain to treat these patients, but Hoopes, a surgeon, acknowledged that "psychotherapy has so far not resolved the problem." The patients themselves desired surgical transition and not psychotherapy. "If the mind cannot be changed to fit the body, then perhaps we should consider changing the body to fit the mind," the Gender Identity Committee concluded in a statement to the press on November 21, 1966.[42] The Hopkins practice of intersex case management, in which surgical fixability of genitals was a main factor in sex assignment and which postulated that gender role/gender identity became indelibly fixed (or imprinted) with time, clearly influenced this recommendation.

At the time, the media and the public were immensely interested in learning about procedures that seemingly transformed men into women and women into men. The media frenzy surrounding Christine Jorgensen's sex-change operation had whetted their appetite for the story of these procedures, which for the first time were officially to happen on US soil at the nation's most prominent hospital.[43] Of course, it was mainly the hospital setting that made the Gender Identity Clinic a first. In actuality, trans people, as the historian Jen Manion shows, were able to medically transition in the United States before the installation of any of these clinics. The example of female-bodied people who could persuade physicians to remove their uterus for medical reasons shows that "the line between gender transition surgeries and other kinds of surgeries" was indeed "blurry."[44]

When Harry Benjamin referred the first patient to Hopkins in February 1965 to undergo a complete sex reassignment procedure from male to female, the Baltimore newspaper the *Afro-American* offered the patient, who was Black, $800 to publish her story with photographs.

The medical personnel were not thrilled. According to the account later written by Money and a colleague, the "patient was admonished that premature release of information was against her best interests . . . and could frustrate any future surgical attempts of the same kind."[45] The newspaper editor agreed to postpone the story. On October 4, 1966, however, the same patient became the object of a gossip column in the *New York Daily News*:

Making the rounds of Manhattan clubs these nights is a stunning girl, who admits she was a male less than a year ago and that she underwent a sex change operation at, of all places, Johns Hopkins Hospital in Baltimore. Surprisingly, the hospital confirms the case, saying surgery followed psychotherapy. Such operations, although rare in this country, are nether illegal nor unethical, according to a Johns Hopkins spokesman. Officials at a number of major hospitals here agreed with Johns Hopkins on the legality and ethics of the operation but none could recall such an operation ever having been performed in New York.[46]

Aware of the controversies that the establishment of a Gender Identity Clinic at the prestigious hospital could generate, and confronted with news inquiries throughout 1966, the newly formed clinical team carefully orchestrated a press release and coverage by prestigious news outlets such as the *New York Times* and *Time* magazine, hoping to set the tone for other publications. In September 1966, Frank Karel, the associate director of the public relations department, wrote to Hoopes that Money had suggested a meeting of the clinic's Gender Identity Committee to "discuss the public implications of the committee's work" in light of recent inquiries from the press.[47] "This new activity through the Gender Identity Clinic is bound to 'leak,'" Karel wrote, and he wanted to be prepared "to react intelligently to inquiries or, better still, head them off with a positive, sensible, and tasteful exposition of the problems with which the Committee and the Clinic deal and the means with which these problems are resolved."[48] Hoopes met several times with Karel to develop "the most efficacious method for presenting [the clinic's] activities to the lay press" and discouraged individual members of the committee from "divulg[ing] information" without Karel's approval.[49] On November 11, Hoopes wrote to the other members of the committee that the *New York Times* was "attempting to accumulate information" and that it appeared "inevitable that a story of some description" would soon be published. The committee would have preferred to "avoid any publicity whatsoever," but since they would not be able to prevent the eventual publication of the story, they devised a news release as a "defensive measure."[50]

On November 21, the Office of Institutional Public Relations issued a statement announcing the establishment of a clinic for transsexuals at the Johns Hopkins Medical Institutions.[51] At this point, the Gender Identity Clinic had already been in operation for a year. The carefully worded six-page release described "the four-step process for screening, evaluating, treating, and following" clinic patients.[52] Twice in the statement, John E. Hoopes, chairman and spokesperson of the Gender Identity Committee, stressed patients' personal happiness as the important outcome and measurement of treatment success. Clinic personnel would measure their success or failure by asking, "Are these people happier and more useful citizens following surgery and other therapy than they were before?" In a plea for respecting the privacy of patients (and presumably sympathetic and favorable press coverage), he emphasized that "these patients wish only to try to build new, happier lives for themselves after leaving Hopkins."[53] Similar to the treatment incentive cited for patients with intersex traits, happiness and "living a happy life" became persistent themes in the argumentation for trans surgery.

The Gender Identity Committee's plan of controlled publicity worked exactly as hoped; coverage included the supportive voices of lay and religious leaders and critics.[54] On November 21, 1966, the *New York Times* reported on its front page that the Johns Hopkins Hospital had "quietly begun performing sex change surgery."[55] "The men and women who seek sex change surgery are called transsexuals," the article explained. "They are almost always physically normal, but they have a total aversion to their biological sex that dates from early childhood. They have the apparently unshakeable conviction that they are either female beings trapped in a male body or males trapped in a female body." The article also stressed a narrative of medical compassion and care, citing Hoopes, who stated, "After exhaustively reviewing the available literature and discussing the problem with people knowledgeable in this area, I arrived at the unavoidable conclusion that these people need and deserve help." The article also deployed the language of gender, referring to "gender confusion, which leads to intense feelings of frustration" and to "the problem of gender identification."[56] *Time* reported in a similar manner a week later, on December 2: "Last week's announcement from Johns Hopkins marked the first time that a prestigious medical center has risked its reputation to give organized help to transsexuals."[57] An accompanying image of Johns Hopkins physicians Knorr, Hoopes, and Edgerton was captioned, "In the hope that society will benefit as well as the individual."

Shortly after Hopkins's 1966 announcement introducing its Gender Identity Clinic, many other clinics and programs opened all over the country. The University of Minnesota Medical School announced its Gender Committee in December 1966; in 1967, Northwestern University Medical School opened a Gender Study and Research Program; in 1968, Stanford University established a Gender Reorientation Program (afterward renamed Gender Identity Clinic); and later that year, the University of Washington, Seattle, created a Gender Identity Research and Treatment Clinic.[58] Hopkins's Gender Identity Clinic was eventually closed in 1979 because of in-house psychiatric opposition to trans surgery, despite the fact that its surgeons had actually performed only 30 such procedures during its short tenure. The main work seems to have consisted of providing about 1,000 surgical consultations as well as many trainings at other hospitals. In the year of the clinic's closure, approximately 15–20 medical centers were performing sex-affirming surgery throughout the United States.[59]

Reports about the opening of these gender identity clinics were at times sensational, but overall they were positive and focused on matters such as the alleviation of suffering, the application of medical expertise, and the advancement of modern biomedicine. But the journalists made little of the fact that the first patient to undergo "a complete sex-reassignment" at the Hopkins Clinic was Black. Nor did reporters note that the first patient (G. L.) referred to the Child Psychiatry Department at the Johns Hopkins Hospital in January 1960 for "the syndrome of transsexuality" was actually a trans child, only thirteen years old at first contact with the institution and seventeen when disappearing from the hospital record without undergoing any "sex-reassignment procedure."[60] In the 1970s, sensationalized yet sympathetic accounts of transsexuality were regular news items, including in the weekly newspaper the *National Observer*, which in 1976 featured a front page with the lead article "What Makes a Person Want to Switch Sexes?"[61] Transsexuality became part of popular culture in that decade and was included in the story lines of movies such as 1970's *Myra Breckinridge* or 1975's *Dog Day Afternoon* and *The Rocky Horror Picture Show*.[62]

Gender, Sex, and the Brain

In the 1960s and early 1970s, gender made yet another transition. It all began with some guinea pigs in 1959. By the late 1940s, the anatomist William C. Young, the psychologist Frank Beach, and the zoologist

Alfred Kinsey had been considered the "Big Three" of sex research.[63] Young and Beach had established the field of behavioral endocrinology; Young's work united the study of physiology and behavior, which would become an important principle of that field.[64] His experiments were considered groundbreaking for understanding the female reproductive cycle, and his work was thought to demonstrate that behavior followed laws and could thus be studied scientifically.[65] In 1959, Young, Charles H. Phoenix, Robert W. Goy, and Arnold A. Gerall, all at the University of Kansas, published a paper on behavioral changes in female guinea pigs after the administration of testosterone.[66] The research that it reported had yielded the first hypothesis of what would subsequently be called Organization Theory (OT). OT postulated that brain structure, as well as genitals and reproductive organs, expressed a person's sex. On the one hand, hormones played a role in the development of sex-specific organs in the originally undifferentiated fetus, presumably after the sixth or seventh week of gestation. Thus, sex was created. On the other hand, hormones also shaped the undifferentiated mammalian brain in a prenatal phase. Thus, "gender" was created. More testosterone shaped the brain into a masculine gender, such that the resulting child would manifest male behavior, desires, cognitive patterns, and above all masculine sexuality—the desire for women. Similarly, the presence of less testosterone initiated a female development of the embryo's brain structures. Put simply, masculinizing hormones shaped the developing brain of either genetic sex to have increased "masculine" traits and decreased "feminine" traits.[67]

At this time, Young was also the new editor of the 1961 edition of *Sex and Internal Secretions*, which included articles by John Money, Joan Hampson, and her husband, John (eventually submitted separately after Money's falling-out with the couple). All three had been the subject of Young's attention for some time. He had organized the November 1954 conference in Amherst, Massachusetts, "Genetic, Psychological and Hormonal Factors in the Establishment and Maintenance of Patterns of Sexual Behavior in Mammals," at which Money and Joan Hampson had presented (discussed in chapter 4).[68] In their 1959 guinea pig article, Young and his colleagues cited a draft chapter that the Hampsons had written for *Sex and Internal Secretions*. Money's contribution was not mentioned in the paper—he might not have submitted yet—but Young would engage with him from there on out.[69]

Young and colleagues' citing researchers who used "human data" reflected the belief that they had had from the beginning: that their hypothesis about brain organization could be applied to humans. Of course, no actual experimental data on humans could be generated for obvious ethical reasons. Instead, they looked to clinical studies. Yet again, patients with intersex traits became of central importance for researchers—this time for those interested in brain organization. Their reasoning went something like this: if genital development was a marker for prenatal hormone exposure, then studying intersex people with genitals that did not fit their genetic sex was the best way to figure out these relationships in humans. Over the next couple of years, Young's group cautiously compared their findings with those of clinician-researchers who were invested in the importance of learning and the environment. In the course of this endeavor, both groups acknowledged each other's work.[70]

It is perhaps ironic, the feminist science studies scholar Rebecca Jordan-Young points out, that given his long-standing commitment to a learned gender role, "Money was actually the first to apply the new brain organization theory to data from humans"; moreover, he became the most prolific researcher in this field.[71] Money started reworking and adjusting his gender concept in 1965, initially in a rather tentative tone, arguing that "the leap from guinea pigs and rats to human beings is a broad one, and there may, in fact, be no similarity."[72] Nevertheless, he used the same group of patients that he had already extensively studied in the early 1950s, girls and women with congenital adrenal hyperplasia (CAH), to rethink gender and brain organization. Because these female patients had been exposed to larger amounts of androgens throughout fetal developments, he thought they might represent an at least partial human parallel to animal experiments with androgen.[73] Yet again, the clinical evidence from his case histories of intersex patients became crucial: they were considered the naturally occurring equivalent to the animal experiments.[74]

In 1955, female (as defined by XX chromosomes and internal reproductive organs) patients with CAH had been Money's prime example for a learned gender role, whether they lived in the male or, after cortisone, in the female sex. In his 1965 article, he suggested that prenatal androgens had organizing effects on these patients' brains, resulting in masculine sexuality, defined as "experiences more typically reported by normal males than by females, namely, erotic arousal with a strong genito-pelvic component from the stimulation of visual and narrative perceptual material."[75] These girls and women, he argued, were aroused more quickly, intensely, and frequently than other women but remained heterosexual in their desires, or, in his words, "suitably feminine."[76] Money also drew from the second group that had been essential in bringing forth his earlier argument for a learned gender role independent of biological factors, chromosomally male patients with testicular feminizing syndrome,[77] all of whom lived as females with female genitalia. Based on the new research on the influence of prenatal hormonal exposure on the brain, Money now speculated that the lack of "a masculinizing principle" actually enhanced these patients' capacity to fulfill the demands of female sex assignment and rearing—rather than, as he had previously claimed, that "their sex assignment and rearing [were] female, in keeping with their genital appearance."[78]

Money's article stands at the beginning of a research program that examined the effects of prenatal hormonal exposure in organizing human brains and consequently human sexual behavior.[79] His approach was certainly cautious. Yes, "hormone effects were real," he insisted, but also "subtle and limited." In the end, "gender and sexuality would develop most seamlessly when sex assignment and rearing were in accord with the hormones that 'primed' the nervous system during fetal life."[80] By the 1960s, Money, together with his collaborator Anke Ehrhardt, a young doctoral candidate from Germany, persistently investigated brain organization in humans.[81] The new team compared hormone-exposed patients (such as girls with CAH or children who had been exposed to progestin during their fetal life) with unexposed or "normal" groups of children and adults. They consistently argued that "girls and women exposed to high levels of androgen exhibited sexual traits and behavior that were more masculine than was expected."[82] Low androgen exposure among boys and men seemed to be the cause of behavior that was more feminine.[83]

The clinician-researchers were studying not only the same syndromes as in the original Hopkins study but also, in many cases, "the same actual patients" from their earlier evaluations at the clinic, as Jordan-Young shows.[84] It turns out that a very small group of patients were at the epicenter of a tremendously varied, new body of research. Interestingly, the definitions of gendered behavior were quite similar to those very normative categories that had been used in the 1955 and 1956 publications on learned gender role. One was sexuality, underwritten by the assumption that sexual orientation was heterosexual by default and that homosexuality was an indication of gender role gone wrong or, in this new understanding, of exposure to the wrong hormone in utero. Just like Money's 1950s definition of proper male and female gendered behavior, the new categories included sex-typed behavior and interests such as play patterns, manner of dress, cognitive skills, career, marriage, and motherhood.

In 1972, Money (fig. 5) and Ehrhardt published *Man and Woman, Boy and Girl* to answer "the ancient question: Is it heredity or environment?"[85] Their book became a classic within a decade, and by 1987 it had been cited in over 460 publications.[86] The *New York Times Book Review* praised it as "the most important volume in the social sciences to appear since the Kinsey reports."[87] In this collaborative work, Money and Ehrhardt balanced the seemingly opposing factors of prenatal hormonal influence and psychosexuality shaped by experiences and learning. Money also showed that he adapted to the new usage of gender identity introduced by Robert Stoller and referred to GR/I (gender role/identity) in his writings.

Man and Woman was a conflicted book. On the one hand, it made a strong case for Money's initial claim of a learned gender role; on the other hand, the authors integrated the new research on prenatal brain organization (OT) throughout the text, shifting toward the return to the biological in the 1970s.[88] Their chapter on fetal hormones and the brain, in which they utilize their research on girls with CAH (who were reared as girls), displays the uneasy integration of OT into Money's previous research on gender role. In this chapter, Money and Ehrhardt asserted that

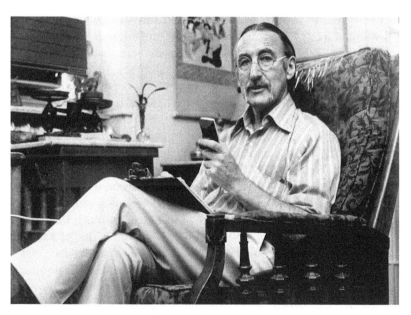

Figure 5   John Money, circa 1970

the childhood behavior of CAH girls was masculinized, and they argued that this was most likely caused by prenatal exposure to androgens. In doing so, they reproduced specific social norms of masculinity in their analysis: active, intelligent, and career oriented. They observed that CAH girls were often tomboys, enjoyed "vigorous outdoor play, games, and sports," "preferred the utilitarian and functional in clothing, rather than the chic, pretty, or fashionably feminine," were "indifferent to dolls" and "turned instead to cars, trucks, and guns," and fantasized about pursuing a career rather than motherhood.[89] Money and Ehrhardt also claimed to have found a lack of interest in romance and boyfriends.[90] This tomboyism was, they argued, "a sequel to a masculinizing effect on the fetal brain."[91] Nonetheless, they were convinced of the importance of postnatal rearing experiences. For example, they still believed that postnatal factors, not prenatal hormones, shaped sexual orientation or choice of sex partner. In their opinion, prenatal hormones shaped the gendered behavior of nonhuman animals much more than that of humans.[92]

The disjunction between postulating a manipulatable gender role/identity shaped by experiences and environment, hypothesizing about the biological basis of difference in male and female, and using very normative gender roles to argue either point arises in the tragic case of David Reimer (né Bruce). At the time of its inclusion in *Man and Woman, Boy and Girl*, this case was anonymized and discussed under the heading "Rearing of a Sex-Reassigned Normal Male Infant after Traumatic Loss of the Penis."[93] It became widely known as the John/Joan case after Milton Diamond and H. Keith Sigmundson published a long-term review article on sex reassignment at birth in 1997.[94] At seven months of age, Bruce and his identical twin brother were taken to a local hospital for a routine circumcision. A malfunction in the electrical cauterizing scalpel caused irreparable damage to Bruce's penis, and it was completely ablated.[95] The upset parents, "young people of rural background and grade school education," were "understandably desperate," Money and Ehrhardt wrote. Finally, a "consultant plastic surgeon who was familiar with the principles of sex reassignment recommended reassignment as a girl." The "sex change" took place at seventeen months; the parents changed Bruce's name to Brenda, and they changed his clothes and hairstyle. At twenty-one months, "the surgical first step of genital reconstruction as a female was undertaken."[96] The plan was to delay vaginoplasty until the child was older and then to regulate puberty and feminization by hormone replacement therapy.

At the time of Brenda's surgery, the family came to Hopkins. Money saw Mr. and Mrs. Reimer in person and counseled them on the management "of their new daughter." After the surgery, the parents kept in close contact and returned for annual follow-up visits "to get psychological support and guidance" (119). Money noted that during those years, the Reimers made every effort to support the development of Brenda's female gender role by focusing on appearance (frilly dresses, feminine hairdos), behavior (neatness, peeing sitting down), rehearsal of the female role (helping with housework), and conversations about the female and male adult reproductive roles (menstruation, pregnancy). Regarding the latter, Money had suggested that they eventually inform their daughter about the possibility of becoming a mother by adoption.

According to Money and Ehrhardt, Brenda had fully embraced the (rather old-fashioned) female gender role. Even more so, thanks to the presence of a male control (her twin brother), the authors could compare the successful assignment in two chromosomally male children. "By the time the twins were five years and nine months of age," they wrote, "they expressed clearly different goals for the future." However, they admitted that Brenda also had "tomboyish traits" and had been "the dominant twin from the beginning" (122). The case gained great publicity at first, as it seemed to demonstrate that the human gender role was learned—given that the chromosomally male child in question was not intersex and had a twin brother who served as the control. In 1975, Money published a write-up of the case in the *Archives of Sexual Behavior*, where, he argued, based on the evidence of intersex patients and this particular case, that "gender identity is sufficiently incompletely differentiated at birth as to permit successful assignment of a genetic male as a girl. Gender identity then differentiates in keeping with the experiences of rearing."[97]

In 1975, Money was optimistic about the outcome of the case: "Her behavior is so normally that of an active little girl, and so clearly different by contrast from the boyish ways of her twin brother, that it offers nothing to stimulate one's conjectures."[98] Initially, only a few scientists challenged his claims, arguing that sex chromosomes only, not rearing, shaped masculinity and femininity.[99] By the late 1990s, significant doubts had arisen about the actual success of this sex reassignment. A decade later, press reports revealed that Brenda had been extremely unhappy with the (heavy-handed) gender identity/role put on her and, when informed of her medical history, had elected to be reassigned as a boy and chosen the name David. These revelations dealt a heavy blow to Money's reputation, since he was portrayed in popular accounts as a ruthless experimenter on children.[100] At the time, the case was deanonymized and widely discussed, and most of these discussions criticized Money's involvement.[101] Many of his critics were inclined, as he himself had been, to utilize David's case to support their own convictions in the nature/nurture debate. Tragically, there was no happy ending to David Reimer's story. In 2004, he died by suicide.

For a good thirty years, however, John Money insisted that the case of Brenda Reimer had been a success, and he and Anke Ehrhardt used this spectacular example to showcase the favorable outcome of consistent gender messaging. Parents only needed to model distinct male and female roles to assure their child's successful gender reassignment. This case was critical evidence for the importance of experience and learning in establishing a person's masculinity and femininity, and it comes as no surprise that for many this was a strong case for nurture over nature.[102] Money also saw himself as an ally of women's liberation, at least initially.[103] The index of *Man and Woman* provided a long list of "quotable material" under the entry "women's liberation." Clearly, Money and Ehrhardt were confidently expecting a particular readership for their volume that went beyond scientists and clinician-researchers.

There is, then, an odd disjunction between the need for the psychological prescription of conventional gender roles to install proper gender identity and Money's recognition that they were just that—conventions. The prescribed male and female roles that would assure proper gender role and identity that Money and Erhardt listed in 1972 seemed very similar to the normative ones that Money and Joan and John Hampson had put forward in the 1950s.[104] In discussing the John/Joan case, for example, Money and Erhardt insisted on the importance of strict and, most important, different gender roles for a successful sex assignment. They wrote, "Of course, girls and boys are not only prepared differently for their future reproductive role as mother and father, but also for their other different roles, such as wife and husband or financial supporter of the family and caretaker of children and house."[105] They presented a description of the Reimer twins' gendered play with dolls and cars, respectively, as a rehearsal for female and male roles, but in the next paragraph they stated that "according to today's standards, not only boys, but also girls pursue a career."[106] This was a recurring contradiction. Once biology was no longer the basis for masculinity and femininity, social norms were at the heart of gender distinction. At the same time, in the 1970s recognition of masculinity and femininity as social artifacts was growing, and feminists argued that gendered behaviors had been socially constructed by a patriarchal society. The tension between social norms being called into question and the need to use behavior and self-identification to indicate gender remained unresolved in *Man and Woman*.

Yet in the 1960s and even more so in the 1970s, journalists and commentators immediately considered both the concept of gender role and the data of the Johns Hopkins team as important assets for feminists and the women's liberation movement. Money himself played an inconsistent role in promoting this understanding of gender, inserting himself into debates about women's role and politics but simultaneously insisting on conventional norms of masculinity and femininity.[107] On December 28, 1972, he gave a talk, "Nativism and Culturalism in Gender Identity Differentiation," for a panel, "Sex-Role Learning in Childhood and Adolescence," at the American Association for the Advancement of Science in Washington, DC.[108] He was the only panelist to use the term *gender* (rather than *sex role*) in his presentation title. Then in January 1973, *Time* magazine published a one-page feature discussing Money, his findings, and *Man and Woman*, which had published months earlier. The article, interestingly titled "Biological Imperatives," described the "dramatic" case of the Reimer twins and reported that it "provides strong support for a major contention of women's liberationists: that conventional patterns of masculine and feminine behavior can be altered." Theories postulating that genes immutably set "major sexual differences, psychological as well as anatomical," at conception were called into question. The *Time* reporter expressed confidence that, as Money had shown in his talk, almost all sex differences were "culturally determined and therefore optional." Money had cautioned that prenatal hormonal exposure programmed the brain in such a way that "some types of behavior may come more naturally to one sex than to the other." In other words, both men and women could "mother" children, Money was saying, every brain had "the necessary circuits," but the "threshold" for releasing this behavior was much higher in males than females.[109]

Despite the use of gendered norms ("to mother"), one could not blame a feminist reader of the *Time* article for thinking that Money was questioning the validity of sexual differences. After all, he was reported to claim that pre- and postnatal hormones mattered less in human beings than the "sex assignment" at birth. The announcement of sex at birth ("It's a boy!" or "It's a girl!") shaped how the infant was treated and set off "a chain of events" that determined whether the child would behave "in traditionally masculine or feminine ways." The article cited Money's clinical data from cases in which "mistakes" in sex assignment had been made at birth, the Reimer twin case, and data from his study of "hermaphrodites" to substantiate the claim. But it ended with Money's caution that "despite his evidence of the importance of environment in molding sex roles," he held out "little hope to feminists" that there could be "any significant breakdown of sex-role stereotypes in the current generation of adults." The reason was quite simply that little change in "male-female attitudes and behavior" was possible after the first four years of life, and change after that critical phase made most people "uncomfortable." Even men who agreed to share household and child care duties hated it, Money explained, and consequently, "a liberated woman today is almost painted into a corner because there are so few liberated men she can marry."[110] Yet by 1973, when the interview with Money was published, the "liberated woman" had already been at work developing her own take on gender.

"In the Air": Early Feminist Engagement with Gender

Gender has deeply intertwined with the history of feminism in the twenty-first century, but most feminists in the 1960s and early 1970s analyzed and contested "sex-role socialization" without ever using the term *gender*. Despite Money's claims, feminists did not need gender to critique biological determinism or social norms. And when gender entered feminist discourse, its usage was at times murky and inconsistent. Indeed, those who engaged with the idea of gender did not attach any single or fixed meaning to it. Some aligned with its use in medical and psychological debates about sex differences, transsexuality, and newly established gender identity clinics in the late 1960s and the 1970s. Many, however, used *gender* without a particular reference to its medical origin, and feminist activists and queer communities applied the term indiscriminately to discuss social and sexual politics and practices. For example, in the 1970s the *Berkeley Barb*, a famous underground newspaper produced between 1965 and 1980, used *gender* mostly instead of *sex*, in combinations such as *opposite gender* or *gender differences*, and very precisely as in *gender role* and *gender identity*.[111]

Also in the 1970s, *New Directions for Women*, which started as a mimeographed newsletter in 1972 but was influential until it ceased publication in 1993, increasingly used *gender* to discuss gender stereotypes, gender roles, and the gender trap, or simply to denote the male or female gender without noting the transition in usage or the distinction. *Chrysalis, a Magazine of Women's Culture*, published between 1977 and 1980 in Los Angeles, sometimes used *gender* in place of *sex*, such as *gender discrimination*, but discussed gender identity and role in articles about psychology, psychoanalysis, or transsexuality. In 1977, for example, in an article titled "Psychoanalysis, Patriarchy, and Power," the psychologist Jean Baker Miller, author of *Toward a New Psychology of Women*, cited as related evidence regarding women's sense of identity that "recent work in several disciplines" suggested "that an individual's basic sense of identity is closely linked to her/his sense of gender identity, and that gender identity becomes firmly established somewhere between the ages of 18 and 36 months." She emphasized that this stable sense of being male or female might be culturally specific to our society.[112]

It was only after gender had already been appropriated and reinterpreted by feminist activists, artists, and the LGBTQ community that academic feminists aimed to define *gender* with more precision and finesse in the late 1970s and early 1980s. It is beyond the scope of this chapter to sketch the complex history of feminist engagement with gender and the role it played in the diverse, global, and intersectional women's liberation movements of the late twentieth century.[113] In this section, I am instead focusing on early feminist discussions of the work of John Money and Robert Stoller, particularly the clinical evidence that they both provide to sustain their concepts of gender role and gender identity. As some of the feminist critique of Money and Stoller overlaps with the critique of Margaret Mead's rejection of radical feminist change, the section will occasionally also engage with her work.

A large segment of feminist activists and scholars saw the idea that gender was culturally inscribed and learned as tremendously liberating.[114] If femininity or masculinity was learned, it could be unlearned or even replaced by something different. Women's (and men's) liberation could be achieved simply by reorganizing social institutions, raising consciousness, and providing education. Gender's alignment with the authority of the Johns Hopkins Hospital, one of the most prominent medical institutions in the nation, strengthened their argumentation against a biological determination of sex and the associated roles women were expected to play in society, even though the link to Hopkins was initially only indirect. Before the publication of Money and Ehrhardt's *Man and Woman, Boy and Girl* in 1972, most feminists had referred to Stoller's concept of gender identity, published in 1968, as a reformulation of Money's gender concept. However, feminists were particularly interested in the clinical data which Stoller had adopted from Money. For example, in 1970 Kate Millett's *Sexual Politics* cited Stoller's concept and Money's data when invoking "important new research" and "fairly concrete positive evidence of the overwhelmingly cultural character of gender, i.e. personality structure in terms of sexual category."[115]

A survey of sociological literature shows that the usage of *gender* was not firmly established until the late 1970s.[116] Yet feminist sociology was an important factor in integrating the concept of gender into sociological discussions of sex, women, equal rights, and the women's movement to a point where it created its own genealogy of gender. Early engagement included the feminist sociologist Jessie Bernard, who referenced Stoller (and indirectly Money and the Hampsons) to point out in her 1971 book *Women and the Public Interest* that "gender, though based on biology, is a social-cultural-sociological-psychological fact."[117] Bernard utilized Money's clinical data to show that some of his patients, despite sharing the "same sex heredity, same prenatal 'error,'" had been given "different gender assignment" at birth and developed gender identities that matched their assignment. Gender was "so thoroughly bred into the infant by the world around it" that it became an unalterable "part of its identity" (19). She also noted that the "constellation of traits suitable for characterizing" feminine gender identity, defined by Stoller as "wanting babies and having a great interest in clothes, cooking, sewing, make-up, ornamentation, and the like," was clearly not biologically defined but was composed of the traits that society "label[s] feminine" (20).[118]

The British feminist sociologist Ann Oakley, whose 1972 book *Sex, Gender and Society* was widely read by US feminists, also played an important role in transmitting Money's and Stoller's gender theories and research to feminist readers.[119] Oakley engaged deeply with Money's and the Hampsons' "invaluable work on intersexuality in America" to base her assumptions about learned gender roles on their clinical data.[120] "Men and women *are* temperamentally different," she wrote, "but what does this 'fact' mean? It means that personality differences between male and female exist within Western society with a certain constancy and stability. But it does not mean that these differences are molded by biology—indeed, it says nothing at all about how much of the difference is due to biology and how much to culture."[121] Much as Bernard had, Oakley argued that Money's intersex patient data indicated cultural learning as the main factor in acquiring gender identity. Further, she reasoned, the fact that men and women were not only taught from birth onward to behave in different ways but also to expect different behavior from the other sex created inequality between the sexes.[122]

By the mid-1970s, gender role had entered broader feminist discourses. When the feminist activist Robin Morgan published the anthology *Sisterhood Is Powerful* in 1970 after two years of collective work, the compilation of "articles, poems, graphics, and sundry papers" engaged with Margaret Mead's work on sex roles (and provided a critique of her politics) but not with gender role or identity.[123] Five years later, authors in the edited volume *Women: A Feminist Perspective* cited Mead as well as Money's publications.[124] For example, in her chapter on sex-role socialization, the sociologist Lenore J. Weitzman quoted the work of "John Money and his associates at Johns Hopkins University" to support her argument about the power of cultural factors in shaping sex differences, right after a section in which she discussed Mead's work.[125]

Like Mead's *sex role*, Money's and Stoller's specific usage of *gender* was not as liberating as it appeared from a feminist point of view. Rather than dismantling and questioning the very categories of masculinity and femininity, the conviction that gender was a social category, shaped by the environment one was raised in and by childhood experiences, could justify the need to fix and uphold a clearly circumscribed gender binary. Hence despite the promise of social and cultural malleability of gender and its precursor sex role, Money, Stoller, and, given her background as a pioneering female anthropologist, Mead most of all, disappointed those who sought immediate change. The feminist push for radical change was on a very different activist timescale from the contemplations and theories of Mead, Money, and Stoller. Mead, for example, thought that radical change was not possible on feminists' timetables. "Cultures" were "wholes" in which change would be either gradual or violent. Radical women who had been inspired by Mead's life and work and who had found *Coming of Age in Samoa* and *Sex and Temperament* formative readings were dismayed by her cautious, conservative, and at times disapproving approach to the women's liberation movement in the 1960s.[126]

Mead was the most prominent representative of a generation of public anthropologists, and she had long been reaching out to a wider audience.[127] For instance, she wrote a monthly column for the women's magazine *Redbook* between 1962 and 1970.[128] In such forums, Mead positioned herself as a champion for abortion and for no-fault divorce and an opponent of laws against homosexuality, but she endorsed very conventional norms. She implied that most women, including college-educated women, wanted to marry, have kids, and stay home. Although she acknowledged increasing workforce participation among women, she suggested that men needed a career and women did not (60). As the anthropologist Paul Shankman notes, Mead had long been "viewed as a pioneer of the sexual revolution by some of her colleagues and cultural liberals," and young feminist activists were shocked by her positions

(58). They saw her claims that socialization was unchangeable as deterministic and thus antithetical to the women's movement.

In 1970, however, Mead's position on the women's liberation movement shifted favorably when she informed *Redbook* readers that it was important to reduce sex-role differences and to promote similar education for men and women. She rejected limitations on women's freedom as a group, but she still was suspicious of the emerging radical feminist movement (60). When she addressed women's liberation in 1970, Mead criticized feminists' "shock tactics" such as the protests at the Miss America pageant in 1968, and she described them as "stormy and obstreperous radicals," and "conspicuously self-centered and hostile women."[129] Though her opposition had softened, she still felt that feminists wanted change too quickly. "The movement has verve, excitement and drama," she acknowledged. But it did not yet have "the potentialities for revolutionary change."[130] Such a radical transition could not be made in one generation. Societies have "heavily reinforced the belief, shared by men and women alike, that maintaining the home and bearing and rearing children are the vital task for women," while feminists wanted changes that were "too superficial to meet the crisis of modern civilization" (64). By this she referred to a widespread concern about the explosive growth of the world's population. Nonetheless, Mead wrote that she understood that the "anger, bitterness and violence of many feminists" (67) was related to real conditions.

Robert Stoller was also concerned with upholding rather than dismantling gender roles. Though for many readers, his book *Sex and Gender* seemed to offer evidence to support that masculinity and femininity were learned, he was far from a feminist or supporter of women's liberation. In his clinical practice, Stoller and his colleagues were deeply invested in instilling traditional gender roles in children;[131] as the historian Joanne Meyerowitz noted, "If gender was mostly socially constructed, then someone, they reasoned, had to repair it when it was improperly built."[132] John Money claimed to support women's liberation, but he, too, insisted on clearly differentiated gender norms to ensure that children with intersex traits learned their proper socially prescribed gender roles. David Reimer and his twin brother were subject to this insistence, and the assessment policies at the new gender identity clinics continued to prescribe stereotypical male and female behavior and normed appearance for trans people.

Over the course of the 1970s, Money for his part seemed to be increasingly on the fence as to whether gender norms could be altered alongside radical social change. In January 1973, he stated in an interview that change of gender norms was not possible within one lifetime, since the gender role would be fixed at an early age.[133] But two months later, in a little-known talk at the Sixth Symposium of the Society of Medical Psychoanalysts (Topic: Sexuality and Psychoanalysis Revisited) held in New York, he seemed to acknowledge and integrate the sweeping changes in gender norms during the 1970s. While discussing innate versus acquired behavior in gender-identity differentiation, Money stressed the danger of dichotomizing the learned and the biological.[134] In the talk's final section, he emphasized that "the majority of gender-divergent roles belong in the optional category"—that is, they were learned. However, "historically" there had been "extensive stereotyping" of roles as masculine and feminine, and these were subsequently "transmitted to each new generation of children as male-female absolutes, and not as optional and ambisexual or gender-shared."[135] "The children of parents with less divergent roles," he added, "more easily learn gender roles that are more sex-shared." Money ended his talk by highlighting that the disparity between the group with divergent gender identity and those who were more flexible in their gendered behavior was "now strong enough itself to be a cultural force in our midst," indicating a sea change in gender norms.[136]

Many feminists noted the discrepancies between gender's apparent promise of the social construction of masculinity and femininity and the stereotypical assessment of these social norms. Money's and Stoller's conservative conception of male and female roles was the most visible in their medical concept of transsexuality, and some feminist critics therefore sought to dismantle that concept. For example, in 1977 Janice Raymond, who at the time taught women's studies and medical ethics at the Five Colleges in Amherst, Massachusetts, critically dissected the gender concepts of "Money and his associates" and of Stoller in an article titled "Transsexualism: The Ultimate Homage to Sex-Role Power," published in *Chrysalis: A Magazine of Women's Culture*.[137] Although the article focused on her particularly hostile definition of "transsexualism" as a symbol of society's persistent antifeminism, it also included a very precise critique of the psychological and clinical concept of gender in Money and Ehrhardt's 1972 book.[138]

Raymond claimed that feminists had widely accepted Money's work, even though in her opinion his claim "to unite biological and environmental factors into a unique, sophisticated gestalt" was just a smokescreen. First, she found his claims of biological sex differences in the brain to be unsubstantiated. Money's assertion, in Raymond's wording, that prenatal hormonal activity set up "certain neural pathways in the brain which provide the biological basis not only for male or female body development, but for gender identity formation (i.e., masculine or feminine behavior)" was, after all, just a hypothesis, and he did not provide any proof for his assumptions. "On the environmental side," Raymond continued, "Money's statements about the effects of socialization or learning are just as deceiving." True, he emphasized that socialization was more significant than biological factors, but he did so by emphasizing that a person's "core" gender identity was "fixed by the age of 18 months" and that the very core of one's consciousness (as being male or female) could not be altered. "Here," Raymond observed, "the theme changes from 'biology is destiny' to 'socialization is destiny.'" She pointed at exactly the same disjunction that feminists had noted earlier with Margaret Mead: that to say socialization cannot be changed, to say that gender identity (or sex role) was absolute and static, was as deterministic as adhering to the point of view that sex differences were natural and thus fixed. But Raymond and other feminists felt that the women's liberation movement had disproved the claim. "One wonders," she mused, "where Money has been during the last decade of feminism. If women had not been able to alter the 'core' of our gender identities, then feminism never could have become a lived reality."[139]

It is unthinkable to write about Raymond without acknowledging the damage her ideas about trans women did to trans women themselves and the women's movement specifically.[140] While critical of Money's and Stoller's normative ideas of masculinity and femininity, she accepted their use of transsexuality as a tool for reinforcing gender stereotypes, in defiance of the lived experience of trans women who were part of feminist and lesbian collectives and who often flouted the narrow and normative medical prescriptions of gender roles. Her call for the exclusion of trans women from feminist, lesbian, and women-centered events and organizations wove narratives of controversies and trans exclusion that now, as the historian Finn Enke writes, "naturalize the separation of trans from feminism" rather than acknowledging the rich history of transfeminism in the 1970s.[141]

While academic feminists criticized Money and Stoller for upholding gender binaries, feminist activists, artists, and the LGBTQ community increasingly used *gender* in the early 1970s, often in combination with provocative terminology, to question and "queer" traditional gender stereotypes. One such term was *gender-fuck*, which described the practice of purposefully confusing and upsetting gender norms, often taking the "form of extended guerilla theater that may, indeed, be effective in changing the stereotypes that cling to social mores."[142] The expression made its appearance in the alternative and LGBTQ press in the early 1970s and was used mostly in reports about various forms of drag shows in which performers caricatured or challenged gender stereotypes. In May 1973, a *Berkeley Barb* article about "the liberated drag queen" featured an interview with Glitters Galore, a member of Manicure ("the new radical transvestite movement in the East Bay"). "I, for instance," Glitters was quoted, "am a glitter queen of the gender-fuck variety. Gender-fuck is confusing genders. You can do that either by dressing so that people are not sure what you are, in neither distinctly male nor female attire, or you can clearly show what you are, say, by wearing a beard, but totally fucking over the sex-role conditioned straight mind by wearing a dress with the beard. . . . Gender-fuck is freedom from sex role playing and very liberating also in a political sense."[143] The same year, an author named "Moon" who penned the "Crazy Ladies" section in the Chicago-based lesbian periodical *Lavender Woman* used the term *gender-fuck* to describe her experiences of being mis-gendered. On her morning paper route, an old man had apologized for mistaking her for a girl, to which she replied "I am." In recounting the hilarious scene, "Moon" asked the readers, maybe somewhat tongue-in-cheek, "Is that gender-fuck?"[144]

In November 1973 the *Great Speckled Bird*, a counterculture underground newspaper based in Atlanta, Georgia, featured a review of the Cosmic Light Show. The star of the show, "bette midler," was "a female drag queen but not a parody of a woman, sexist but not macho, tacky but full of grace, a kitsch kewpie doll but a very real presence." One scene, the review continued, was "hotbed of hysteria, with cosmic, gender-fuck, drag, and evening wear contributing to a glitter/lurex dervish, fun to ruin the staid vibes of the civic center with a cluster of cherries, glitter hose, rhinestones, maribou, and tutti-fruitti headdresses!"[145] Articles in 1975 and 1976 featured the "Cycle Sluts"—"male 'gender-fuck' singing group whose members perform wearing mixed 'drag queen' and 'leatherman' costumes."[146] In an interview, one of "the reigning queens of the Sunset Strip," a Miss Humility (Lola), explained, "We're not drag queens. We're genderfucks. We're exploiting what we hate. In men, women, S&M freaks, straights, squares. We know that we start out scaring the audience, but that doesn't last. They start laughing with us right away."[147]

Gender was up for grabs, and as *gender* became ubiquitous, there were significant divergences among the ways clinician-researchers, psychologists, social scientists, feminists, activists, transgender individuals, and queer communities deployed the term. For example, the anthropologist Gayle Rubin in her highly influential 1975 essay "The Traffic in Women," written from an activist's perspective when she was in her early twenties, first applied the term *sex/gender system* to describe "the set of arrangements by which a society transforms biological sexuality into products of human activity."[148] She attached gender to notions of biological sex and to the assumption of heterosexuality. "It is important— even in the face of a depressing history," Rubin wrote, "to maintain a distinction between the human capacity and necessity to create a sexual world, and the empirically oppressive ways in which sexual worlds have been organized. Patriarchy subsumes both meanings into the same term. Sex/gender system, on the other hand, is a neutral term which refers to the domain and indicates that oppression is not inevitable in that domain, but is the product of the specific social relations which organize it."[149] Though Rubin had read John Money and Anke Ehrhardt's *Man and Woman*, she did not reference the book or any of Money's other writings in the essay, which was a deep engagement with the theories of Karl Marx, Sigmund Freud, and Claude Lévi-Strauss. As she later stated in an interview, her motivation for writing the essay also stemmed from a rejection of the biological determinism that simmered in feminist debates about transsexuality in the mid-1970s.[150]

The term *gender* and its many usages offered new ways of speaking and thinking about sex. In a personal communication with me, Rubin indicates that by the time she was thinking about "The Traffic in Women" (starting around 1968 and into the early 1970s), *gender* had been "around and a term that quickly caught on." As she puts it, "*gender* was just kind of in the air, in the water, and in the intense conversations taking place in my early feminist group(s) and among my feminist friends. To many, it seemed more potent and more promising than *sex role*."[151] In the late 1970s, *gender* became part of feminist discourse and was increasingly scrutinized and defined. In the next two decades, academic feminists advanced a set of epistemological debates about the meaning of the sex/gender binary while theorizing bodies and sexual difference. Gender had become a feminist creation, increasingly separated from its clinical origins.

Epilogue

Can anyone fully inhabit a gender without a degree of horror? How could someone be a woman "through and through," make a final home in that classification
without suffering claustrophobia?

There is no essence of womanhood (or of manhood) to provide a stable subject
for our histories; there are only successive iterations of a word that doesn't have
a fixed referent and so doesn't always mean the same thing.

Gender matters. The genealogy of gender that we encountered in this book continues to shape our current engagement with the concept. There is an ongoing struggle about
who owns the idea of gender, who may instill it with meaning, define its implications, and judge its importance. For
some, it is just a polite way to say *sex*, as evident in the surge
of gender reveal parties which are in reality just a celebration
of whether a child's genital sex appears to be male or female
on a sonogram. Others fear that current theories and practices of gender carry radical implications. Such concerns are
expressed in debates about public bathrooms or fears about
the destruction of the nuclear family and proper binary gender roles. These multiple variations in the meanings and
uses of *gender* should be of little surprise, given the history
I laid out in this book. Our diverse understandings of gender all address the relation between biology and culture, between nature and nurture, but they do not easily map onto
each other. These formulations share the legacy of gender's
normative origins in the clinic, but they have been adapted
to different uses and translated into different disciplines.

Gender, in its conception and birth at the clinic, was an inherently normative concept. The sex/gender binary developed at the John Hopkins Hospital in the 1950s proposed that gender role was learned and (relatively) independent of biology, but it was nonetheless "real." That is, a person's gender role not only became fixed (through a somewhat opaque process of imprinting) and ultimately indelible, but it also did so according to agreed-on cultural norms of masculinity and femininity. In reformulating the relation between biology and culture, nature and nurture, the team at Hopkins judged the latter to be as deterministic as the former. Here we must remember the medical context in which gender role was formulated in the 1950s: clinicians sought to develop protocols for assigning sex to children with intersex traits. These intersex bodies represented a medical "problem," while an increase in hospital births contributed to early diagnosis and new developments in endocrinology, and surgery allowed for the creation of a malleable body. The gender concept developed at Hopkins accounted for the observation that psychological sex was simultaneously malleable and fixed. That is, it could be detached from the body to some extent, and yet it became fixed over time.

This legacy of normative gender roles is probably the most pronounced in the ongoing medical management of children with intersex traits, whose genitals are still surgically "fixed" to fit their assigned sex. The Hopkins optimum gender of rearing model, which recommended early sex assignment and surgical intervention on infants' genitals, maintained unquestioned hegemony in intersex case management (ICM) until the 1990s.[1] These forty years of ICM, mainly based on John Money's publications, give an "impression of a consensus that is rarely encountered in science." As the sociologist Suzanne Kessler found in 1990, "Even though psychologists fiercely argue issues of gender identity and gender role development, doctors who treat intersexed infants seem untouched by these debates. There are no renegade voices either from within the medical establishment or, thus far, from outside."[2] Indeed, this hegemonic application of the Hopkins model coincided with a shift toward biological essentialism in the life sciences and an increasing dominance of Organization Theory (OT) in explaining sexual differences in behavior.[3] As I have shown in chapter 7, OT hypothesized that prenatal hormonal exposure predestined model animals to male or female typical behavior, a theory quickly expanded to humans. While Money was an important figure in the application of these findings to humans, he still insisted that gender role was mostly learned. And while most physicians might have disagreed with Money's gender theory, they still uniformly applied the standardized optimum gender of rearing model.

The first fundamental critique of ICM came not from medicine but from feminists, gender scholars, and activists, many of them individuals with intersex traits who had been subjected to invasive ICM in their childhoods. These procedures had been performed on them at an age when they were incapable of consent, and they only learned about their diagnosis and these procedures much later in adulthood. Kessler's 1990 essay, based on interviews with medical experts (three women and three men) in the field of "pediatric intersexuality," was one of the first critiques of the Hopkins recommendations. In 1993, the feminist biologist Anne Fausto-Sterling published two articles in the *New York Times* and *Sciences* in which she criticized the binary framework into which individuals with intersex traits were forced. She proposed broader, more inclusive categorizations of sex.[4] Cheryl Chase wrote a letter in response to the *Sciences* article in which she described the immensely destructive effect intersex surgery has on sexual sensation and the sense of bodily integrity. She denounced the "monstrous 'treatment'" of children, who could not consent. Also in this letter, Chase announced the formation of the Intersex Society of North America and encouraged "intersexuals and those close to them" to get in touch.[5] In 1998, the historian Alice Dreger became engaged in intersex scholarship and activism. Her work analyzed the emergence of Western medicine's preoccupation with sex and the enforcement of "normative" notions of masculinity and femininity in nineteenth-century Europe, and it explored the ethics of intersex treatment.[6]

In the decades that followed, intersex activists, feminists, bioethicists, and gender scholars formed a new alliance to confront ICM and improve medical and social attitudes toward people with intersex.[7] Multiple statements that condemn the medicalization of variations in sex and consider nonconsensual genital surgery a human rights violation, as well as new regulations that allow for a sex category other than male or female on the birth certificate, have been put forth in the United States and in other, mainly European countries.[8] Yet ICM continues to be the main approach to children born with intersex traits.[9]

Feminists who started to use gender as part of a political critique of patriarchy in the 1970s also struggle with the legacy of the Hopkins gender concept. Feminists addressed the question of whether gender was real: if as a group women share similar cultural experiences, does that mean they have some shared characteristic features? In other words, gender role might be learned, but it was "real" at the same time that all women grew up in the face of sexist stereotyping, prescription of approved behaviors, and sexual objectification. This position, exemplified by Betty Friedan's *The Feminine Mystique*, often neglected taking into account racial and class differences in the socialization of females into women.[10] White Western middle- and upper-class feminists simply presumed that the social and cultural experiences that shaped their gender represented womanhood. They neglected to consider that if gender was learned, then females became particular kinds of women—including Black women, women of color, queer women, or white working-class women, to name just a few.[11]

The assumption that gender was real in the sense that it had a social meaning raised further questions. If gender was socially constructed and different from sex, this implied that sex was solely biologically determined. Money had rejected binaries of body/mind, biology/culture, nature/nurture in his gender concept and proposed a somewhat opaque unity in which gendered experiences became indelibly imprinted through a process of learning. In contrast, feminists acknowledged the full consequences of a learned gender role and argued that the difference between sex and gender was that the first is a biological and the second a cultural category. This opened up the seemingly liberating possibility that gender can be different from sex. However, as many feminists have pointed out since then, distinguishing *biological* sex from *social* gender is problematic, since it neglects how the sexed body is a historically contingent and deeply social formation. Historians have shown that our current understanding of incommensurable male and female bodies is fairly recent and that cultural assumption, material conditions, and scientific practices as well as politics and economics shape scientific definitions of sex differences. Take something that today seems as essential as sex chromosomes. As the historian Sarah Richardson has shown, geneticists resisted calling the X and the Y sex chromosomes for three decades, preferring to refer to them by structure. Sexing the chromosomes to carry the essence of masculinity and femininity was a cultural process rather than a scientific discovery.[12]

Many gender scholars have suggested abandoning the sex/gender binary entirely. As Judith Butler pointed out in her critique of gender, "If the immutable character of sex is contested, perhaps this construct called 'sex' is as culturally constructed as gender; indeed, perhaps it was always already gender, with the consequence that the distinction between sex and gender turns out to be no distinction at all."[13] In other words, our bodies are the material foundations on which our gender is constructed, yet our sexed bodies are constructs themselves.[14] Culture also shapes our bodies in very material ways as we see through their crafting by dieting and exercising, and medical phenomena like menopause have social causes directly related to expectations about or limitations by gender.[15]

In a moment when some are calling for the dissolution of gender, the number of individuals who identify as trans or gender nonbinary has risen significantly (or merely become more visible) in the twenty-first century. The medical definition of gender this book has explored has had a tremendous impact on the lives of trans individuals after the 1960s. This is not to say, as the rich repertoire of recent trans and gender nonbinary histories has shown, that individuals who challenged or transcended the male/female binary did not exist before the 1960s or that transgender individuals have not found a way to affirm their gender outside or in opposition to the medical paradigm of trans.[16] Yet in the dominant medical formulation of "transsexuality" dating from the 1960s, the idea of gender identity was defined as one's innermost concept of self as male or female based on the very normative concepts that feminists (and trans feminists alike) challenged in the 1970s and 1980s. John Money and his colleagues at the Gender Identity Clinic rejected applicants who sought to affirm their gender yet did not fit the narrow categories of stereotypical gender role (including heterosexuality).

As we live through the latest debates about what gender is and how real it is, it seems timely to ask whether gender is salvageable as a concept. Is it, to quote Joan Scott again, still a "useful category"?[17] Gender, as I have shown, has distinct and historically shifting meanings that are far from settled; "who counted as a woman, and for whose sake" remains a live question in gender history.[18] To know gender's history and to acknowledge that current usage is diverse—that we do not always mean the same thing when we talk about gender—allow us to grapple with complex questions and their dilemmas rather than shutting them off or simplifying. Most important, gender matters because it is still a concept that organizes the world we live in. As the history of gender I have laid out in this book has shown, gender is constantly remade through medical, social, cultural, economic, and political practices. In its original conception, it was introduced into medicine to solve a particular clinical problem, and in the context of 1950s norms of masculinity and femininity became a restrictive practice of enforcing strict gender roles. When gender was up for grabs in the context of 1970s feminism, it carried the promise of being a liberating tool to dismantle prescribed gender roles.

Discrimination by sex or gender, including gender identities outside the male/female binary, remains a live issue. We are still asked to "fully inhabit a gender," and *man* and *woman* are deployed as if they possessed indelible essences in ways that have real-world consequences. In other words, gender is still a language of power linked to perceived differences between men and women, and the social consequences of what it means to be a woman or a man continue to be contentious.[19] As long as being male, female, or nonbinary provokes social and cultural differences, gender surely remains a useful concept to address resulting inequalities. This does not prevent us from imagining a world where gender has no social meaning or consequence and is merely an expression of human behavior, potential, and creativity.

Acknowledgments

So many people and institutions made it possible for me to write this book. First, I must thank Nathaniel Comfort at the Institute of the History of Medicine at Johns Hopkins School of Medicine, who helped me find my own voice and whom I am glad to call not only my mentor but also a friend. I am indebted to Dan Todes, Mary Fissell, Gianna Pomata, Graham Mooney, Marta Hanson, and Jeremy Greene at the institute and to Judith Walkowitz, Mary Ryan, and the participants of the Johns Hopkins Gender Colloquium for their support and stimulating comments.

Flurin Condrau welcomed me to the Institute and Museum of the History of Medicine at the University of Zurich and supported me every step of the way. The friendship, support, and insights of my colleagues there, especially Janina Kehr, Niklaus Ingold, and Mark Honigsbaum ("the dream team"), made my time in Zurich not only academically fruitful but also very enjoyable. Warm thanks also go to Lorraine Daston and Christine von Oertzen for offering me a fellowship at the Max Planck Institute for the History of Science in Berlin.

I found a new academic home at the University of California, Berkeley. Not only have my colleagues in the Department of History made me feel extremely welcomed, but they have also supported me in countless ways since my arrival in fall 2015. Their advice and support as well as the feedback I received on various draft chapters were invaluable. I am especially indebted to Mark Brilliant, Margarete Chowning, Brian DeLay, Victoria Frede, David Henkin, Carla Hesse, Stefan-Ludwig Hoffmann, Stefanie Jones-Rogers, Waldo Martin,

Rebecca McLennan, Maureen C. Miller, Caitlin Rosenthal, Daniel Sargent, Elena Schneider, Ronit Stahl, and Peter Zinoman. Special thanks go to Thomas Laqueur for his unwavering encouragement and his insightful comments and to James Vernon for the support he has given to me as I completed this project. James has been immensely gracious with his time and was a tremendously kind and inspiring intellectual interlocutor. I would also like to thank the staff of the History Department, especially Marianne Bartholomew-Couts, for their support and patience.

The Center for Science, Technology, Medicine, and Society at UC Berkeley has become a second home for me; I extend my gratitude to Massimo Mazzotti, Cathryn Carson, and Morgan Aimes. I am also grateful to the members of the Medicine Working Group at the center, especially Elena Conis, Aimee Medeiros, John (Jack) Lesch, Laura Nelson, Ian Read, and Caroline Jean Acker, who provided valuable feedback and an inspiring and supportive community of medical historians. In addition, the UC Consortium for the Study of Women's, Gender, and Sexuality Histories in the Americas offered a community of like-minded scholars.

I am particularly indebted to Dorothy Porter, Rebecca Lemov, and Lisa Materson, who generously agreed to participate in my manuscript conference, reading the first draft of my manuscript and providing invaluable feedback. It was a truly inspiring day. I owe many thanks to Laura Nelson, Leslie Salzinger, Rebecca Kluchin, Sarah Stoller, and Lisa Materson, who at such short notice read and provided beneficial comments on chapter 7. Lisa has supported and advised me in innumerable ways and provided feedback on several chapters. She has been a true role model in academic mentoring. The manuscript also greatly benefited from the comments of two anonymous reviewers selected by my editor at the University of Chicago Press, Karen Darling. Early on, Karen saw the potential of the book and skillfully guided me through the review and publication process.

Over the years, I have met a number of outstanding scholars whose advice, insights, and friendship helped me develop my ideas and clarify my arguments. I am particularly grateful to Alice Dreger, Elizabeth Reis, Sarah B. Rodriguez, and Ellen Feder. Special thanks go to Rebecca Jordan-Young, who first inspired me as a student to study sexuality and science. I would also like to thank Gayle Rubin, who kindly and patiently answered my queries during the pandemic summer of 2020 and shared her recollections about writing *The Traffic of Women*.

It seems impossible to list all the people who have supported and inspired me along the way as I worked on this book. The comments and questions I received from panels at the American Historical Association, the American Association of Historians of Medicine, and the Berkshire Conference of Women Historians were crucial for thinking through the project. I am grateful for the opportunity to discuss chapters at the Generation to Reproduction Seminar in the Department of History and Philosophy of Science at Cambridge University; the Surgical ReConstruction of Sex Workshop in the Gender Studies Department at the University of Zurich; the Cross-Cultural Women's and Gender History research cluster at the University of California, Davis; the New Direction in Modern US History Seminar at Boston University; the History of Science, Medicine, and Technology Colloquium at Johns Hopkins University; and the History of Science Colloquium at the University of California, Los Angeles.

Thanks are also in order to the wonderful staff at the Alan Mason Chesney Medical Archives of Johns Hopkins Medicine, Nursing, and Public Health for their support, help, and advice, especially Phoebe Evans Letocha, Andrew Harrison, Timothy Wisniewski, and Nancy McCall, who patiently responded to all my requests and questions. I am indebted to the staff at the Johns Hopkins Medical Record Services, who provided me with invaluable assistance in finding the Harriet Lane Home patient records and locating the microfilmed records. Without these records, this project would not be what it is now, so I am deeply grateful for the opportunity to use these sources. I was touched by the lives of the patients to whom I tried to do justice. I am grateful as well for the opportunity to use the archives at the Kinsey Institute at Indiana University and for the generous assistance Shawn C. Wilson gave me there. Ali Clarke in the Hocken Collections at the University of Otago, New Zealand, went above and beyond in helping me explore the Money collection from across the world, and she made it possible for me to receive hundreds of scans of primary sources I would otherwise not have been able to access.

I would like to acknowledge funding from the following institutions at UC Berkeley that helped me finish my book. The Berkeley Regents' Junior Faculty Fellowship financed my summer research, and the Institute of International Studies provided the generous funds for a manuscript workshop. A Humanities Research Fellowship allowed me to revise my manuscript, and the Doreen B. Townsend Center for the Humanities offered me a fellowship during my leave year.

None of my work would have been possible without the support of my friends and family. I wish my parents were still with me so that I could thank them in person. They always believed in me and deserve more gratitude than I could ever express in words. This project would not have happened without the friendship and support of Hester Betlem and Angelika Hoelger. Finally, I want to thank my partner, Christoph Hermann, for his unwavering and steadfast intellectual and emotional support through challenging times. The book is dedicated to our child, Noah Mpho.

Abbreviations

HLH   Records of the Harriet Lane Home, Office of Medical Records, the Johns Hopkins Hospital, Baltimore

JMC   John Money Collection, Alan Chesney Mason Archives, the Johns Hopkins Hospital, Baltimore

JMK   John Money Collection, Kinsey Institute, Bloomington, Indiana

JMH   John Money Papers (1915–2004), Hocken Collections—Uare Taoka o Hākena, University of Otago, Dunedin, New Zealand

StAZH Records of the University Children's Hospital Zurich, State Archives of Zurich

Note: Certain archival collections are subject to strict privacy conventions concerning the protection of the Personal Health Information of individuals described therein. In conformity with federal regulations under the Health Insurance Portability and Accountability Act (HIPAA) and to preserve the confidentiality of those records, these materials are identified by research code and collection abbreviation. A copy of the HLH code has been deposited at the Alan Chesney Mason Medical Archives, the Johns Hopkins Hospital, Baltimore.

Notes

All patient names and Personal Health Information in this book have been anonymized and replaced with pseudonyms, and family names have been anonymized. Names of medical staff having a publication record have been left unchanged.

1. Patient record, Q5CT4 (Charles), HLH. I discuss this case in more detail in chapter 5.
2. The classification via gonads dates back to Theodor Albrecht Klebs, who distinguished between true hermaphrodites and pseudohermaphrodites and who believed that a person's sex should be entirely based on the nature of the gonads. See E. Klebs, *Handbuch der pathologischen Anatomie* (Berlin: Hirschwald, 1876). On Klebs, see also Alice Domurat Dreger, *Hermaphrodites and the Medical Invention of Sex* (Cambridge, MA: Harvard University Press, 1998), 145–46.
3. Today, many patients with CAH reject being defined as intersex, but at the time physicians referred to them as female pseudohermaphrodites. The new term *disorders of sex development* (DSD) is controversial, as many consider the inclusion of the word *disorders* pathologizing. Some scholars and activists have suggested using *differences or divergence of sex development* instead. See Elizabeth Reis, *Bodies in Doubt: An American History of Intersex* (Baltimore: Johns Hopkins University Press, 2009), 153–62. In this book, I use the historical terminology when citing or paraphrasing primary sources, and I use *intersex, intersex traits,* or *differences of sex development* (DSD) otherwise. On DSD, see Ellen K. Feder and Katrina Karkazis, "What's in a Name?: The Controversy over 'Disorders of Sex Development,'" *Hastings Cent Rep* 38, no. 5 (September–October 2008): 33–36.

4. Some scholars have consequently argued for expanding our categories of sex beyond the binary of male and female; see Anne Fausto-Sterling, "The Five Sexes: Why Male and Female Are Not Enough," *Sciences* 33, no. 2 (March–April 1993): 20–24; Anne Fausto-Sterling, "How Many Sexes Are There?," editorial, *New York Times*, March 12, 1993.

5. Murray Barr introduced the Barr body test in 1949. Using scrapings from the lining of the cheeks, the test visualizes the second inactive X chromosome. In humans with two X chromosomes (such as XX or XXY), one Barr body will be visible; humans with one X chromosome (such as XY or XO) will have no Barr body. See Murray L. Barr and Ewart G. Bertram, "A Morphological Distinction between Neurones of the Male and Female, and the Behaviour of the Nucleolar Satellite during Accelerated Nucleoprotein Synthesis," *Nature* 163, no. 4148 (1949): 676–77.

6. "Gender and Health," Health Topics, World Health Organization, accessed September 13, 2021, https://www.who.int/gender-equity-rights /understanding/gender-definition/en/.

7. Joan Wallach Scott, "Gender: A Useful Category of Historical Analysis," *American Historical Review* 91, no. 5 (1986): 1053–75.

8. Anne Fausto-Sterling's groundbreaking book *Sexing the Body*, for example, only mentions Wilkins once and in passing; see Anne Fausto-Sterling, *Sexing the Body: Gender Politics and the Construction of Sexuality* (New York: Basic Books, 2000), 205. Joanne Meyerowitz's account of the emergence of a transsexual identity also centralizes the emergence of the modern usage of *gender* in the 1950s; see Joanne J. Meyerowitz, *How Sex Changed: A History of Transsexuality in the United States* (Cambridge, MA: Harvard University Press, 2002). One exception is Alison Redick's dissertation, which situates Wilkins as an influential figure; see Alison Redick, "American History XY: The Medical Treatment of Intersex, 1916–1955" (PhD diss., New York University, 2004).

9. On John Money and his theories, see Jennifer Germon, *Gender: A Genealogy of an Idea* (New York: Palgrave Macmillan, 2009); Lisa Downing, Iain Morland, and Nikki Sullivan, *Fuckology: Critical Essays on John Money's Diagnostic Concepts* (Chicago: University of Chicago Press, 2015); Terry Goldie, *The Man Who Invented Gender: Engaging the Ideas of John Money*, Sexuality Studies Series (Vancouver: UBC Press, 2014).

10. See for example Julia Epstein, "Either/Or-Neither/Both: Sexual Ambiguity and the Ideology of Gender," *Genders* 7 (1990):99–142; Morgan Holmes, *Intersex: A Perilous Difference* (Selinsgrove, PA: Susquehanna University Press, 2008); Ellen K. Feder, *Making Sense of Intersex: Changing Ethical Perspectives in Biomedicine* (Bloomington: Indiana University Press, 2014).

11. Simone de Beauvoir, *The Second Sex*, trans. and ed. H. M. Parshley (London: J. Cape, 1956), 273. See also Joan Riviere, "Womanliness as a Masquerade," in *Female Experience: Three Generations of British Women Psychoanalysts on*

Work with Women, ed. Joan Raphael-Leff and Rosine Jozef Perelberg (London: Routledge, 1997), 228–36.

12. On the science of human behavior, see for example Rebecca M. Lemov, *World as Laboratory: Experiments with Mice, Mazes, and Men* (New York: Hill and Wang, 2005).

13. See Marga Vicedo, "Cold War Emotions: Mother Love and the War over Human Nature," in *Cold War Social Science: Knowledge Production, Liberal Democracy, and Human Nature*, ed. Mark Solovey and Hamilton Cravens (New York: Palgrave Macmillan, 2012), 233–50; Rebecca Jo Plant, *Mom: The Transformation of Motherhood in Modern America* (Chicago: University of Chicago Press, 2010).

14. Joanne Meyerowitz describes popular ideas that transsexuality was caused by hormones or maladjustment: Meyerowitz, *How Sex Changed*. On the importance of instinct and behavior based on biology in the post–World War II period, see for example Marga Vicedo, *The Nature and Nurture of Love: From Imprinting to Attachment in Cold War America* (Chicago: University of Chicago Press, 2013). See also Erika Lorraine Milam, *Creatures of Cain: The Hunt for Human Nature in Cold War America* (Princeton, NJ: Princeton University Press, 2019).

15. For a history of American sexuality, see John D'Emilio and Estelle B. Freedman, *Intimate Matters: A History of Sexuality in America* (New York: Harper and Row, 1988).

16. The most prominent homophile groups of the 1950s were the Mattachine Society and the Daughters of Bilitis; see for example Jonathan Katz, *Gay American History: Lesbians and Gay Men in the U.S.A.; A Documentary History*, rev. ed. (New York: Meridian, 1992); Stuart Timmons, *The Trouble with Harry Hay: Founder of the Modern Gay Movement* (Boston: Alyson, 1990); John D'Emilio, *Sexual Politics, Sexual Communities: The Making of a Homosexual Minority in the United States, 1940–1970* (Chicago: University of Chicago Press, 1983).

17. Alfred C. Kinsey, Wardell Baxter Pomeroy, and Clyde Eugene Martin, *Sexual Behavior in the Human Male* (Philadelphia: W. B. Saunders, 1948); Institute for Sex Research and Alfred C. Kinsey, *Sexual Behavior in the Human Female* (Philadelphia: Saunders, 1953). On Kinsey's new quantitative notion of sexual normality, see Paul A. Robinson, *The Modernization of Sex: Havelock Ellis, Alfred Kinsey, William Masters, and Virginia Johnson* (New York: Harper and Row, 1976). On Kinsey's methodology, see also Donna J. Drucker, *The Classification of Sex: Alfred Kinsey and the Organization of Knowledge* (Pittsburgh: University of Pittsburgh Press, 2014). On the public perception of Kinsey and his lasting influence on American sexuality, see Miriam G. Reumann, *American Sexual Character: Sex, Gender, and National Identity in the Kinsey Reports* (Berkeley: University of California Press, 2005).

18. On the Kinsey scale, see Donna J. Drucker, "Male Sexuality and Alfred Kinsey's 0–6 Scale: Toward 'a Sound Understanding of the Realities of Sex,'"

J Homosex 57, no. 9 (2010): 1105–23. Kinsey, who found himself under attack and without funding by the mid-1950s, shared a panel with John Money and Joan Hampson in 1954. See John Money, "Once upon a Time I Met Alfred C. Kinsey," *Arch Sex Behav* 31, no. 4 (2002): 319–22.

19. On Jorgensen and the transformation of sex in the mid-twentieth century, see Meyerowitz, *How Sex Changed.*

20. On the history of the conceptual framework for distinguishing gender identity, sex, and sexuality, see for example Geertje, *Doubting Sex: Inscriptions, Bodies and Selves in Nineteenth-Century Hermaphrodite Case Histories* (Manchester: Manchester University Press, 2012), 10.

21. Havelock Ellis and John Addington Symonds, *Sexual Inversion*, Studies of the Psychology of Sex (London: Wilson and Macmillan, 1897).

22. Hirschfeld collaborated with Viennese physiologist Eugen Steinach, who produced sex changes in guinea pigs through gonad transplantation experiments; see Chandak Sengoopta, *The Most Secret Quintessence of Life: Sex, Glands, and Hormones, 1850–1950* (Chicago: University of Chicago Press, 2006). On sex hormones, see also Nelly Oudshoorn, *Beyond the Natural Body: An Archaeology of Sex Hormones* (New York: Routledge, 1994).

23. See Reis, *Bodies in Doubt*, 39.

24. On the long history of the racialization of bodies in medicine, see for example Keith Wailoo, "Historical Aspects of Race and Medicine: The Case of J. Marion Sims," *JAMA* 320, no. 15 (2018): 1529–30; Deirdre Cooper Owens, *Medical Bondage: Race, Gender, and the Origins of American Gynecology* (Athens, GA: University of Georgia Press, 2017); Todd Lee Savitt, *Race and Medicine in Nineteenth- and Early-Twentieth-Century America* (Kent, OH: Kent State University Press, 2007); Harriet A. Washington, *Medical Apartheid: The Dark History of Medical Experimentation on Black Americans from Colonial Times to the Present* (New York: Doubleday, 2006); Keith Wailoo, *Dying in the City of the Blues: Sickle Cell Anemia and the Politics of Race and Health*, Studies in Social Medicine (Chapel Hill: University of North Carolina Press, 2001).

25. See Hugh Hampton Young, *Genital Abnormalities: Hermaphroditism and Related Adrenal Diseases* (Baltimore: Williams and Wilkins, 1937); Lawson Wilkins, *The Diagnosis and Treatment of Endocrine Disorders in Childhood and Adolescence* (Springfield, IL: Thomas, 1950); Howard Wilbur Jones and William Wallace Scott, *Hermaphroditism, Genital Anomalies and Related Endocrine Disorders* (Baltimore: Williams and Wilkins, 1958).

26. See Campbell Gibson and Kay Jung, *Historical Census Statistics on Population Totals by Race, 1790 to 1990, and by Hispanic Origin, 1790 to 1990, for the United States, Regions, Divisions, and States* (Washington, DC: US Census Bureau, 2002), 98, 103.

27. See the discussion by the now-defunct Intersex Society of North America: https://isna.org/faq/frequency/, archived from the original on August 22, 2009; accessed September, 13, 2021. See also Melanie Blackless et al., "How

Sexually Dimorphic Are We? Review and Synthesis," *Am J Hum Biol* 12, no. 2 (2000): 151–66.

28. The relationship between the Johns Hopkins Hospital and its surrounding Black neighborhoods was (and remains) complicated and thorny. See Antero Pietila, *The Ghosts of Johns Hopkins: The Life and Legacy That Shaped an American City* (Lanham, MD: Rowman and Littlefield, 2018).

29. See Johns Hopkins Hospital, *Administrative and Statistical Report: Sixth Report of the Superintendent of the Johns Hopkins Hospital* (Baltimore: Johns Hopkins Hospital, 1894–1900), 7; Johns Hopkins Hospital, *Administrative and Statistical Report: Thirty-Fourth Report of the Director of the Johns Hopkins Hospital* (Baltimore: Johns Hopkins Hospital, 1921–1924), 21. For the Harriet Lane Home, see Edwards A. Park, *The Harriet Lane Home: A Model and a Gem* (Baltimore: Department of Pediatrics, School of Medicine, Johns Hopkins University, 2006).

30. One cause of this mistrust was certainly the practice of using poor and Black bodies for dissection at medical schools; see Michael Sappol, *A Traffic of Dead Bodies: Anatomy and Embodied Social Identity in Nineteenth-Century America* (Princeton, NJ: Princeton University Press, 2002). Rebecca Skloot also addresses the distrust the Baltimorean Black community had of Hopkins doctors; see Rebecca Skloot, *The Immortal Life of Henrietta Lacks* (New York: Crown, 2010).

31. See Saidiya Hartman, *Wayward Lives, Beautiful Experiments: Intimate Histories of Social Upheaval* (New York: W. W. Norton, 2019), 7.

32. See also Reis, *Bodies in Doubt*.

33. Zine Magubane, "Spectacles and Scholarship: Caster Semenya, Intersex Studies, and the Problem of Race in Feminist Theory," *Signs* 39, no. 3 (2014): 761–85; quotation is from p. 768.

34. Magubane, 782.

35. See for example bell hooks's critique of white liberal feminism: bell hooks, *Feminist Theory: From Margin to Center* (London: Pluto Press, 2000).

36. See Dreger, *Hermaphrodites*; Bernice L. Hausman, *Changing Sex: Transsexualism, Technology, and the Idea of Gender* (Durham, NC: Duke University Press, 1995); Fausto-Sterling, *Sexing the Body*; Meyerowitz, *How Sex Changed*; Reis, *Bodies in Doubt*; Mak, *Doubting Sex*.

37. See for example Fausto-Sterling, "The Five Sexes"; Suzanne J. Kessler, *Lessons from the Intersexed* (New Brunswick, NJ: Rutgers University Press, 1998); Katrina Alicia Karkazis, *Fixing Sex: Intersex, Medical Authority, and Lived Experience* (Durham, NC: Duke University Press, 2008); Iain Morland, "What Can Queer Theory Do for Intersex?," *GLQ: A Journal of Lesbian and Gay Studies* 15, no. 2 (2009): 285–312; Sarah M. Creighton et al., "Intersex Practice, Theory, and Activism: A Roundtable Discussion," *GLQ: A Journal of Lesbian and Gay Studies* 15, no. 2 (2009): 249–60; Feder, *Making Sense of Intersex*; Morgan Holmes, ed., *Critical Intersex* (London: Routledge, 2016).

38. Meyerowitz, *How Sex Changed*.
39. Charles E. Rosenberg, "Disease in History: Frames and Framers," *Milbank Quarterly* 67 (1989): 1–15; quotations are from pp. 1–2.
40. Anne Fausto-Sterling, *Myths of Gender: Biological Theories about Women and Men* (New York: Basic Books, 1985), 9. Historians have explored how the sexed body is a scientific construct rather than a natural phenomenon; see for example Thomas Walter Laqueur, *Making Sex: Body and Gender from the Greeks to Freud* (Cambridge, MA: Harvard University Press, 1990); Londa Schiebinger, *Nature's Body: Gender in the Making of Modern Science* (Boston: Beacon Press, 1993); Oudshoorn, *Beyond the Natural Body*; Sarah S. Richardson, *Sex Itself: The Search for Male and Female in the Human Genome* (Chicago: University of Chicago Press, 2013).
41. Jack David Pressman, *Last Resort: Psychosurgery and the Limits of Medicine* (Cambridge: Cambridge University Press, 1998), 5.
42. Pressman, 8.
43. Annemarie Mol proposes a praxiographic approach to medical practice in Annemarie Mol, *The Body Multiple: Ontology in Medical Practice*, Science and Cultural Theory (Durham, NC: Duke University Press, 2002). Historian Geertje Mak has applied Mol's approach to the complex practices of physicians who doubted patients' sex in nineteenth-century Europe; see Geertje Mak, "Doubting Sex from Within: A Praxiographic Approach to a Late Nineteenth-Century Case of Hermaphroditism," *Gender and History* 18, no. 2 (2006): 332–56; Mak, *Doubting Sex*.
44. Guenter B. Risse and John Harley Warner, "Reconstructing Clinical Activities: Patient Records in Medical History," *Soc Hist Med* 5, no. 2 (1992): 183–205; quotation is from pp. 189–90. On patient history and patient narrative, see for example N. D. Jewson, "The Disappearance of the Sick-Man from Medical Cosmology, 1770–1870," *Sociology* 10, no. 2 (1976): 225–44; D. Armstrong, "The Patient's View," *Soc Sci Med* 18, no. 9 (1984): 737–44; Roy Porter, "The Patient's View: Doing Medical History from Below," *Theory and Society* 4 (1985): 175–98; Sheila M. Rothman, *Living in the Shadow of Death: Tuberculosis and the Social Experience of Illness in America* (New York: Basic Books, 1994); John Harley Warner, "The Uses of Patient Records by Historians—Patterns, Possibilities, and Perplexities," *Health History* 1 (1999):101–11; Flurin Condrau, "The Patient's View Meets the Clinical Gaze," *Soc Hist Med* 20, no. 3 (2007): 525–40.
45. See Mak, "Doubting Sex from Within," 332–33.
46. See Mak, 334.
47. On the specific nature of pediatric patient records, see Jonathan Gillis, "Taking a Medical History in Childhood Illness: Representations of Parents in Pediatric Texts since 1850," *Bull Hist Med* 79 (2005): 393–429, 417. On the construction of the patient body through patient records, see Marc Berg and Paul Harterink, "Embodying the Patient: Records and Bodies in Early 20th-Century US Medical Practice," *Body and Society* 10, nos. 2–3 (2004): 13–41.

48. Jewson describes this loss of power in the patient-physician relationship in Jewson, "Disappearance of the Sick-Man."
49. See Berg and Harterink, "Embodying the Patient," 16.
50. Berg and Harterink, 21–22.

CHAPTER ONE

1. Patient record, PS0WO (Mary), HLH.
2. Patient record, UKC0T (Shirley), HLH.
3. For a description of symptoms, see Wilkins, *Diagnosis and Treatment of Endocrine Disorders*, 221–27.
4. At the time, Wilkins used deoxycorticosterone, a steroid hormone produced by the adrenal glands that acts as a precursor to aldosterone, to counter her loss of electrolytes.
5. C. J. Migeon, "Lawson Wilkins and My Life: Part 3," *Int J Pediatr Endocrinol* (2014): suppl. 1, "Remembering Doctor Lawson Wilkins: A Pioneer of Pediatric Endocrinology," S4.
6. See Park, *Harriet Lane Home*.
7. On Park, see B. Childs, "Park, Edwards A.," *J Pediatr* 125, no. 6 (December 1994): 1009–13.
8. Edwards A. Park, "Lawson Wilkins," *J Pediatr* 57, no. 3 (1960): 317–22, esp. 319.
9. Lawson Wilkins, "Acceptance of the Howland Award," pt. 2, *J Pediatr* 63, no. 4 (October 1963): 808–11; quotation is from p. 808.
10. Park, "Lawson Wilkins," 317.
11. Park, *Harriet Lane Home*, 180.
12. See Park, "Lawson Wilkins," 317–18. See also Robert M. Blizzard, "Pediatric Profiles: Lawson Wilkins (1894–1963)," *J Pediatr* 133, no. 4 (1998): 577–80, esp. 578.
13. Park, "Lawson Wilkins," 318.
14. Park, *Harriet Lane Home*, 180. Wilkins published the results of these collaborations in 1937; see Lawson Wilkins, "Epilepsy in Childhood: I. A Statistical Study of Clinical Types," *J Pediatr* 10, no. 3 (March 1937): 317–28; Lawson Wilkins, "Epilepsy in Childhood: II. The Incidence of Remissions," *J Pediatr* 10, no. 3 (March 1937): 329–40; Lawson Wilkins, "Epilepsy in Childhood: III. Results with the Ketogenic Diet," *J Pediatr* 10, no. 3 (March 1937): 341–57.
15. On specialization in US medicine, see G. Weisz, "Medical Directories and Medical Specialization in France, Britain, and the United States," *Bull Hist Med* 71, no. 1 (1997): 23–68; G. Weisz, "The Emergence of Medical Specialization in the Nineteenth Century," *Bull Hist Med* 77, no. 3 (Fall 2003): 536–75; George Weisz, *Divide and Conquer: A Comparative History of Medical Specialization* (Oxford: Oxford University Press, 2006).
16. On the history of hormones, see John Henderson, "Ernest Starling and 'Hormones': An Historical Commentary," *J Endocrinol* 184, no. 1 (2005): 5–10.

17. Medvei refers to the first forty years of the twentieth century as troubled and exciting years; see Victor Cornelius Medvei, *A History of Endocrinology* (Lancaster, UK: MTP Press, 1982). On the history of the endocrine society, see Hans Lisser, "The Endocrine Society—the First 40 Years (1917–1957)," *Endocrinology* 80, no. 7 (1967): 5–28. For a discussion of the most important findings during this period, see Arthur F. Hughes, "A History of Endocrinology," *J Hist Med Allied Sci* 32, no. 3 (1977): 292–313.

18. Sengoopta describes the obsession with rejuvenation and with transformative power of "sex hormones" in Sengoopta, *Most Secret Quintessence of Life*. On testosterone, see John M. Hoberman, *Testosterone Dreams: Rejuvenation, Aphrodisia, Doping* (Berkeley: University of California Press, 2005); Rebecca M. Jordan-Young and Katrina Karkazis, *Testosterone: An Unauthorized Biography* (Cambridge, MA: Harvard University Press, 2019). For a critique of sex antagonism, see also Oudshoorn, *Beyond the Natural Body*; Diana Long Hall, "Biology, Sex Hormones and Sexism in the 1920s," *Philosophical Forum* 5, nos. 1–2 (1974): 81–96. For insulin, see John Christopher Feudtner, *Bittersweet: Diabetes, Insulin, and the Transformation of Illness*, Studies in Social Medicine (Chapel Hill: University of North Carolina Press, 2003).

19. See Delbert A. Fisher, "A Short History of Pediatric Endocrinology in North America," *Pediatr Res* 55, no. 4 (2004): 716–26, esp. 717. On the history of pediatrics, see Sydney A. Halpern, *American Pediatrics: The Social Dynamics of Professionalism, 1880–1980* (Berkeley: University of California Press, 1988); Sydney A. Halpern, "Medicalization as Professional Process: Postwar Trends in Pediatrics," *J Health Soc Behav* 31 (March 1990): 28–42; Janet Golden, Richard A. Meckel, and Heather Munro Prescott, *Children and Youth in Sickness and in Health: A Historical Handbook and Guide*, Children and Youth: History and Culture (2004); Alexandra Minna Stern and Howard Markel, *Formative Years: Children's Health in the United States, 1880–2000* (Ann Arbor: University of Michigan Press, 2009).

20. See Fisher, "Short History of Pediatric Endocrinology."

21. Wilkins's textbook went through several editions; see Wilkins, *Diagnosis and Treatment of Endocrine Disorders*; N. B. Talbot et al., *Functional Endocrinology from Birth through Adolescence* (Cambridge, MA: Harvard University Press, 1952).

22. Bartolomeo Eustachi published his treatise on the kidneys in his *Opuscula anatomica* in 1564.

23. See for example Charles-Edouard Brown-Séquard, "Recherches expérimentales sur la physiologie des capsules surrénales," *Comptes rendus de l'Académie des Sciences* 43 (1856): 422.

24. See Claude Bernard, A. Dastre, and Muséum national d'Histoire naturelle, *Leçons sur les phenomenes de la vie, communs aux animaux et aux vegetaux* (Paris: J.-B. Bailliere, 1878).

25. On the early years of adrenal research, see for example T. R. Elliott, "The Sidney Ringer Memorial Lecture on the Adrenal Glands: Delivered at Uni-

versity College Hospital Medical School, June, 1914," *Br Med J* 1, no. 2791
(June 27, 1914): 1393–97. On endocrinology, especially clinical endocrinology, see Medvei, *A History of Endocrinology*; Victor Cornelius Medvei, *The
History of Clinical Endocrinology: A Comprehensive Account of Endocrinology
from Earliest Times to the Present Day* (Carnforth, UK: Parthenon, 1993).
26. See for example Adele E. Clarke, "Research Material and Reproductive
Science in the United States, 1910–1940," in *Physiology in the American Context, 1850–1940* (Baltimore: American Physiological Society, 1987; distributed by Williams and Wilkins), 323–50; Nelly Oudshoorn, "On the Making
of Sex Hormones. Research Material and the Production of Knowledge,"
Social Studies of Science 20 (1990): 5–33.
27. L. De Crecchio, "Sopra un caso di apparenze virili in una donna," *Morgagni*
7 (1865): 151–89.
28. W. Bulloch and J. H. Sequeira, "On the Relation of the Suprarenal Capsules
to the Sexual Organs," *Transactions of the Pathological Society of London* 56
(1905): 189–208.
29. See Oudshoorn, *Beyond the Natural Body*; Long Hall, "Biology, Sex Hormones and Sexism"; Diana Long Hall and Thomas F. Glick, "Endocrinology: A Brief Introduction," *J Hist Biol* 9, no. 2 (Autumn 1976): 229–33;
Clarke, "Research Material and Reproductive Science."
30. See for example Richard Goldschmidt, *Mechanismus und Physiologie der Geschlechtsbestimmung* (Berlin: Gebr. Borntraeger, 1920); Richard Goldschmidt
and William J. Dakin, *The Mechanism and Physiology of Sex Determination*
(London: Methuen, 1923). On the interplay between hormones and genetics, see Frank R. Lillie, "The Free-Martin: A Study of the Action of Sex Hormones in the Foetal Life of Cattle," *J Exp Zool* 308, no. 3 (1917): 371–452.
For a discussion of the debates, see Sengoopta, *Most Secret Quintessence of
Life*, 64–67. See also Nathan Q. Ha, "The Riddle of Sex: Biological Theories
of Sexual Difference in the Early Twentieth-Century," *J Hist Biol* 44, no. 3
(2011): 505–46. Sarah Richardson shows how the sex binary that framed
hormones was also mapped onto chromosomes, despite alternative models
and contradicting scientific evidence; see Richardson, *Sex Itself.*
31. In 1913, for example, the British zoologist and embryologist Walter Heape
published his book *Sex Antagonism*, an anthropological study claiming that
women's biological destiny was the opposite of men's and that women's
role was entirely shaped and restricted by their biology. See Walter Heape,
Sex Antagonism (New York: G. P. Putnam's Sons, 1913).
32. See Sengoopta, *Most Secret Quintessence of Life.*
33. See Heape, *Sex Antagonism*. For a reaction to Heape, see for example "Sex
Antagonism; a Scientist's View of the Woman Movement," *New York Times*,
October 19, 1913.
34. See Long Hall, "Biology, Sex Hormones and Sexism," 87–88. We find
these debates in the United States and in Europe; see for example Carroll
Smith-Rosenberg and Charles Rosenberg, "The Female Animal: Medical and

Biological Views of Woman and Her Role in Nineteenth-Century America," *Journal of American History* (1973): 332–56; Lesley A. Hall, "Hauling down the Double Standard: Feminism, Social Purity and Sexual Science in Late Nineteenth-Century Britain," *Gender and History* 16, no. 1 (2004): 36–56; Lesley A. Hall, *Sex, Gender and Social Change in Britain since 1880*, Gender and History (New York: Palgrave Macmillan, 2012). On the emergence of a two-sex system, see Laqueur, *Making Sex*.

35. See Bernhard Zondek, "Mass Excretion of Oestrogenic Hormones in the Urine of the Stallion," *Nature* 133 (February 10, 1934): 209–10.

36. See Oudshoorn, *Beyond the Natural Body*.

37. Sengoopta, *Most Secret Quintessence of Life*, 5. See Carl R. Moore and Dorothy Price, "Gonad Hormone Functions, and the Reciprocal Influence between Gonads and Hypophysis with Its Bearing on the Problem of Sex Hormone Antagonism," *Am J Anat* 50, no. 1 (March 1932): 13–71.

38. Knud H. Krabbe, "The Relation between the Adrenal Cortex and Sexual Development," *New York Medical Journal* 114 (1921): 4–8; quotation is from p. 5.

39. Krabbe, 4–8.

40. Arthur Grollman, *The Adrenals* (Baltimore: Williams and Wilkins, 1936), 339.

41. Young, *Genital Abnormalities*.

42. Young, 112.

43. See Stephanie Hope Kenen, "Scientific Studies of Human Sexual Difference in Interwar America" (PhD diss., University of California, Berkeley, 1998), 90–93.

44. See Redick, "American History XY," 26.

45. See Kenen, "Scientific Studies of Human Sexual Difference" 209. Further citations of this work are given in the text.

46. L. Wilkins, W. Fleischmann, and J. E. Howard, "Macrogenitosomia Precox Associated with Hyperplasia of the Androgenic Tissue of the Adrenal and Death from Corticoadrenal Insufficiency," *Endocrinology* 26 (March 1940): 385–95, esp. 385.

47. Lawson Wilkins and Curt P. Richter, "A Great Craving for Salt by a Child with Cortico-Adrenal Insufficinecy," *JAMA* 114, no. 10 (March 9, 1940): 866–68, esp. 866.

48. Wilkins and Richter, 868.

49. See patient statistics in Wilkins, *Diagnosis and Treatment of Endocrine Disorders*; Lawson Wilkins, "The Diagnosis of the Adrenogenital Syndrome and Its Treatment with Cortisone," *J Pediatr* 41, no. 6 (1952): 860–74.

50. A. W. Jacobsen et al., "The Adrenal Gland in Health and Disease," *Pediatrics* 3, no. 4 (1949): 515–48, esp. 548.

51. Wilkins had published only a few articles on his trials with various substances before cortisone. Most evidence about such trials, often consisting of a single patient at a time, can be found in the HLH patient records.

52. See Roger A. Lewis and Lawson Wilkins, "The Effect of Adrenocorticotrophic Hormone in Congenital Adrenal Hyperplasia with Virilism and in Cushing's Syndrome Treated with Methyl Testosterone," *J Clin Investig* 28, no. 2 (1949): 394–400; L. Wilkins, R. Klein, and R. A. Lewis, "The Response to ACTH in Various Types of Adrenal Hyperplasia," in *Proceedings of the First Clinical ACTH Conference*, ed. John R. Mote (Philadelphia: Blakiston, 1950), 184–92.
53. See Young, *Genital Abnormalities*.
54. Jacobsen et al., "Adrenal Gland in Health and Disease," 548.
55. The entire panel presentation and discussion was published in Jacobsen et al. Further citations of this work are given in the text.
56. Nathan B. Talbot, A. M. Butler, and R. A. Berman, "Adrenal Cortical Hyperplasia with Virilism: Diagnosis, Course and Treatment," *J Clin Invest* 21 (1942): 559, 569.
57. This approach is evident in Wilkins's textbook, which he was writing and compiling around this time—the first textbook of pediatric endocrinology. See especially Wilkins, *Diagnosis and Treatment of Endocrine Disorders*, 147–49. Further citations of this work are given in the text.
58. On Young, see Kenen, "Scientific Studies of Human Sexual Difference," 63–65.
59. Moore and Price, "Gonad Hormone Functions." On endocrine research and sexuality, especially the concept of sex antagonism, see Sengoopta, *Most Secret Quintessence of Life*.
60. Wilkins, *Diagnosis and Treatment of Endocrine Disorders*, 274.
61. Wilkins, 274.
62. This phallic standard was the most important criteria for assigning sex to an intersex child. See for example Kessler, *Lessons from the Intersexed*, 25–26; Fausto-Sterling, *Sexing the Body*, 57–60. Recently, Karkazis has claimed that the importance of penis size is diminishing; see Karkazis, *Fixing Sex*, 100–105.
63. Wilkins, *Diagnosis and Treatment of Endocrine Disorders*, 274.
64. Wilkins, 224.
65. See Sarah B. Rodriguez, *Female Circumcision and Clitoridectomy in the United States: A History of a Medical Treatment*, Rochester Studies in Medical History (Rochester, NY: University of Rochester Press, 2014).
66. Rodriguez, 30.
67. See Christina Matta, "Ambiguous Bodies and Deviant Sexualities: Hermaphrodites, Homosexuality, and Surgery in the United States, 1850–1904," *Perspect Biol Med* 48, no. 1 (Winter 2005): 74–83; quotation is from p. 76.
68. See Kessler, *Lessons from the Intersexed*, 25–26.
69. Wilkins, *Diagnosis and Treatment of Endocrine Disorders*, 224.
70. See Redick, "American History XY," 26ff.
71. Reis, *Bodies in Doubt*, 88.

72. See for example Wendy Kline, *Building a Better Race: Gender, Sexuality, and Eugenics from the Turn of the Century to the Baby Boom* (Berkeley: University of California Press, 2001).

73. Jacobsen et al., "Adrenal Gland in Health and Disease," 548.

74. Jacobsen et al., 548.

75. See P. S. Hench, "Potential Reversibility of Rheumatoid Arthritis," *Ann Rheum Dis* 8, no. 2 (June 1949): 90–96.

76. In 1950, E. C. Kendall, P. S. Hench, and T. Reichstein shared the Nobel Prize for their work with adrenal cortical hormones. See Edward C. Kendall, "The Development of Cortisone as a Therapeutic Agent," *Indian Med J* 45, no. 10 (October 1951): 239–41.

77. Waldemar Kaempfferz, "Hormone Treatment for Arthritis Promises to Bring a Baffling Disease under Control," *New York Times*, June 5, 1949.

78. "The 'Elixir of Life,'" *New York Times*, August 21, 1949.

79. Viviane Quirke, "Making British Cortisone: Glaxo and the Development of Corticosteroids in Britain in the 1950s–1960s," *Stud Hist Philos Sci C* 36, no. 4 (2005): 645–74; quotation is from p. 648.

80. David Cantor describes how the dramatic image of cortisone's beneficial effects in the treatment of rheumatoid arthritis was transformed by the persistent shortages of the drug and its harmful side effects; see David Cantor, "Cortisone and the Politics of Drama, 1949–55," in *John V. Pickstone, Hg., Medical Innovations in Historical Perspective* (London: Macmillan, 1992), 167. Chris Feudtner offers an insightful perspective on the transmutation of a disease from an acute to a chronic condition, using the example of diabetes. See Feudtner, *Bittersweet*.

81. Edward C. Kendall, "The Development of Cortisone as a Therapeutic Agent," Nobel Lecture, December 11, 1950, NobelPrize.org., https://www.nobelprize.org/prizes/medicine/1950/kendall/lecture/; quotation is from p. 272.

82. Kendall, 271. Rumor had it that the Germans' Luftwaffe was experimenting with these drugs. See Nicolas Rasmussen, "Steroids in Arms: Science, Government, Industry, and the Hormones of the Adrenal Cortex in the United States, 1930–1950," *Med Hist* 46, no. 3 (2002): 299–324.

83. Quirke, "Making British Cortisone," 649. Cantor describes the politics of drama in the introduction of cortisone between 1949 and 1955 in Cantor, "Cortisone and the Politics of Drama."

84. Harry M. Marks, "Cortisone, 1949: A Year in the Political Life of a Drug," *Bull Hist Med* 66, no. 3 (Fall 1992): 419–39, esp. 420.

85. Lea Haller, *Cortison: Geschichte eines Hormons, 1900–1955* (Zurich: Chronos, 2012), 192–93.

86. Marks, "Cortisone, 1949," 437.

87. See Roy Gibbons, "Science Gets Synthetic Key to Rare Drug. Discovery Is Made in Chicago," *Chicago Daily Tribune*, September 30, 1949. In 1954, Julian switched from soybeans to wild yams. On Julian, see G. Weissmann,

"Cortisone and the Burning Cross: The Story of Percy Julian," *Pharos Alpha Omega Alpha Honor Med Soc* 68, no. 1 (Winter 2005): 13–16.

88. Lawson Wilkins et al., "The Suppression of Androgen Secretion by Cortisone in a Case of Congenital Adrenal Hyperplasia," *Bulletin of the Johns Hopkins Hospital* 86 (1950): 249–52. Further citations of this work are given in the text.

89. Wilkins, "Diagnosis of the Adrenogenital Syndrome," 868–70.

90. Wilkins, 868.

91. Lawson Wilkins et al., "Further Studies on the Treatment of Congenital Adrenal Hyperplasia with Cortisone: II. The Effects of Cortisone on Sexual and Somatic Development, with an Hypothesis concerning the Mechanism of Feminization," *J Clin Endocrinol Metab* 12 (1952): 277–307. However, even in the short-duration studies the team always looked for signs of changes in virilization. L. Wilkins et al., "Treatment of Congenital Adrenal Hyperplasia with Cortisone," *J Clin Endocrinol* 11 (1951): 1–25.

92. Wilkins et al., "Further Studies on the Treatment of Congenital Adrenal Hyperplasia with Cortisone: II.," 281.

93. Wilkins et al., 281. Wilkins also reports on this method in Wilkins et al., "Treatment of Congenital Adrenal Hyperplasia," 20.

94. Howard Wilbur Jones and Georgeanna Seegar Jones, "The Gynecological Aspects of Adrenal Hyperplasia and Allied Disorders," *Am J Obstet Gynecol.* 68, no. 5 (1954): 1330–65, 1348.

95. Wilkins, "Diagnosis of the Adrenogenital Syndrome," 869–70.

96. Wilkins et al., "Further Studies on the Treatment of Congenital Adrenal Hyperplasia with Cortisone: II.," 291.

97. While the introduction of cortisone in 1949 created a public uproar, CAH was not at the forefront of conditions that gained media attention for the drug's success. Only one of the major East Coast newspapers mentions Wilkins's therapeutic achievements: "Cortisone Helps to Restore Sex Balance, Survey Shows," *Washington Post*, March 30, 1952. Neither the *Baltimore Sun* nor the *New York Times* reported on Wilkins's new cortisone treatment, though his 1963 obituary in the *NYT* mentions it; see "Dr. Lawson Wilkins, Endocrinologist, 69," *New York Times*, September 29, 1963.

98. "Cortisone Helps to Restore Sex Balance."

99. See Feudtner, *Bittersweet*, 64–65.

100. For earlier examples of this practice, see Dreger, *Hermaphrodites*, 159–66. Another example is H. H. Young's practice; see Kenen, "Scientific Studies of Human Sexual Difference," 34–109.

ROBERT

Epigraph: N. Rose, "Beyond Medicalisation," *Lancet* 369, no. 9562 (February 24, 2007): 700–702; quotation is from p. 702.

1. Gillis, "Taking a Medical History," 395.

2. Patient record, GYI1K (Robert), HLH.
3. Names of doctor, hospital, and location omitted to protect patient privacy.
4. Name of social worker changed to protect patient privacy.
5. On the "golden age" of medicine, see Allan M. Brandt and Martha Gardner, "The Golden Age of Medicine?," in *Medicine in the Twentieth Century*, ed. Roger Cooter and John V. Pickstone (Amsterdam: Harwood Academic, 2000), 21–38.
6. Name of social worker changed to protect patient privacy.
7. *Facies* is the medical term for distinctive facial expressions associated with specific medical conditions.

CHAPTER TWO

1. Jacob E. Finesinger, Joe V. Meigs, and Hirsh W. Sulkowitch, "Clinical, Psychiatric and Psychoanalytic Study of a Case of Male Pseudohermaphroditism," *Am J Obstet Gynecol* 44, no. 2 (1942): 310–17; quotation is from p. 310. Further citations of this work are given in the text.
2. Young, *Genital Abnormalities*. Kenen used Young's patient records to show how his clinical practice at times contradicted his theoretical stance on sex determination; see Kenen, "Scientific Studies of Human Sexual Difference."
3. Finesinger, Meigs, and Sulkowitch, "Clinical, Psychiatric and Psychoanalytic Study," 310.
4. Finesinger, Meigs, and Sulkowitch, 316.
5. Reis discusses the fear of deception in her *Bodies in Doubt*.
6. See Sengoopta, *Most Secret Quintessence of Life*.
7. William Henry Mikesell, *Psychology of Adjustment*, The Van Nostrand Series in Psychology (New York: Van Nostrand, 1952).
8. Charles Louis Crawford Burns, *Maladjusted Children* (London: Hollis and Carter, 1955), ix.
9. Bert Pierce, "Automobiles: Drivers; Study Shows Most Accident Repeaters Suffer Personality Maladjustments," *New York Times*, April 10, 1949.
10. Arthur Miller, *Death of a Salesman* (New York: Viking, 1949).
11. See Vicedo, *Nature and Nurture of Love*.
12. Jack David Pressman, "Psychiatry and Its Origins," *Bull Hist Med* 71, no. 1 (1997): 129–39, esp. 138.
13. Pressman, 131.
14. On Meyer, see Ruth Leys, "Types of One: Adolf Meyer's Life Chart and the Representation of Individuality," *Representations*, no. 34 (1991): 1–28; S. D. Lamb, *Pathologist of the Mind: Adolf Meyer and the Origins of American Psychiatry* (Baltimore: Johns Hopkins University Press, 2014).
15. Lamb, *Pathologist of the Mind*, 4.
16. Gerald N. Grob, "Presidential Address: Psychiatry's Holy Grail; The Search for the Mechanisms of Mental Diseases," *Bull Hist Med* 72, no. 2 (1998): 189–219; quotation is from p. 202.

17. Pressman, "Psychiatry and Its Origins," 132.
18. See Theresa R. Richardson, *The Century of the Child: The Mental Hygiene Movement and Social Policy in the United States and Canada* (Albany: SUNY Press, 1989).
19. Redick, "American History XY," 423.
20. Matta, "Ambiguous Bodies and Deviant Sexualities," 82.
21. See Matta, 494. On the practice of relating the shape of genitals to homosexuality, see Reis, *Bodies in Doubt*, 56.
22. Matta, "Ambiguous Bodies and Deviant Sexualities," 502.
23. Mak, *Doubting Sex*. On the general adaptation of anesthesia in the nineteenth-century United States, see Martin S Pernick, *A Calculus of Suffering: Pain, Professionalism, and Anesthesia in Nineteenth-Century America* (New York: Columbia University Press, 1985).
24. Mak, *Doubting Sex*, 148.
25. The historian Charlotte Borst shows how by the 1930s, physicians had replaced midwives and taken over childbirth among white families; see Charlotte G. Borst, *Catching Babies: The Professionalization of Childbirth, 1870–1920* (Cambridge, MA: Harvard University Press, 1995).
26. Grob, "Presidential Address," 211.
27. Finesinger, Meigs, and Sulkowitch, "Clinical, Psychiatric and Psychoanalytic Study," 310.
28. Eugene B. Brody, "Jacob E. Finesinger, M.D.," *Am J Psychiatry* 116, no. 4 (1959): 383–84; quotation is from p. 383.
29. Brody, 383–84.
30. Finesinger, Meigs, and Sulkowitch, "Clinical, Psychiatric and Psychoanalytic Study." Further citations of this work are given in the text.
31. Even though many sexologists postulated same-sex desire as caused by some form of sexual or gender inversion, it was the British physician Havelock Ellis who popularized the term (and idea of) *sexual inversion*; see Ellis and Symonds, *Sexual Inversion*.
32. Kenen, "Scientific Studies of Human Sexual Difference," 209.
33. Finesinger, Meigs, and Sulkowitch, "Clinical, Psychiatric and Psychoanalytic Study," 316. Further citations of this work are given in the text.
34. F. M. Ingersoll and J. E. Finesinger, "A Case of Male Pseudohermaphroditism, the Importance of Psychiatry in the Surgery of This Condition," *Surg Clin North Am* 27 (1947): 1218–25; quotation is from p. 1218. Further citations of this work are given in the text.
35. See E. C. Dodds et al., "Oestrogenic Activity of Certain Synthetic Compounds," *Nature* 141, no. 3562 (February 1, 1938): 247–48.
36. Ingersoll and Finesinger, "Case of Male Pseudohermaphroditism," 1224. Further citations of this work are given in the text.
37. Albert Ellis, "Reviews, Abstracts, Notes, and Correspondence: The Sexual Psychology of Human Hermaphrodites," *Psychosom Med* 7, no. 2 (1945): 108–25; quotation is from p. 108.

38. In the nineteenth century, the desire of adults to live in a sex other than their gonadal sex had often been interpreted as an attempt to mask homosexual desire and behavior; see for example Dreger, *Hermaphrodites*.
39. Albert Ellis and Shawn Blau, *The Albert Ellis Reader: A Guide to Well-Being Using Rational Emotive Behavior Therapy* (New York: Citadel Press, 1998), 95.
40. Ellis, "Reviews, Abstracts, Notes, and Correspondence," 120. Further citations of this work are given in the text.
41. Sigmund Freud, "Three Essays on the Theory of Sexuality (1905)," in *A Case of Hysteria, Three Essays on Sexuality and Other Works*, translated from the German under the general editorship of James Strachey, in collaboration with Anna Freud and with the assistance of Alix Strachey and Alan Tyson, 123–246; vol. 7 (1901–1905) of *The Standard Edition of the Complete Psychological Works of Sigmund Freud* (London: Hogarth Press and the Institute of Psychoanalysis, 1953). See Ronald Bayer, *Homosexuality and American Psychiatry: The Politics of Diagnosis* (New York: Basic Books, 1981), 21–27.
42. See Bayer, *Homosexuality and American Psychiatry*, 28–29.
43. Bayer, 77. On the medical and scientific engagement with homosexuality in modern America, see Jennifer Terry, *An American Obsession: Science, Medicine, and Homosexuality in Modern Society* (Chicago: University of Chicago Press, 1999). For Ellis homosexuality studies, see Albert Ellis, *Homosexuality: Its Causes and Cure* (New York: Lyle Stuart, 1965).
44. Ellis, "Reviews, Abstracts, Notes, and Correspondence," 119.
45. On the perspective on homosexuality in the culture and personality school, see Joanne Meyerowitz, "'How Common Culture Shapes the Separate Lives': Sexuality, Race, and Mid-Twentieth-Century Social Constructionist Thought," *Journal of American History* 96, no. 4 (2010): 1057–84.
46. Ellis, "Reviews, Abstracts, Notes, and Correspondence," 119.
47. Ellis, 108.
48. "In Memory," *San Francisco Chronicle*, May 27, 2011.
49. Frank Hinman Jr., "Advisability of Surgical Reversal of Sex in Female Pseudohermaphroditism," *J Am Med Assoc* 146, no. 5 (1951): 423–29.
50. Hinman, 425.
51. In his paper, Hinman did not cite the two similar articles published by Finesinger and Ingersoll in 1942 and 1947. He might have been unfamiliar with them.
52. Hinman, "Advisability of Surgical Reversal," 423. Further citations of this work are given in the text.
53. See Matta, "Ambiguous Bodies and Deviant Sexualities"; Reis, *Bodies in Doubt*.
54. See Wilkins, "Diagnosis of the Adrenogenital Syndrome."
55. Hinman, "Advisability of Surgical Reversal," 426.
56. Hinman, 426.
57. Wilkins et al., "Suppression of Androgen Secretion."
58. Hinman, "Advisability of Surgical Reversal," 427.

59. Hinman, 427. Further citations of this work are given in the text. In 1955, the psychiatrist Joan Hampson proposed an even shorter critical phase of 18 months to 2.5 years.

60. This tragic incident is published as case 25 in Young, *Genital Abnormalities*, 347.

61. Patient Record LEJN7 (Carol), HLH.

62. "Dr. Jacob H. Conn, 86, a Psychiatrist, Is Dead," *New York Times*, July 10 1990.

63. Patient record, LEJN7 (Carol), HLH.

64. See for example this article published in the *New York Medical Journal* in 1900 discussing how women's emancipation produced effeminate boys and masculine girls: William Lee Howard, "Effeminate Men and Masculine Women," *New York Medical Journal* 71 (May 5, 1900): 686–87. Cited in Jennifer Terry, "'Momism' and the Making of Treasonous Homosexuals," in *"Bad" Mothers: The Politics of Blame in Twentieth-Century America*, ed. Molly Ladd-Taylor and Lauri Umansky (New York: New York University Press, 1998), 169.

65. Philip Wylie, *Generation of Vipers* (New York: Rinehart, 1942). On Momism, see Elaine Tyler May, *Homeward Bound: American Families in the Cold War Era* (New York: Basic Books, 1988), 64–65 and 100–142. On Wylie and Momism, see Rebecca Jo Plant, "The Repeal of Mother Love: Momism and the Reconstruction of Motherhood in Philip Wylie's America" (PhD diss., Johns Hopkins University, 2001); Plant, *Mom*, 19–54.

66. Plant, *Mom*. 20. On Wylie and motherhood, see also Vicedo, *Nature and Nurture of Love*, 32–33.

67. See Talcott Parsons quoted in Deborah Weinstein, *The Pathological Family: Postwar America and the Rise of Family Therapy* (Ithaca, NY: Cornell University Press, 2013), 14.

68. Weinstein, 15.

69. Name changed to protect patient privacy.

70. Patient record, IZOA9 (Karen), HLH. I discuss Karen's experience in more detail in the following chapter.

71. Patient record, IZOA9 (Karen), HLH.

72. Passing, that is, convincingly appearing as man or woman, has been addressed by scholars of the history of homosexuality and of gender nonbinary individuals. See for example Harold Garfinkel, "Passing and the Managed Achievement of Sex Status in an 'Intersexed' Person," in *The Transgender Studies Reader*, ed. Susan Stryker and Stephen Whittle (New York: Routledge, 2006), 58–93; Sandy Stone, "The Empire Strikes Back: A Posttranssexual Manifesto," in ibid., 221–35.

KAREN

Epigraph: Shigehisa Kuriyama, *The Expressiveness of the Body and the Divergence of Greek and Chinese Medicine*, 1st pbk. ed. (New York: Zone Books, 2002), 9.

1. Patient record, IZOA9 (Karen), HLH.
2. This encounter took place in 1959.

CHAPTER THREE

1. See the "Rangitiki Letters," August–December 1947, box 503603, JMC.
2. Most of his peers in New Zealand chose to go to Great Britain, where their citizenship made immigration easier. The period after World War II was marked by a profound exchange and circulation of persons and knowledge, mainly across the Atlantic from Europe to the United States; see for example Jean-Paul Gaudillière, "Paris–New York Roundtrip: Transatlantic Crossings and the Reconstruction of the Biological Sciences in Post-War France," *Stud Hist Philos Sci C* 33, no. 3 (2002): 389–417.
3. Camille Paglia cited in Goldie, *The Man Who Invented Gender*, 3.
4. Goldie, 4.
5. See for example the depiction of Money in John Colapinto, *As Nature Made Him: The Boy Who Was Raised as a Girl* (New York: HarperCollins, 2000); Jeffrey Eugenides, *Middlesex* (New York: Picador / Farrar, Straus and Giroux., 2003).
6. Meyerowitz, "'How Common Culture Shapes,'" 1057–58. On cultural relativism, see also David A. Hollinger, *Cosmopolitanism and Solidarity: Studies in Ethnoracial, Religious, and Professional Affiliation in the United States* (Madison: University of Wisconsin Press, 2006).
7. Richard Handler, "Boasian Anthropology and the Critique of American Culture," *AQ* 42, no. 2 (1990): 252–73; quotation is from p. 253.
8. Carl N. Degler, *In Search of Human Nature: The Decline and Revival of Darwinism in American Social Thought* (New York: Oxford University Press, 1991).
9. On scientific racism, see Melissa N. Stein, *Measuring Manhood: Race and the Science of Masculinity, 1830–1934* (Minneapolis: University of Minnesota Press, 2015); Michael Yudell, *Race Unmasked: Biology and Race in the Twentieth Century* (New York: Columbia University Press, 2014); Nancy Leys Stepan, "Race, Gender, Science and Citizenship," *Gender and History* 10, no. 1 (1998): 26–52; Cynthia Eagle Russett, *Sexual Science: The Victorian Construction of Womanhood* (Cambridge, MA: Harvard University Press, 1989). On Boasian anthropology, see Handler, "Boasian Anthropology."
10. See Franz Boas, *The Mind of Primitive Man: A Course of Lectures Delivered before the Lowell Institute, Boston, Mass., and the National University of Mexico, 1910–1911* (New York: Macmillan, 1911).
11. The first statement issued in 1949 to counter irrational racial doctrine was quickly revised by 1951. For a history of postwar antiracism, see Michelle Brattain, "Race, Racism, and Antiracism: UNESCO and the Politics of Presenting Science to the Postwar Public," *American Historical Review* 112, no. 5 (2007): 1386–1413.

12. Margaret Mead, *Coming of Age in Samoa: A Psychological Study of Primitive Youth for Western Civilisation* (New York: William Morrow, 1928).

13. Peter Mandler, "One World, Many Cultures: Margaret Mead and the Limits to Cold War Anthropology," *History Workshop Journal*, no. 68 (2009): 149–72, esp. 151.

14. Philip Gleason, "Americans All: World War II and the Shaping of American Identity," *Review of Politics* 43, no. 4 (1981): 483–518, esp. 487.

15. Margaret Mead, *Sex and Temperament in Three Primitive Societies* (New York: William Morrow, 1935), ix.

16. Mead first analyzed what constitutes American culture in 1942: Margaret Mead, *And Keep Your Powder Dry: An Anthropologist Looks at America* (New York: William Morrow, 1942).

17. Margaret Mead, *Male and Female: A Study of the Sexes in a Changing World* (New York: William Morrow, 1949). On Mead's depiction of American identity, see Gleason, "Americans All," 506–7.

18. See Degler, *In Search of Human Nature*, 199–200.

19. Mead, *Male and Female*, 185.

20. Mandler, "One World, Many Cultures," 152.

21. Meyerowitz, "'How Common Culture Shapes,'" 1072.

22. See Meyerowitz, 1072.

23. Mead, *And Keep Your Powder Dry*.

24. Gleason, "Americans All."

25. Eugenics gained traction by widespread fears that hereditary traits such as feeblemindedness and other undesirable characteristics would be passed on from one generation to another as single-unit characters. The prevailing concern about the racial deterioration of the US population led to a series of sterilization laws in many states targeting mostly poor women and women of color as well as those already institutionalized.

   As a consequence, as many as sixty thousand to seventy thousand people were sterilized in the United States, the majority without their consent. See Daniel J. Kevles, *In the Name of Eugenics: Genetics and the Uses of Human Heredity* (Berkeley: University of California Press, 1986); Kline, *Building a Better Race*; Alexandra Stern, *Eugenic Nation: Faults and Frontiers of Better Breeding in Modern America*, 2nd ed., American Crossroads 17 (Oakland: University of California Press, 2016). After World War II, eugenic practices fell out of favor, even though the "science of human perfection" persisted in other fields and guises. See for example Nathaniel C. Comfort, *The Science of Human Perfection: How Genes Became the Heart of American Medicine* (New Haven, CT: Yale University Press, 2012). For the continuance of eugenic practices of sterilization, see Alexandra Minna Stern, "Sterilized in the Name of Public Health," *Am J Public Health* 95, no. 7 (July 1, 2005): 1128–38; Johanna Schoen, *Choice and Coercion: Birth Control, Sterilization, and Abortion in Public Health and Welfare* (Chapel Hill: University of North Carolina Press, 2005).

26. Mead was strongly influenced by Ruth Benedict's notion of cultures as integrated wholes, which she viewed as an analogy for individual personality. Benedict had published *Patterns of Culture*, one of the most widely read anthropological studies, in 1934. She viewed culture holistically rather than as an assembly of disconnected parts, personalities, and behaviors and argued that any given culture structured what was considered normal and abnormal. Most individuals, she wrote, were "plastic to the moulding force of the society into which they are born": Ruth Benedict, "Anthropology and the Abnormal," *J Gen Psychology* 10, no. 1 (January 1, 1934): 59–82, esp. 74. On Benedict, see also Gleason, "Americans All," 486.

27. Most famously, Ruth Benedict's work on Japan; see Ruth Benedict, *The Chrysanthemum and the Sword: Patterns of Japanese Culture* (Boston: Houghton Mifflin, 1946). See also Raymond Augustine Bauer, *How the Soviet System Works: Cultural, Psychological, and Social Themes*, Russian Research Center Studies (Cambridge, MA: Harvard University Press, 1956).

28. Gleason, "Americans All."

29. Meyerowitz, "'How Common Culture Shapes,'" 1059. On the application of science in postwar "Kulturkämpfe" and the trope of the cosmopolitan intellectual, see David A. Hollinger, "Science as a Weapon in Kulturkampfe in the United States during and after World War II," *Isis* 86, no. 3 (1995): 440–54; Hollinger, *Cosmopolitanism and Solidarity*. On behaviorist human engineering during the Cold War, see Lemov, *World as Laboratory*.

30. Meyerowitz in her discussion of the psychoanalyst Abram Kardiner, another participant in the culture and personality networks; see Meyerowitz, "'How Common Culture Shapes,'" 1078.

31. United States Children's Bureau, *The Story of the White House Conferences on Children and Youth* (Washington, DC: US Department of Health, Education, and Welfare, Social Rehabilitation Service, Children's Bureau, 1967), 16.

32. Richardson, *Century of the Child*, 2. On the history of childhood science, expert advice, family, motherhood, and children, see Julia Grant, *Raising Baby by the Book: The Education of American Mothers* (New Haven, CT: Yale University Press, 1998); Barbara Beatty, Emily D. Cahan, and Julia Grant, *When Science Encounters the Child: Education, Parenting, and Child Welfare in 20th-Century America*, Reflective History Series (New York: Teachers College Press, 2006).

33. Goldie, *The Man Who Invented Gender*, 21; Michael King and Eastern Southland Gallery, Gore, NZ, *Splendours of Civilisation: The John Money Collection at the Eastern Southland Gallery* (Dunedin, NZ: Eastern Southland Gallery in association with Longacre Press, 2006), 25.

34. On Money's childhood and upbringing, see Goldie, *The Man Who Invented Gender*.

35. John Money, "Explorations in Human Behavior," in *The History of Clinical Psychology in Autobiography*, ed. C. Eugene Walker (Pace Grove, CA: Thomson Brooks / Cole, 1991), 2:238.

36. During that period, Money notably counseled a celebrated New Zealand author, the then unknown Janet Frame. Money, 2:240. See also Goldie, *The Man Who Invented Gender.*
37. James Ritchie and Jane Ritchie, "Beaglehole, Ernest," orig. pub. 2000 in *The Dictionary of New Zealand Biography,* which is now online as part of *Te Ara—the Encyclopedia of New Zealand,* accessed September 13, 2021, https://teara.govt.nz/en/biographies/5b15/beaglehole-ernest.
38. Money, "Explorations in Human Behavior," 233. See Goldie, *The Man Who Invented Gender,* 24–25.
39. Letter dated March 19, 1947, JMH.
40. Letter dated June 5, 1947, JMH.
41. The dodo bird hypothesis is a "reference to Lewis Carroll's 1865 book, *Alice in Wonderland,* in which a dodo bird declares: 'Everybody has won and all must have prizes.'" See the obituary by Gerry Everding, "Saul Rosenzweig, 97, Professor Emeritus in Arts & Sciences," *Newsroom,* August 26, 2004, accessed September, 13, 2021, http://news.wustl.edu/news/Pages/3669.aspx.
42. Money, "Explorations in Human Behavior," 240.
43. Money, 242.
44. Unable to afford living in Cambridge, he moved into a run-down apartment across the Charles River in Boston's West End. The apartment was behind Massachusetts General Hospital, at 104 Brighton Street on the first floor of a nineteenth-century tenement house. Brighton Street no longer exists. It was roughly located where Emerson Place is today. See D. A. Sanborn, *Insurance Map of Boston,* vol. 1 (New York: D. A. Sanborn, 1867), accessed September 14, 2021, http://hdl.loc.gov/loc.gmd/g3764bm.g03693001.
45. Gordon W. Allport and Edwin G. Boring, "Psychology and Social Relations at Harvard University," *Am Psychol* 1, no. 4 (1946): 119.
46. The committee consisted of Talcott Parsons, who became the chairman, G. W. Allport, E. G. Boring, Donald Scott, A. M. Tozzer, and C. C. Zimmerman. It had proposed "that Harvard adopt, and thus help establish, the term Social Relations to characterize the emerging discipline which deals not only with the body of fact and theory traditionally recognized as the subject-matter of sociology, but also with that portion of psychological science that treats the individual within the social system, and that portion of anthropological science that is particularly relevant to the social and cultural patterns of literate societies." Allport and Boring, 119.
47. See Joel Isaac, *Working Knowledge: Making the Human Sciences from Parsons to Kuhn* (Cambridge, MA: Harvard University Press, 2012), 158. On Cold War science, see Lemov, *World as Laboratory;* Jamie Cohen-Cole, *The Open Mind: Cold War Politics and the Sciences of Human Nature* (Chicago: University of Chicago Press, 2014); Mark Solovey and Hamilton Cravens, eds., *Cold War Social Science: Knowledge Production, Liberal Democracy, and Human Nature* (New York: Palgrave Macmillan, 2012); Vicedo, *Nature and Nurture of Love.*

48. Isaac, *Working Knowledge*, 159.
49. Isaac, 160.
50. Talcott Parsons and Edward Shils, *Toward a General Theory of Action* (Cambridge, MA: Harvard University Press, 1951).
51. Talcott Parsons, *The Social System* (Glencoe, IL: Free Press, 1951).
52. Parsons, 17. Germon suggests that Parsons's understanding of role shaped Money's conceptualization of "gender role"; see Germon, *Gender*, 31–32. Iain Morland argues that Germon overstates sociology's influence on Money's thought. Instead, he credits the contemporaneous discipline of cybernetics (and homeostasis as its signature concern) as the essential factor for how Money would conceptualize gender as a self-regulating system; see Morland's chapter "Cybernetic Sexology" in Downing, Morland, and Sullivan, *Fuckology*, 101–32.
53. Allport and Boring, "Psychology and Social Relations," 119.
54. Arthur J. Vidich, "The Department of Social Relations and 'Systems Theory' at Harvard: 1948–50," *International Journal of Politics, Culture, and Society* 13, no. 4 (2000): 607–48; quotation is from p. 616. Further citations of this work are given in the text.
55. Murray's tenure review was a matter of much contestation and controversy in 1936, and though he was promoted to associate professor in 1937, he was not given tenure but rather a ten-year appointment. See Rodney G. Triplet, "Henry A. Murray: The Making of a Psychologist?," *Am Psychol* 47, no. 2 (1992): 299–307.
56. See Triplet, 299–307.
57. Triplet, 299.
58. Gordon W. Allport, *Personality: A Psychological Interpretation* (New York: Henry Holt, 1937).
59. Allport, 48.
60. Triplet, "Henry A. Murray," 304.
61. Christiana D. Morgan and Henry A. Murray, "A Method for Investigating Fantasies: The Thematic Apperception Test," *Arch Neurol Psychiatry* 34, no. 2 (1935): 289–306.
62. Henry A. Murray and Harvard Psychological Clinic, Harvard University, *Explorations in Personality: A Clinical and Experimental Study of Fifty Men of College Age* (New York: Oxford University Press, 1938). See Clifford Thomas Morgan, *Introduction to Psychology* (New York: McGraw-Hill, 1956).
63. Money, "Explorations in Human Behavior," 243.
64. Kluckhohn had followed a trajectory similar to many of his cultural relativist colleagues. In the 1930s, he conducted research on Navajo Indians, followed by a stint at the Foreign Morale Analysis Division of the Office of War Information, where he studied Japanese culture during World War II. After the war, Kluckhohn became increasingly interested in national character studies. He wrote about Soviet cultural patterns, but he never visited

the Soviet Union, and he never learned to speak Russian. Nevertheless, the study of culture at a distance was considered a successful application of anthropology to the needs of the nation. See David C. Engerman, "Social Science in the Cold War," *Isis* 101, no. 2 (2010): 393–400, esp. 397. For the culture at a distance approach in the social sciences, see Margaret Mead and Rhoda Métraux, *The Study of Culture at a Distance* (Chicago: University of Chicago Press, 1953); Clyde Kluckhohn, *Mirror for Man: The Relation of Anthropology to Modern Life* (New York: Whittlesey House, 1949).

65. Clyde Kluckhohn and Henry A. Murray, *Personality in Nature, Society, and Culture* (New York: A. A. Knopf, 1948). Further citations of this work are given in the text.

66. Money, "Explorations in Human Behavior," 244.

67. Redick, "American History XY," 176.

68. John Money, "Hermaphroditism: An Inquiry into the Nature of a Human Paradox" (PhD diss., Harvard University, 1952), 2.

69. S. Robert Snodgrass, "Stanley Cobb, the Rockefeller Foundation and the Evolution of American Psychiatry," *History of Psychiatry* 29, no. 4 (2018): 438–55.

70. Stanley Cobb, *Borderlands of Psychiatry*, Harvard University Monographs in Medicine and Public Health (Cambridge, MA: Harvard University Press, 1943), 19.

71. Money, "Explorations in Human Behavior," 247.

72. Money, 248.

73. Money, "Hermaphroditism: An Inquiry."

74. See Redick, "American History XY," 18.

75. Money, "Hermaphroditism: An Inquiry," 201–2. Further citations of this work are given in the text.

76. Most famously Neugebauer; see Franz Ludwig Von Neugebauer, *Hermaphroditismus beim Menschen*, vol. 2 (Leipzig: Klinkhardt, 1908).

77. The French psychologist Alfred Binet and the psychiatrist Theodore Simon first produced a measuring scale of intelligence in 1908 and 1911 to test schoolchildren. In the United States, uptake was initially slow until Lewis Terman, psychologist at Stanford University, revised the test by changing the age range to include adulthood. Terman also introduced an intelligence quotient, or IQ, as a measurable result of the test, which came to be called the Stanford-Binet test. The psychologist Robert Yerkes pushed to include the test to measure the mental abilities of army recruits as the United States entered World War I, and by 1918 the US Army began mass intelligence testing. See Daniel J. Kevles, "Testing the Army's Intelligence: Psychologists and the Military in World War I," *Journal of American History* 55, no. 3 (1968): 565–81. Ability, ethnicity, race, and class were often connected in the study of intelligence, and intelligence tests were strongly skewed toward particular forms of education and white middle-class Anglo-American

culture. Lewis Terman, for example, wrote in *The Measurement of Intelligence* that a low level of intelligence was "very, very common among Spanish-Indian and Mexican families of the Southwest and also among negroes. Their dullness seems to be racial, or at least inherent in the family stocks from which they come." He predicted that "new experimental methods would discover enormously significant racial differences in general intelligence, differences which cannot be wiped out by any scheme of mental culture." Lewis Madison Terman, *The Measurement of Intelligence: An Explanation of and a Complete Guide for the Use of the Stanford Revision and Extension of the Binet-Simon Intelligence Scale* (Boston: Houghton Mifflin, 1916).

78. Wechsler had revised his adult test for children using one hundred white male and one hundred white female subjects at each age from five to fifteen years: David Wechsler and Psychological Corporation, *Wechsler Intelligence Scale for Children: Manual* (New York: Psychological Corporation, 1949). On the development of the test, see Corwin Boake, "From the Binet-Simon to the Wechsler-Bellevue: Tracing the History of Intelligence Testing," *J Clin Exp Neuropsychol* 24, no. 3 (2002): 383–405.

79. Florence Laura Goodenough, *Measurement of Intelligence by Drawings* (New York: World Book, 1926).

80. Money, "Hermaphroditism: An Inquiry," i.

81. Kinsey, Pomeroy, and Martin, *Sexual Behavior in the Human Male*; Institute for Sex Research and Kinsey, *Sexual Behavior in the Human Female*.

82. On the quantification of sex, see Robinson, *Modernization of Sex*.

83. A major inspiration for Kinsey's research was his realization that many of the undergraduate students he taught in his marriage course at the University of Indiana suffered from a lack of knowledge about sexuality. His biographers, however, make much of Kinsey's prudish upbringing and experience of guilt and ignorance; see James H. Jones, *Alfred C. Kinsey: A Public/Private Life* (New York: W. W. Norton, 1997); Jonathan Gathorne-Hardy, *Alfred C. Kinsey: Sex the Measure of All Things; A Biography* (London: Chatto and Windus, 1998). On Kinsey's methods and motivation, see Donna J. Drucker, "'A Noble Experiment': The Marriage Course at Indiana University, 1938–1940," *Indiana Magazine of History* (2007): 231–64; Donna J. Drucker, "Keying Desire: Alfred Kinsey's Use of Punched-Card Machines for Sex Research," *Journal of the History of Sexuality* 22, no. 1 (2013): 105–25; Drucker, *Classification of Sex*; Donna J. Drucker, "The Machines of Sex Research," in *The Machines of Sex Research* (Heidelberg, Springer, 2014), 1–18. On the effect of the Kinsey Reports on American sexuality, see Reumann, *American Sexual Character*.

84. Money, "Explorations in Human Behavior," 254.

85. Cited in Goldie, *The Man Who Invented Gender*, 29. On the history of masturbation, see Thomas Walter Laqueur, *Solitary Sex: A Cultural History of Masturbation* (New York: Zone Books, 2003).

86. Money, "Hermaphroditism: An Inquiry," 33, 49, 72. Further citations of this work are given in the text.

87. Margaret Mead, for example, ended her 1942 book, meant to boost morale and promote democracy and tolerance, by encouraging Americans to have "faith in the power of science"; Mead, *And Keep Your Powder Dry*, 262. The value, historical specificity, and attainability of the ideal of objectivity has been the subject of much debate and criticism in the history and philosophy of science; see for example Ludwik Fleck, *Genesis and Development of a Scientific Fact*, trans. Fred Bradley and Thaddeus J. Trenn (Chicago: University of Chicago Press, 1979); Thomas S. Kuhn, *The Structure of Scientific Revolutions* (Chicago: University of Chicago Press, 1962); Donna Haraway, "Situated Knowledges: The Science Question in Feminism and the Privilege of Partial Perspective," *Feminist Studies* 14, no. 3 (1988): 575–99; Lorraine Daston and Peter Galison, *Objectivity* (New York: Zone Books, 2007; distributed by MIT Press).

88. On the persecution of homosexuals in the 1950s and on the formation of the first homophile movements in the same period, see D'Emilio, *Sexual Politics, Sexual Communities*; Robert J. Corber, *Homosexuality in Cold War America: Resistance and the Crisis of Masculinity*, New Americanists (Durham, NC: Duke University Press, 1997); David K. Johnson, *The Lavender Scare: The Cold War Persecution of Gays and Lesbians in the Federal Government* (Chicago: University of Chicago Press, 2004); Margot Canaday, *The Straight State: Sexuality and Citizenship in Twentieth-Century America*, Politics and Society in Twentieth-Century America (Princeton, NJ: Princeton University Press, 2009). There was also renewed interest in the scientific study of homosexuality, its causes, and its relation to gender; see Stephanie H. Kenen, "Who Counts When You're Counting Homosexuals? Hormones and Homosexuality in Mid-Twentieth Century America," in *Science and Homosexualities*, ed. Vernon A. Rosario (New York: Routledge, 1997), 197–218; Terry, *An American Obsession*; Roel van den Oever, *Mama's Boy: Momism and Homophobia in Postwar American Culture* (New York: Palgrave Macmillan, 2012).

89. See Kinsey, Pomeroy, and Martin, *Sexual Behavior in the Human Male*, 639.

90. Edward Sagarin's *The Homosexual in America*, published under the pseudonym Donald Webster Cory in 1951, was among the first homophile publications stating that homosexuals were an unrecognized minority group and deserved civil rights; Donald Webster Cory, *The Homosexual in America: A Subjective Approach* (New York: Greenberg, 1951). For Cory and homophile movements before Stonewall, see Vern L. Bullough, *Before Stonewall: Activists for Gay and Lesbian Rights in Historical Context*, Haworth Gay and Lesbian Studies (New York: Harrington Park Press, 2002). Historians also argue that among other factors, the experiences of young gay and lesbian Americans during World War II, in which they found themselves in sex-segregated environments in the military, allowed for the development

of a group identity; see D'Emilio, *Sexual Politics, Sexual Communities*; Allan Berube, *Coming Out under Fire: The History of Gay Men and Women in World War Two* (New York: Free Press, 1990).

91. Of his own sex life, Money wrote in 1991 that he had "sexual visitations and friendly companionships with compatible partners, some women, some men, some briefly, and some with continuity." See Money, "Explorations in Human Behavior," 254.

92. Money, "Hermaphroditism: An Inquiry," 82.

93. Money, 75.

94. On sexual inversion, see George Chauncey, "From Sexual Inversion to Homosexuality: Medicine and the Changing Conceptualization of Female Deviance," *Salmagundi* (1982): 114–46; Matt T. Reed, "Historicizing Inversion: Or, How to Make a Homosexual," *History of the Human Sciences* 14, no. 4 (2001): 1–29.

95. See for example the "Rangitiki Letters," August–December 1947, box 503603, JMC. See also letter dated July 16, 1949, JMH.

96. Historians of childhood have shown that a particular American version of childhood, which differentiated American youth from European children, stressed independence, self-definition, and individual success; see Paula S. Fass, *The End of American Childhood: A History of Parenting from Life on the Frontier to the Managed Child* (Princeton, NJ: Princeton University Press, 2016).

97. Mandler argues that once the war broke out, Mead and Bateson referred to their work as studies of national character rather than "culture and personality." See Mandler, "One World, Many Cultures," 153.

98. Mead, *And Keep Your Powder Dry*. On Mead's war effort, see Gleason, "Americans All," 506–7. Further citations of the Gleason work are given in the text.

99. Mead, *And Keep Your Powder Dry*, 262.

100. Money, "Hermaphroditism: An Inquiry," 179.

101. See Julia Grant, "A 'Real Boy' and Not a Sissy: Gender, Childhood, and Masculinity, 1890–1940," *Journal of Social History* 37, no. 4 (2004): 829–51; Beatty, Cahan, and Grant, *When Science Encounters the Child*.

102. Money, "Hermaphroditism: An Inquiry," 179.

103. Money, 154–55.

104. Few cases of African-American children and adults are given in the published literature on intersex. On race and intersex, see Magubane, "Spectacles and Scholarship."

105. Money, "Hermaphroditism: An Inquiry," 101.

106. Money, 113.

107. Money, "Explorations in Human Behavior," 249.

108. Letter by George E. Gardner, November 21, 1951, JMK.

109. Letter by George E. Gardner, November 21, 1951, JMK.

110. Money, "Hermaphroditism: An Inquiry."

CHAPTER FOUR

1. Press release dated May 2, 1956, JMK; my emphasis.
2. By 1958, the team was no longer on speaking terms, and the Hampsons left Hopkins soon afterward; see John Money, *The Hampsons Leave the Johns Hopkins Hospital Psychohormonal Research Unit*, vol. 1, 1953–1966, JMK.
3. See Wilkins et al., "Treatment of Congenital Adrenal Hyperplasia"; Wilkins et al., "Suppression of Androgen Secretion."
4. Sandra Eder, "From 'Following the Push of Nature' to 'Restoring One's Proper Sex'—Cortisone and Sex at Johns Hopkins's Pediatric Endocrinology Clinic," *Endeavour* 36, no. 2 (2012): 69–76.
5. See "Joan Gannon Hampson, MD," *Seattle Times*, August 7, 2005. While Money's life is well documented, this is not the case with Joan Hampson or her husband, John.
6. John Money, *Venuses Penuses: Sexology, Sexosophy, and Exigency Theory* (Buffalo, NY: Prometheus Books, 1986), 8. Money interviewed some of Wilkins's patients to develop case studies for fulfilling part of the requirements for receiving the PhD; see Money, "Hermaphroditism: An Inquiry."
7. John Money, *The Adam Principle: Genes, Genitals, Hormones and Gender; Selected Readings in Sexology* (Buffalo, NY: Prometheus Books, 1993), 95; Money, *Venuses Penuses*, 8.
8. These three meetings were later published with verbatim transcripts of the discussions. See P. György et al., "Inter-University Round Table Conference by the Medical Faculties of the University of Pennsylvania and Johns Hopkins University: Psychological Aspects of the Sexual Orientation of the Child with Particular Reference to the Problem of Intersexuality," *J Pediatr* 47, no. 6 (1955): 771–90; Lytt I. Gardner, ed., *Adrenal Function in Infants and Children: A Symposium* (New York: Grune and Stratton, 1956); Joan Hampson, "Human Hermaphroditism: Establishment of Gender Role and Erotic Practices," in *Symposium: Genetic, Psychological and Hormonal Factors in the Establishment and Maintenance of Patterns of Sexual Behavior in Mammals; November 17–19, 1954, the Lord Jeffrey, Amherst, Massachusetts*, comp. William C. Young (Lawrence, KS, 1954), 292–308; unpublished conference proceedings bound and held at the University of Kansas.
9. György et al., "Inter-University Round Table Conference," 786.
10. György et al., 788.
11. See Dreger, *Hermaphrodites*, 29.
12. See Eder, "From 'Following the Push.'" On finding the "best sex" rather than determining somebody's "true sex," see also Redick, "American History XY."
13. György et al., "Inter-University Round Table Conference," 779. Further citations of this work are given in the text.
14. See for example Redick, "American History XY," 224. See also Fausto-Sterling, *Sexing the Body*, 72.

15. György et al., "Inter-University Round Table Conference," 774. Further citations of this work are given in the text.
16. Joanne Meyerowitz revises the history of 1950s gender conformity and domestic ideology by showing that the gender scripts of the 1950s were more complex than, for example, their depiction in Betty Friedan's feminist classic *The Feminine Mystique* (1963); see Joanne Meyerowitz, "Beyond the Feminine Mystique: A Reassessment of Postwar Mass Culture, 1946–1958," *Journal of American History* 79, no. 4 (1993): 1455–82.
17. György et al., "Inter-University Round Table Conference," 779–80. Further citations of this work are given in the text.
18. For Young's clinical practice in assessing sex, see Kenen, "Scientific Studies of Human Sexual Difference," 34–108.
19. Kenen, 90–93.
20. György et al., "Inter-University Round Table Conference," 789. For a history of the Macy Jr. Foundation and the extraordinary role of Frank Fremont-Smith in organizing interdisciplinary conferences, see Christopher Tudico, *The History of the Josiah Macy Jr. Foundation*, ed. George E. Thibault, MD (New York: Josiah Macy Jr. Foundation, September 2012), https://macyfoundation.org/assets/img/macy-history-book--final-2012.pdf; Tara H. Abraham, "Transcending Disciplines: Scientific Styles in Studies of the Brain in Mid-Twentieth Century America," *Studies in History and Philosophy of Science Part C: Studies in History and Philosophy of Biological and Biomedical Sciences* 43, no. 2 (2012): 552–68.
21. György et al., "Inter-University Round Table Conference," 790. Further citations of this work are given in the text.
22. John C. Burnham, "American Medicine's Golden Age: What Happened to It?," *Science* 215, no. 4539 (1982): 1474–79, esp. 1474. For the golden age of medicine, see also Brandt and Gardner, "The Golden Age of Medicine?" The 1910 *Flexner Report* concerning medical education in the United States and Canada standardized that education on a scientific footing but also led to the exclusion of many Black, female, or indigent practitioners from medical education and practice.
23. The 1966 Henry Beecher report on ethics and clinical research provoked serious debates about research protocols, practices, and ethics and led to landmark changes; see Henry K. Beecher, "Ethics and Clinical Research," in *Biomedical Ethics and the Law*, ed. James M. Humber (Boston: Springer, 1966), 215–27. For an analysis of this internal critique, see David J. Rothman, *Strangers at the Bedside: A History of How Law and Bioethics Transformed Medical Decision Making* (New York: Basic Books, 1991). For the women's health movement, see Wendy Kline, *Bodies of Knowledge: Sexuality, Reproduction, and Women's Health in the Second Wave* (Chicago: University of Chicago Press, 2010).
24. The meeting at Syracuse resembled a pediatric family reunion. Wilkins had brought young colleague Claude Migeon, along with John Money and Joan

Hampson. Several of the other participants had previously been fellows at his clinic (Alfred M. Bongiovanni, Walter H. Eberlein, Lytt I. Gardner, Melvin M. Grumbach, Robert Klein). Edna H. Sobel and Nathan B. Talbot from Mass General were also working on a cortisone treatment.

25. John Money, "Hermaphroditism, Gender and Precocity in Hyperadrenocorticism: Psychologic Findings," in *Adrenal Function in Infants and Children: A Symposium*, ed. Lytt I. Gardner (Syracuse: Public Relations Office, Upstate Medical Center, State University of New York, 1954), 15.

26. Joan G. Hampson, "Hermaphroditic Genital Appearance, Rearing and Eroticism in Hyperadrenocorticism: Psychologic Findings," in *Adrenal Function in Infants and Children: A Symposium*, ed. Lytt I. Gardner (Syracuse: Public Relations Office, Upstate Medical Center, State University of New York, 1954), 18.

27. Lytt I. Gardner, ed., *Adrenal Function in Infants and Children: A Symposium* (New York: Grune and Stratton, 1956).

28. Joan G. Hampson, "Hermaphroditic Genital Appearance, Rearing and Eroticism in Hyperadrenocorticism," in *Adrenal Function in Infants and Children: A Symposium*, ed. Lytt I. Gardner (New York: Grune and Stratton, 1956), 129. Further citations of this work are given in the text.

29. For Wilkins's focus on genitals, see Redick, "American History XY."

30. See John Money, Joan G. Hampson, and John L. Hampson, "Hermaphroditism: Recommendations concerning Assignment of Sex, Change of Sex and Psychological Management," *Bulletin of the Johns Hopkins Hospital* 97, no. 4 (1955): 284–300, esp. 294. For a discussion of the "phallic standard," see Fausto-Sterling, *Sexing the Body*, 57–61.

31. This aspect was also emphasized in the foreword of the 1956 publication, in which Lytt I. Gardner, editor of the published proceedings, highlighted the usefulness of "an important new concept of the ontogenetic factors influencing the human sex role, as described by Hampson and Money"; see Gardner, foreword to *Adrenal Function in Infants and Children* (Grune and Stratton, 1956), v.

32. Hampson, "Hermaphroditic Genital Appearance," 131. Further citations of this work are given in the text.

33. This data is from Hampson's 1955 publication, on which this chapter was based; see Joan G. Hampson, "Hermaphroditic Genital Appearance, Rearing and Eroticism in Hyperadrenocorticism," *Bulletin of the Johns Hopkins Hospital* 96, no. 6 (1955): 265–73, esp. 270–71.

34. Hampson, "Hermaphroditic Genital Appearance" (Grune and Stratton, 1956), 126. Further citations of this work are given in the text.

35. György et al., "Inter-University Round Table Conference," 773.

36. Hampson, "Hermaphroditic Genital Appearance," 131. Further citations of this work are given in the text.

37. Hampson, "Human Hermaphroditism."

38. Kinsey and his coworkers had been scheduled to go first but requested to change places. Money and Hampson gave the only specifically human and

clinical paper—other than Kinsey's, which by his request was off the record
and not included in the conference report. On Kinsey's talk, see Money,
"Once upon a Time I Met Alfred C. Kinsey." There was, of course, one other
woman present at conference: the typist who produced the transcript of
the event.

39. Hampson, "Human Hermaphroditism," 309. Further citations of this work
are given in the text.

40. The *Bulletin* had been established in 1889 and was published monthly
until 1982. Money and the Hampsons might have decided to publish in it
because it had a quick turnaround between submission and publication,
and all its articles were published within two to three months of their
submission.

41. John Money, "Hermaphroditism, Gender and Precocity in Hyperadrenocorticism: Psychological Findings," *Bulletin of the Johns Hopkins Hospital*
96, no. 6 (1955): 253–64, esp. 258–64; Hampson, "Hermaphroditic Genital
Appearance." The authors paid special attention to precocity and somatic
virilization, both typical symptoms of hyperadrenocorticism (CAH) in boys
and girls. The second half of Money's article was focused on IQ and precocity in boys and girls with CAH.

42. John L. Hampson, Joan G. Hampson, and John Money, "The Syndrome of
Gonadal Agenesis (Ovarian Agenesis) and Male Chromosomal Pattern in
Girls and Women: Psychologic Studies," *Bulletin of the Johns Hopkins Hospi-
tal* 97, no. 3 (September 1955): 207–26.

43. Money, Hampson, and Hampson, "Hermaphroditism: Recommendations";
John Money, Joan G. Hampson, and John L. Hampson, "An Examination
of Some Basic Sexual Concepts: The Evidence of Human Hermaphroditism," *Bulletin of the Johns Hopkins Hospital* 97, no. 4 (October 1955): 301–19.

44. John Money, Joan G. Hampson, and John L. Hampson, "Sexual Incongruities and Psychopathology: The Evidence of Human Hermaphroditism,"
Bulletin of the Johns Hopkins Hospital 98, no. 1 (1956): 43–57. Though the
papers are structured and published by a group of authors, Money maintained that the ideas and conceptual framework were predominantly his
own. See also Redick, "American History XY," 196.

45. Today, we understand *sexual orientation* to indicate sexual preference. At the
time, Money and the Hampsons used the term to designate masculinity or
femininity.

46. Hampson, "Hermaphroditic Genital Appearance" (*Bulletin*, 1955), 266.

47. Money, Hampson, and Hampson, "An Examination," 310.

48. Money, Hampson, and Hampson, 308.

49. Parsons, *Social System*.

50. Parsons, 17. See also Germon, *Gender*.

51. For an analysis of Wilkins's focus on genitalia as determining the sex variable, see Redick, "American History XY."

NOTES TO PAGES 130–133

52. A paper on how the Barr test was used to detect chromosomal sex in hermaphrodites via this new technique was published in 1953; see K. L. Moore, M. A. Graham, and M. L. Barr, "The Detection of Chromosomal Sex in Hermaphrodites from a Skin Biopsy," *Surg Gynecol Obstet* 96, no. 6 (1953): 641–48. For the Hopkins study, the chromosomal determinations of these and other patient groups was done by Dr. M. L. Barr and Dr. K. L. Moore at the University of Western Ontario; see Hampson, Hampson, and Money, "Syndrome of Gonadal Agenesis," 207n3; Money, Hampson, and Hampson, "An Examination," 302.

53. Fiona Alice Miller argues that this discovery allowed scientists and clinicians to "see" something that was otherwise invisible, and for a decade it was, as Miller shows, "good enough" science to be used to determine the sex of intersexuals, transsexuals, and homosexuals. See Fiona Alice Miller, "'Your True and Proper Gender': The Barr Body as a *Good Enough* Science of Sex," *Stud Hist Philos Biol Biomed Sci* 37 (2006): 449–83, esp. 460. As I show in the following chapter, the Barr body test required a particular skill set.

54. Hampson, Hampson, and Money, "Syndrome of Gonadal Agenesis," 218.

55. Money, Hampson, and Hampson, "An Examination," 305–6.

56. Money, Hampson, and Hampson, 308.

57. Money, "Hermaphroditism, Gender and Precocity," 253.

58. Money, Hampson, and Hampson, "An Examination," 301.

59. Redick, "American History XY," 164ff. See John Money, "Delusion, Belief and Fact," *Psychiatry* 11 (1948): 33–38; John Money, "Unanimity in the Social Sciences with Reference to Epistemology, Ontology and Scientific Method," *Psychiatry* 12 (1949): 211–21; John Money, *A First Person History of Pediatric Psychoendocrinology, 1951–2000* (New York: Kluwer Academic / Plenum, 2002); John Money, "An Examination of the Concept of Psychodynamics," *Psychiatry* 17 (1954): 325–30.

60. John Money, *The Psychologic Study of Man* (Springfield, IL: Charles C. Thomas, 1957).

61. Money, 5.

62. Money, Hampson, and Hampson, "Hermaphroditism: Recommendations," 258.

63. Money applied the language metaphor and the word *imprinting* in Money, "Examination of the Concept of Psychodynamics," 310. In his 1957 textbook, Money also specifically referred to language acquisition; see Money, *Psychologic Study of Man*, 51.

64. See Money, "Examination of the Concept of Psychodynamics," 310; Money, *Psychologic Study of Man*, 51.

65. See Vicedo, *Nature and Nurture of Love*, 55. For the term *Prägung*, see Konrad Z. Lorenz, "The Companion in the Bird's World," *Auk* 54, no. 3 (1937): 245–73. The literal translation from the German is "stamped in."

66. On Lorenz's influence in Cold War America, see also Milam, *Creatures of Cain*.

67. Vicedo, *Nature and Nurture of Love*, 56.
68. Milam discussed the popularization of animal behavior studies, including the work of Lorenz, in Milam, *Creatures of Cain*. See Niko Tinbergen, *The Study of Instinct* (Oxford: Clarendon Press, 1951); Konrad Lorenz, *King Solomon's Ring; New Light on Animal Ways* (New York: Crowell, 1952); Konrad Lorenz, *Man Meets Dog* (London: Methuen, 1954); Konrad Lorenz, *On Aggression* (London: Methuen, 1966).
69. See for example Morgan, *Introduction to Psychology*.
70. Money, Hampson, and Hampson, "An Examination," 309–10.
71. Money addressed Lorenz specifically in John Money, Joan G. Hampson, and John L. Hampson, "Imprinting and the Establishment of Gender Role," *Arch Neurol Psychiatry* 77 (1957): 333–36. There he cited Lorenz's *King Solomon's Ring* as a reference; see Lorenz, *King Solomon's Ring*. In his 1957 textbook, Money also referred to Lorenz, *Man Meets Dog*. See Money, *Psychologic Study of Man*, 50–51.
72. Money, Hampson, and Hampson, "Imprinting," 335.
73. Lorenz, "Companion in the Bird's World," 266. Although Lorenz insisted that this kind of behavior only occurred in birds, he later suggested that it might appear in humans as well.
74. Vicedo, *Nature and Nurture of Love*, 56.
75. Money, *Psychologic Study of Man*, 48.
76. Money, 49.
77. Redick, "American History XY," 8.
78. Money, *Psychologic Study of Man*, 50–51.
79. Money, 52.
80. Hampson, "Hermaphroditic Genital Appearance" (*Bulletin*, 1955), 267.
81. Hampson, Hampson, and Money, "Syndrome of Gonadal Agenesis," 224.
82. Hampson, "Hermaphroditic Genital Appearance," 265, 271.
83. Money, Hampson, and Hampson, "Hermaphroditism: Recommendations," 288.
84. Money, Hampson, and Hampson, 301.
85. Hampson, "Hermaphroditic Genital Appearance," 272.
86. Money, Hampson, and Hampson, "Sexual Incongruities and Psychopathology," 52.
87. Money, Hampson, and Hampson, "Hermaphroditism: Recommendations," 285.
88. Money, Hampson, and Hampson, 285.
89. See D'Emilio, *Sexual Politics, Sexual Communities*; Berube, *Coming Out under Fire*; Corber, *Homosexuality in Cold War America*; Terry, *An American Obsession*; Johnson, *Lavender Scare*; Canaday, *Straight State*.
90. See Alfred C. Kinsey, "Homosexuality: Criteria for a Hormonal Explanation of the Homosexual," *J Clin Endocrinol* 1, no. 5 (1941): 424–28; Kinsey, Pomeroy, and Martin, *Sexual Behavior in the Human Male*. On homosexuals as a minority, see Cory, *Homosexual in America*. On the Kinsey research and

its historical significance, see Drucker, "Male Sexuality"; Reumann, *American Sexual Character*; Drucker, *Classification of Sex*.

91. Money, Hampson, and Hampson, "Hermaphroditism: Recommendations," 291–92.

92. Hampson, "Hermaphroditic Genital Appearance" (*Bulletin*, 1955), 269n.

93. Money, Hampson, and Hampson, "An Examination," 315.

94. Hampson, "Human Hermaphroditism," 311–12. Suzanne J. Kessler noted this stress on "happiness" in her 1985 interviews with six medical experts in New York on the treatment of intersex patients. One urologist put it this way: "Happiness is the biggest factor. Anatomy is part of happiness." See Kessler, *Lessons from the Intersexed*, 26.

CHAPTER FIVE

An earlier version of this chapter was published as Sandra Eder, "The Volatility of Sex: Intersexuality, Gender and Clinical Practice in the 1950s," Gender & History 22, no. 3 (2010): 692–707.

1. Patient record, GQ2L4 (Ann/Andy), HLH.

2. Wilkins et al., "Suppression of Androgen Secretion"; Wilkins et al., "Treatment of Congenital Adrenal Hyperplasia."

3. See Georges Canguilhem, *On the Normal and the Pathological*, trans. Carolyn R. Fawcett, Studies in the History of Modern Science, vol. 3 (Dordrecht: D. Reidel, 1978).

4. See Charles E. Rosenberg and Janet Lynne Golden, *Framing Disease: The Creation and Negotiation of Explanatory Schemes*, the Milbank Quarterly (New York: Published for the Milbank Memorial Fund by Cambridge University Press, 1989); Charles E. Rosenberg, Janet Lynne Golden, and Francis Clark Wood Institute for the History of Medicine, *Framing Disease: Studies in Cultural History*, Health and Medicine in American Society (New Brunswick, NJ: Rutgers University Press, 1992).

5. See for example Nancy Tomes's discussion of household products and cleaning regimes in Nancy Tomes, *The Gospel of Germs: Men, Women, and the Microbe in American Life* (Cambridge, MA: Harvard University Press, 1998).

6. See Mak, "Doubting Sex from Within."

7. See Park, *Harriet Lane Home*.

8. R. W. Fraser et al., "Colorimetric Assay of 17-Ketosteroids in Urine—a Survey of the Use of This Test in Endocrine Investigation, Diagnosis and Therapy," *J Clin Endocrinol* 1, no. 3 (1941): 234–56.

9. For a description and images of such devices, see for example Thelma Reynolds, "A Metabolism Bed," *American Journal of Nursing* 43, no. 2 (1943): 183–85; Fraser et al., "Colorimetric Assay."

10. Patient record, QB9LE (James), HLH.

11. Mak, "Doubting Sex from Within," 340.

12. Patient record, LEJN7 (Carol), HLH.
13. Richard W. TeLinde was professor of gynecology at Johns Hopkins from 1939 to 1960; see Howard Wilbur Jones, Georgeanna Seegar Jones, and William E. Ticknor, *Richard Wesley TeLinde* (Baltimore: Williams and Wilkins, 1986).
14. For the introduction of the Barr test into clinical practice, see Miller, "'Your True and Proper Gender.'"
15. Moore, Graham, and Barr, "Detection of Chromosomal Sex."
16. Miller, "'Your True and Proper Gender,'" 460. On the sexing of sex chromosomes, see also Richardson, *Sex Itself.*
17. Miller, "'Your True and Proper Gender,'" 465.
18. Patient record, 16UU6 (Richard), HLH.
19. See Moore, Graham, and Barr, "Detection of Chromosomal Sex."
20. Patient record, 16UU6 (Richard), HLH.
21. Patient record, Q5CT4 (Charles), HLH.
22. Postcortisone, chromosomally female children with CAH were usually raised as girls; see also Karkazis, *Fixing Sex,* 57.
23. For the HLH patient statistics, see Wilkins, *Diagnosis and Treatment of Endocrine Disorders,* 9–10.
24. Patient record, GQ2L4 (Ann/Andy), HLH.
25. Wilkins, "Diagnosis of the Adrenogenital Syndrome." For the first patient treated and published on, see Wilkins et al., "Suppression of Androgen Secretion."
26. Howard Jones and William Scott mainly performed these operations. See Jones and Scott, *Hermaphroditism, Genital Anomalies and Related Endocrine Disorders.* On the history of clitoral anatomy, see Laqueur, *Making Sex*; Lisa Jean Moore and Adele E. Clarke, "Clitoral Conventions and Transgressions: Graphic Representations in Anatomy Texts, c1900–1991," *Feminist Studies* 21, no. 2 (1995): 255–301; Darlaine Claire Gardetto, "Engendered Sensations: Social Construction of the Clitoris and Female Orgasm, 1650–1975" (PhD diss., University of California, Davis, 1992).
27. For earlier practices, see Young, *Genital Abnormalities.* For a more cautious approach, see Talbot et al., *Functional Endocrinology,* 234. For a discussion of experiences with clitoridectomy, see Karkazis, *Fixing Sex,* 148–49.
28. See Rodriguez, *Female Circumcision and Clitoridectomy.*
29. Rodriguez, 30.
30. Karkazis, *Fixing Sex,* 158–59. On genital variability, see Kessler, *Lessons from the Intersexed,* 8–10.
31. Patient record, ZN34O (Linda), HLH.
32. Eustace Chesser and Zoe Dawe, *The Practice of Sex Education: A Plain Guide for Parents and Teachers* (New York: Roy, 1946), 24. Chesser cites a recent publication about child sexuality by Anna Freud in chapter 2: Anna Freud, "Sex in Childhood," *Health Educ J* 2, no. 1 (1944): 2–6. See also Edith Hale Swift, *Step by Step in Sex Education* (New York: Macmillan, 1948), 18–22.

On masturbation as "one stage of normal sexual development," see Roy M. Dorcus and G. Wilson Shaffer, *Textbook of Abnormal Psychology*, 4th ed. (Baltimore: Williams and Wilkins, 1950), 259. On parental concerns about masturbation, see Jessica Martucci, "'A Habit That Worries Me Very Much': Raising Good Boys and Girls in the Postwar Era," In *Pink and Blue: Gender, Culture, and the Health of Children*, ed. Elena Conis, Sandra Eder, and Aimee Madeiros (New Brunswick, NJ: Rutgers University Press, 2021), 31–50.

33. Chesser and Dawe, *Practice of Sex Education*, 23.
34. Chesser and Dawe, 24; Dorcus and Shaffer, *Textbook of Abnormal Psychology*, 259.
35. Dorcus and Shaffer, *Textbook of Abnormal Psychology*, 259.
36. Wilkins—being an endocrinologist and not a surgeon—might have also relied on existing surgical practices and the judgment of the surgeons he worked with.
37. On the practice of making a "cosmetic clitoris," see Howard W. Jones, "Female Hermaphroditism without Virilization," *Obstet Gynecol Surv* 12, no. 4 (1957): 433–60.
38. Patient record, JDCUV (Betty), HLH.
39. Patient record, V73QC (Dorothy), HLH.
40. See Hampson, "Hermaphroditic Genital Appearance" (*Bulletin*, 1955). Further citations of this work are given in the text.
41. Patient record, IJZQY (Donna), HLH.
42. Patient record, SBQFW (Kathleen), HLH.
43. Patient record, 16UU6 (Richard), HLH.
44. See for example Wilkins, "Diagnosis of the Adrenogenital Syndrome."
45. Jones and Jones, "Gynecological Aspects of Adrenal Hyperplasia," 1348. One must note that the clitoral amputation did not seem to count in this setting.
46. Jones and Jones, 1351.
47. Patient records: CEY66 (Barbara), HLH; JDCUV (Betty), HLH; 8A4YN (Janet), HLH; 3FGGT (Carolyn), HLH; V73QC (Dorothy), HLH; IJZQY (Donna), HLH.
48. On the practice of vaginal dilations, see Karkazis, *Fixing Sex*, 223–24.
49. Patient record, 3FGGT (Carolyn), HLH.
50. Carolyn's previous hospital record had been lost, so her story was reconstructed through her patient narrative.
51. Patient record, Q5CT4 (Charles), HLH.

CHAPTER SIX

1. Money, *The Hampsons Leave*, vol. 1, JMK.
2. "Storm Dumps up to 2 Feet of Snow on State, Leaves Thousands of Homes without Electricity, Heat or Telephone Service; at Least Five Die," *Sun* (Baltimore), March 21, 1958.

3. Money, *The Hampsons Leave*, vol. 1, JMK.
4. Money, vol. 1.
5. Money, vol. 1.
6. See Meyerowitz, *How Sex Changed*, 222.
7. The team remained protective of their work. For example, all three signed a letter to the editor of the *Canadian Psychiatric Association Journal*, published in April 1960, protesting the finding of a 1959 article which contradicted the Hopkins study; see John Money, John L. Hampson, and Joan G. Hampson, "Hermaphroditism: Psychology and Case Management," *Can Psychiatr Assoc J* 5, no. 2 (1960): 131–33.
8. See chaps. 22 and 23 in William C. Young and Edgar Allen, eds., *Sex and Internal Secretions*, 3rd ed. (Baltimore: Williams and Wilkins, 1961).
9. See Fisher, "Short History of Pediatric Endocrinology," 720.
10. Fisher, 719–20.
11. Melvin Grumbach discusses this rivalry in 1998, on the occasion of *Pediatrics*'s republication of Wilkins's 1952 paper; see M. M. Grumbach, "Further Studies on the Treatment of Congenital Adrenal Hyperplasia with Cortisone: IV. Effect of Cortisone and Compound B in Infants with Disturbed Electrolyte Metabolism, by John F. Crigler Jr., MD, Samuel H. Silverman, MD, and Lawson Wilkins, MD, *Pediatrics*, 1952; 10: 397–413," pt. 2, *Pediatrics* 102, no. 1 (1998): 215–21, esp. 215.
12. Lawson Wilkins's group reported preliminary treatment success with cortisone in 1950 in the *Bulletin of the Johns Hopkins Hospital* and published an expanded study in the *Journal of Clinical Endocrinology* in 1951. Bartter, Fuller Albright, and others presented their results in 1950 at the annual spring meeting of the American Society of Clinical Investigation. They published a full-length paper in 1951 in the *Journal of Clinical Investigation*. See F. C. Bartter et al., "The Effects of Adrenocorticotropic Hormone and Cortisone in the Adrenogenital Syndrome Associated with Congenital Adrenal Hyperplasia: An Attempt to Explain and Correct Its Disordered Hormonal Pattern," *J Clin Investig* 30, no. 3 (1951): 237–51.
13. Talbot's *Functional Endocrinology, from Birth through Adolescence*, very much like Wilkins's textbook, briefly mentioned the promise of cortisone treatment for CAH. It went through only one edition, while Wilkins's textbook went through four. Nathan B. Talbot, *Functional Endocrinology, from Birth through Adolescence* (Cambridge, MA: Harvard University Press, 1952).
14. Talbot, *Functional Endocrinology, from Birth through Adolescence*, 366.
15. Talbot, 234.
16. A longer version of the Zurich case study was published as Sandra Eder, "Gender and Cortisone: Clinical Practice and Transatlantic Exchange in the Medical Management of Intersex in the 1950s," *Bull Hist Med* 92, no. 4 (2018): 604–33.
17. Elizabeth Wilkins McMaster, "Lawson Wilkins: Recollections by His Daughter," *Int J Pediatr Endocrinol* suppl. 1 (May 2014): S1.

18. See Fisher, "Short History of Pediatric Endocrinology," 719. For the conference program, see *Comptes-rendus du Sixième congrès international de pédiatrie/Transactions of the Sixth International Congress of Pediatrics* (Zurich, Switzerland, July 24-28, 1950), 377.

19. Fanconi in Andrea Prader, "Pseudohermaphroditismus Femininus mit kongenitaler Nebennierenrinden-Insuffizienz: Günstige Wirkung Von Cortison, Desoxycorticosteronacetat Und Kochsalz," *Helvet Paediatr Acta* 5 (1950): 426–33. Translations from German are my own, unless otherwise indicated. Further citations of this work are given in the text.

20. See Wolfgang G. Sippell, ed., *ESPE—the First 50 Years: A History of the European Society for Paediatric Endocrinology* (Basel: S. Karger, 2011), 6; Milo Zachmann, "Andrea Prader 1919–2001," *Horm Res Paediatr* 56, nos. 5–6 (2001): 205–7.

21. Andrea Prader, "Cortison Dauerbehandlung des kongenitalen adrenogenitalen Syndroms," *Helv Paediatr Acta* 5 (1953): 368–423. Compare with Wilkins, "Diagnosis of the Adrenogenital Syndrome."

22. Patient record, MOQ91 (Bernard), StAZH.

23. Patient record, NIW82 (Verena), StAZH.

24. Marks, "Cortisone, 1949," 420.

25. On cortisone in Switzerland, see Haller, *Cortison*, esp. 220–30.

26. Prader, "Cortison Dauerbehandlung," 417.

27. Patient record, MOQ91 (Bernard), StAZH.

28. Patient record, BRU73 (Anna), StAZH.

29. Patient record, BRU73 (Anna), StAZH.

30. See Andrea Prader, "Gonadendysgenesie und testikuläre Feminisierung," *Schweiz Med Wochenschr* 87 (1957): 278–85, 281.

31. Patient record, VYE64, Erika.

32. The panel was part of the Eighth International Congress of Paediatrics, Copenhagen, July 22–27, 1956.

33. Lawson Wilkins et al., "Hermaphroditism: Classification, Diagnosis, Selection of Sex and Treatment," *Pediatrics* 16 (1955): 287–302, esp. 297.

34. Such case exchanges can be found, for example, in Wilkins et al., "Treatment of Congenital Adrenal Hyperplasia," p. 12; Lawson Wilkins and Jose Cara, "Further Studies on the Treatment of Congenital Adrenal Hyperplasia with Cortisone: V. Effects of Cortisone Therapy on Testicular Development," *J Clin Endocrinol Metab* 14, no. 3 (1954): 287–96, quotation is is from p. 292; Lawson Wilkins et al., "Virilizing Adrenal Hyperplasia: Its Treatment with Cortisone and the Nature of the Steroid Abnormalities," *Ciba Foundation Colloquia on Endocrinology* 8 (1955): 460–86, quotations are from pp. 482 and 484.

35. *The Rockefeller Foundation Annual Report 1950* (N.p.: Rockefeller Foundation, 1950), 93–94.

36. W. Züblin, "Zur Psychiatrie des adrenogenitalen Syndroms bei kongenitaler Nebennierenrinden-Hyperplasie," *Helv Paediatr Acta* 8 (1953): 117–35.

Money cites Züblin as "additional reference" in Money, "Hermaphroditism, Gender and Precocity."

37. Züblin cited Ellis and Hinman as two examples of the environmental approach; see Ellis, "Reviews, Abstracts, Notes, and Correspondence"; Hinman, "Advisability of Surgical Reversal"; Frank Hinman Jr., "Sexual Trends in Female Pseudohermaphrodism," *J Clin Endocrinol Metab* 11, no. 5 (1951): 477–86.

38. Züblin, "Zur Psychiatrie des adrenogenitalen Syndroms," 121.

39. Andrea Prader, *Intersexualität: Habilitationsschrift*, Labhart, Klinik der inneren Sekretion (Berlin: Springer, 1957), 372.

40. Prader, 666.

41. See Ulrike Klöppel, *XXOXY Ungelöst: Hermaphroditismus, Sex und Gender in der deutschen Medizin; Eine historische Studie zur Intersexualität*, vol. 12 (Bielefeld: Transcript 2010), 492.

42. Prader, *Intersexualität*, 666.

43. In the literature section on psychosexuality and intersexes, Prader listed Money, Hampson, and Hampson, "Hermaphroditism: Recommendations." In the section on the adrenogenital syndrome, he referred to the Joan Hampson's and John Money's talks given at the 1954 symposium on adrenal health in Syracuse, New York; see Gardner, *Adrenal Function in Infants and Children* (State University of New York, 1954).

44. Wilkins's textbook went through four editions (1950, 1957, 1967, and 1994); see Wilkins, *Diagnosis and Treatment of Endocrine Disorders in Childhood and Adolescence*. Howard Jones and William Scott's textbook had two editions (1958 and 1971); see Jones and Scott, *Hermaphroditism, Genital Anomalies and Related Endocrine Disorders*.

45. L. Emmett Holt Jr., Rustin MacIntosh, and L. Emmett Holt, *Holt Pediatrics*, 12th ed. (New York: Appleton-Century-Crofts, 1953); Waldo E. Nelson, ed., *Textbook of Pediatrics*, 7th ed. (Philadelphia: W. B. Saunders, 1959).

46. Wilkins, *Diagnosis and Treatment of Endocrine Disorders in Childhood and Adolescence*, xi.

47. Wilkins, 284.

48. Lawson Wilkins, *The Diagnosis and Treatment of Endocrine Disorders in Childhood and Adolescence*, with the assistance of Robert M. Blizzard and Claude J. Migeon, 3rd ed. (Springfield, IL: Thomas, 1965), xi.

49. Joe Hin Tjio and Albert Levan, "The Chromosome Number of Man," *Hereditas* 42, nos. 1–2 (1956): 1–6.

50. Jones and Scott, *Hermaphroditism, Genital Anomalies and Related Endocrine Disorders*. Further citations of this work are given in the text.

51. Rodriguez, *Female Circumcision and Clitoridectomy*, 3. Masters and Johnson proposed a four-stage model of sexual response and emphasized the importance of clitoral stimulation; see William H. Masters, Virginia E. Johnson, and Reproductive Biology Research Foundation (USA), *Human Sexual Response* (Boston: Little, Brown, 1966).

52. Rodriguez, *Female Circumcision and Clitoridectomy*, 4.
53. Jones and Scott, *Hermaphroditism, Genital Anomalies and Related Endocrine Disorders*, 57.
54. Lytt I. Gardner, *Endocrine and Genetic Diseases of Childhood* (Philadelphia: Saunders, 1969); Lytt I. Gardner, *Endocrine and Genetic Diseases of Childhood and Adolescence*, 2nd ed. (Philadelphia: Saunders, 1975). See Gardner, *Endocrine and Genetic Diseases of Childhood*, 539–44. He did not refer to any of the articles Money (and the Hampsons) published in the 1950s, only Money's publication from 1965.
55. Holt, MacIntosh, and Holt, *Holt Pediatrics*. In 1953, the classic was first published under the new title *Holt Pediatrics*.
56. L. Emmett Holt Jr. et al., *Pediatrics*, 13th ed. (New York: Appleton-Century-Crofts, 1962); Henry L. Barnett and L. Emmett Holt, *Pediatrics*, 14th ed. (New York: Appleton-Century-Crofts, 1968); Henry L. Barnett and L. Emmett Holt, *Pediatrics*, 15th ed. (New York: Appleton-Century-Crofts, 1972). Grumbach is listed as author in the 1962 edition. The 1968 edition does not list his name, but the entry is practically identical. He is listed again as author in the 1972 edition.
57. Holt et al., *Pediatrics*, 870.
58. Holt et al., 870–71.
59. Nelson, *Textbook of Pediatrics*, 1203.
60. Nelson, 1203.
61. Waldo E. Nelson, ed., *Textbook of Pediatrics*, 8th ed. (Philadelphia: Saunders, 1964), 1150. Nelson cited Wilkins's textbook.
62. Daniel Cappon, Calvin Ezrin, and Patrick Lynes, "Psychosexual Identification (Psychogender) in the Intersexed," *Can Psychiatr Assoc J* 4, no. 2 (1959): 90–106; quotation is from p. 95.
63. Cappon, Ezrin, and Lynes, 99. Further citations of this work are given in the text. Cappon and his colleagues, similar to Money, only cited Lorenz's popular 1952 book; see Lorenz, *King Solomon's Ring*.
64. Money, Hampson, and Hampson, "Hermaphroditism: Psychology," 131.
65. Cappon, Ezrin, and Lynes, "Psychosexual Identification," 90. Further citations of this work are given in the text.
66. Money, Hampson, and Hampson, "Hermaphroditism: Psychology," 131, 33. Further citations of this work are given in the text. In 1972, Money yet again criticized Cappon and others for becoming "instrumental in wrecking the lives of unknown numbers of hermaphroditic youngsters, by authorizing or denying sex reassignment"; see John Money and Anke A. Ehrhardt, *Man and Woman, Boy and Girl: Differentiation and Dimorphism of Gender Identity from Conception to Maturity* (Baltimore: Johns Hopkins University Press, 1972), 154.
67. In this comment, Money and the Hampsons were referring to patients with Turner's and Klinefelter's syndromes. In 1959, researchers determined that the sex chromosomes in Turner's syndrome were XO and not XY, and in Klinefelter's syndrome they were determined as XXY and not XX. One of the

references the Hopkins team cited was listed as "in press" and thus not generally available at the time of their response. This was certainly another aspect of their privileged access to information; see M. A. Ferguson-Smith, "Cytogenetics in Man," *Arch Intern Med* 105, no. 4 (1960): 627–39. See also C. E. Ford et al., "A Sex-Chromosome Anomaly in a Case of Gonadal Dysgenesis (Turner's Syndrome)" *Lancet* 273, no. 7075 (April 4, 1959): 711–13; Patricia A. Jacobs and John Anderson Strong, "A Case of Human Intersexuality Having a Possible XXY Sex-Determining Mechanism," *Nature* 183, no. 4657 (1959): 302–3.

68. Bernard Zuger, "Gender Role Determination: A Critical Review of the Evidence from Hermaphroditism," *Psychosom Med* 32, no. 5 (1970): 449–63; quotation is from p. 449.

69. John Money, "Critique of 'Gender Role Determination: A Critical Review of the Evidence from Hermaphroditism,' by B. Zuger," *Psychosom Med* 32, no. 5 (1970): 463–65; quotation is from p. 463.

70. Money, 465.

71. Bernard Zuger, "Rebuttal," *Psychosom Med* 32, no. 5 (September–October 1970): 465–67, esp. 465.

72. Zuger, 467.

73. Milton Diamond, "A Critical Evaluation of the Ontogeny of Human Sexual Behavior," *Q Rev Biol* 40, no. 2 (1965): 147–75; Milton Diamond, "Genetic-Endocrine Interactions and Human Psychosexuality," *Perspectives in Reproduction and Sexual Behavior* (1968): 417–43.

74. Diamond, "Critical Evaluation," 169.

75. Charles H. Phoenix et al., "Organizing Action of Prenatally Administered Testosterone Propionate on the Tissues Mediating Mating Behavior in the Female Guinea Pig," *Endocrinology* 65 (1959): 369–82. Organization theory (OT) would become one of the most dominant theories over the next decades, and as I show in chapter 7, Money became an important figure in the application of this theory to humans. For a history of OT, see Rebecca M. Jordan-Young, *Brain Storm: The Flaws in the Science of Sex Differences* (Cambridge, MA: Harvard University Press, 2010). Milton Diamond would over time become Money's most vocal opponent, especially in the case of sex reassignment in the Joan/John case, which I also discuss in chapter 7. Zuger stressed that recent studies of Money and his associates showed "the possible masculinizing of the brains of early fetuses by androgens in some mothers with the adrenogenital syndrome." Zuger, "Gender Role Determination," 451. Zuger is referring here to Anke A. Ehrhardt, Ralph Epstein, and John Money, "Fetal Androgens and Female Gender Identity in the Early-Treated Adrenogenital Syndrome," *Johns Hopkins Med J* 122, no. 3 (1968): 160; Anke A. Ehrhardt, Kathryn Evers, and John Money, "Influence of Androgen and Some Aspects of Sexually Dimorphic Behavior in Women with the Late-Treated Adrenogenital Syndrome," *Johns Hopkins Med J* 123, no. 3 (1968): 115–22.

76. Money, "Critique of 'Gender Role Determination,'" 464.

77. Zuger, "Gender Role Determination," 460. Zuger also stressed that even though Money still insisted that any change of sex after the age of about two years was hazardous, Wilkins, "however, in the latest edition of his book, recommended that sex change in the adrenogenital syndrome be considered even in later childhood and early adulthood"; Zuger, 462. As we have seen, after cortisone became available Wilkins recommended raising as girls those girls whose CAH had been diagnosed in their infancy. Initially, he had advised against changing the sex of the girls who had already been raised as boys and recommended keeping them in the male sex. By the 1965 edition of the textbook, Wilkins wrote that "with cortisone therapy such completely femi-nine development and fertility can be assured that we believe now that the advisability of a change of sex should be considered even in later childhood or early adult life. This should be undertaken only after prolonged psychological consultations in order to obtain complete assurance that both the patient and the parents truly desire it." This change was underwritten by the notion that girls with CAH who were treated with cortisone could get pregnant, some-thing Wilkins had initially not believed to be possible; see Wilkins, *Diagnosis and Treatment of Endocrine Disorders in Childhood and Adolescence*, 3rd ed., 420.
78. Zuger, "Gender Role Determination," 458–59.
79. Money, "Critique of 'Gender Role Determination,'" 464.
80. See Fausto-Sterling, *Sexing the Body*, 78.

JANET

Epigraph: Geoffrey H. Bourne, *An Introduction to Medical History and Case Taking* (Edinburgh: E. and S. Livingstone, 1931), 18; cited in Armstrong, "Patient's View," 738.

1. Patient record, 8A4YN (Janet), HLH.
2. Arthur Kleinman, *Writing at the Margin: Discourse between Anthropology and Medicine* (Berkeley: University of California Press, 1995), 32; emphasis in the orginal.
3. For a description and images of such devices, see for example Reynolds, "Metabolism Bed."
4. On the use of dilators, see my discussion in chapter 5. See also Karkazis, *Fixing Sex*, 223–24; Kessler, *Lessons from the Intersexed*, 49, 59, 63–64.
5. See Berg and Harterink, "Embodying the Patient."

CHAPTER SEVEN

1. Joanne Meyerowitz, "A History of 'Gender,'" *Am Hist Rev* 113, no. 5 (2008): 1346–56, esp. 1354.
2. In 1963, Stoller and his colleague Ralph Greenson first used his version of gender at the International Psychoanalytic Congress in Sweden, and in

1964 they published their talk in the *International Journal of Psychoanalysis*; see Robert J. Stoller, "Gender-Role Change in Intersexed Patients," *JAMA* 188 (1964): 684–85; Robert J. Stoller, "A Contribution to the Study of Gender Identity," *Int J Psychoanal* 45 (1964): 220–26; Robert J. Stoller, "A Further Contribution to the Study of Gender Identity," *Int J Psychoanal* 49 (1968): 364. See also Robert J. Stoller, *Sex and Gender: On the Development of Masculinity and Femininity* (New York: Science House, 1968).

3. Stoller, "Contribution to the Study of Gender Identity," 220.
4. Money, Hampson, and Hampson, "An Examination"; Money, Hampson, and Hampson, "Imprinting."
5. Stoller, "Contribution to the Study of Gender Identity," 220. Further citations of this work are given in the text.
6. Pseudonym used by Harold Garfinkel in 1967; see Garfinkel, "Passing." See also Hausman, *Changing Sex*, 1–8.
7. Garfinkel, "Passing," 60.
8. Stoller, "Contribution to the Study of Gender Identity," 225.
9. Garfinkel, "Passing," 61.
10. See also Germon, *Gender*, 74–76.
11. Stoller, "Further Contribution to the Study of Gender Identity," 366. Further citations of this work are given in the text.
12. See Grant, *Raising Baby by the Book*; Plant, "Repeal of Mother Love"; Plant, *Mom*; Vicedo, "Cold War Emotions."
13. Stoller, "Contribution to the Study of Gender Identity," 225.
14. Stoller, "Further Contribution to the Study of Gender Identity," 366n4.
15. Stoller, "Contribution to the Study of Gender Identity," 225.
16. Marcel Heiman, "Comment on Dr Stoller's Paper," *Int J Psychoanal* 49 (1968): 368.
17. Stoller, *Sex and Gender*. See Meyerowitz, "History of 'Gender,'" 1354.
18. Germon, *Gender*, 66.
19. Stoller, "Contribution to the Study of Gender Identity," 220.
20. See Germon, *Gender*, 66.
21. Germon, 63–82.
22. See Joanne Meyerowitz, "Sex Change and the Popular Press: Historical Notes on Transsexuality in the United States, 1930–1955," *GLQ: A Journal of Lesbian and Gay Studies* 4, no. 2 (1998): 159–87; Meyerowitz, *How Sex Changed*.
23. On terminology, see Harry Benjamin, "Clinical Aspects of Transsexualism in the Male and Female," *Am J Psychother* 18, no. 3 (1964): 458–69. On "eonism," see Havelock Ellis, *Studies in the Psychology of Sex*, vol. 7, *Eonism and Other Supplementary Studies* (Philadelphia: F. A. Davis, 1928). On "contrasexism," see John Money, "Hermaphroditism," in *The Encyclopedia of Sexual Behavior*, ed. Albert Ellis and Albert Abarbanel (New York: Hawthorn Books, 1961), 472–84.

24. David O. Cauldwell, "Psychopathia Transexualis," *Sexology* 16 (1949): 274–80; quotations are from p. 274.
25. Cauldwell, 280.
26. Albert Ellis was one of the cofounders and first president of the Society for the Scientific Study of Sex (1958–60). John Money was its president from 1972 to 1974. Leah Cahan Schaefer and Connie Christine Wheeler, "Harry Benjamin's First Ten Cases (1938–1953): A Clinical Historical Note," *Arch Sex Behav* 24, no. 1 (1995): 73–93, esp. 74.
27. Harry Benjamin gave a talk on these patients before the Association for the Advancement of Psychotherapy on December 18, 1953, which published in 1954 and republished in 1961. Harry Benjamin, "Transsexualism and Transvestism—a Symposium: Transsexualism and Transvestism as Psycho-somatic and Somato-Psychic Syndromes," *Am J Psychother* 8, no. 2 (1954): 219–30.
28. Benjamin, "Clinical Aspects of Transsexualism."
29. Benjamin, 462. Richard Green, who worked with all three, described them as the "three sexological kings"; see Richard Green, "The Three Kings: Harry Benjamin, John Money, Robert Stoller," *Arch Sex Behav* 38, no. 4 (2009): 610–13, esp. 610.
30. Benjamin, "Clinical Aspects of Transsexualism," 468–69.
31. Benjamin, 469.
32. Harry Benjamin, *The Transsexual Phenomenon* (New York: Julian Press, 1966), 18n9.
33. Benjamin, 21–24.
34. See Meyerowitz, *How Sex Changed*, 209–11. On trans activism, see Susan Stryker, *Transgender History*, Seal Studies (Berkeley, CA: Seal Press, 2008; distributed by Publishers Group West).
35. Money, "Hermaphroditism."
36. John Money and Florence Schwartz, "Public Opinion and Social Issues in Transsexualism: A Case Study in Medical Sociology," in *Transsexualism and Sex Reassignment*, ed. Richard Green and John Money (Baltimore: Johns Hopkins University Press, 1969), 255.
37. Memorandum, December 9, 1965, box 503600, JMC.
38. Money and Schwartz, "Public Opinion and Social Issues," 255. The staff of the Gender Identity Committee included Dr. Dietrich P. Blumer, assistant professor of psychiatry; Dr. Milton T. Edgerton, professor and plastic-surgeon-in-charge; Dr. Howard W. Jones Jr., associate professor of gynecology and obstetrics; Dr. Norman J. Knorr, assistant professor of psychiatry and plastic surgery; Dr. Claude J. Migeon, associate professor of pediatrics; Dr. Eugene Mater, professor of psychiatry; Dr. Horst K. Schirmer, associate professor of urology; and M. C. Frank Velkas, a psychologist and associate of John Money's; see Johns Hopkins University, Office of Institutional Public Relations, "Statement of the Establishment of a Clinic for Transsexuals at

the Johns Hopkins Medical Institutions," November 21, 1966, box 503600, JMC.

39. Letter to John Money, June 29, 1966, box 503600, JMC.

40. Money and Schwartz, "Public Opinion and Social Issues," 257. See Meyerowitz, *How Sex Changed*, 220.

41. Johns Hopkins University, Office of Institutional Public Relations, "Statement of the Establishment of a Clinic for Transsexuals at the Johns Hopkins Medical Institutions," November 21, 1966, box 503600, JMC.

42. Johns Hopkins University, Office of Institutional Public Relations, "Statement of the Establishment of a Clinic."

43. On Jorgensen, see Joanne Meyerowitz, "Transforming Sex: Christine Jorgensen in the Postwar Us," *OAH Magazine of History* 20, no. 2 (2006): 16–20.

44. Jen Manion, "Transgender Representations, Identities, and Communities," in *The Oxford Handbook of American Women's and Gender History*, ed. Ellen Hartigan-O'Connor and Lisa G. Materson (New York: Oxford University Press, 2018), 311–31; quotation is from p. 324.

45. Money and Schwartz, "Public Opinion and Social Issues," 255–56.

46. Cited in Money and Schwartz, 256.

47. Letter to Hoopes, September 19, 1966, box 503600, JMC.

48. Letter to Hoopes.

49. Letter to John Money, November 10, 1966, box 503600, JMC.

50. Memorandum, November 11 1966, box 503600, JMC.

51. Johns Hopkins University, Office of Institutional Public Relations, "Statement of the Establishment of a Clinic for Transsexuals at the Johns Hopkins Medical Institutions," November 21, 1966, box 503600, JMC.

52. Johns Hopkins University, Office of Institutional Public Relations, "Statement of the Establishment of a Clinic."

53. Johns Hopkins University, Office of Institutional Public Relations, "Statement of the Establishment of a Clinic."

54. Money and Schwartz, "Public Opinion and Social Issues," 257.

55. Thomas Buckley By, "A Changing of Sex by Surgery Begun at Johns Hopkins: Johns Hopkins Becomes First U.S. Hospital to Undertake Program of Sex Change through Surgery," *New York Times*, November 21, 1966.

56. By, "Changing of Sex."

57. "A Body to Match the Mind," *Time*, December 22, 1966, 52–57.

58. See Meyerowitz, *How Sex Changed*, 222. The latter was headed by a former member of the Hopkins team: John Hampson.

59. See C. Siotos et al., "Origins of Gender Affirmation Surgery: The History of the First Gender Identity Clinic in the United States at Johns Hopkins," *Ann Plast Surg* 83, no. 2 (August 2019): 132–36. On the Hopkins Gender Identity Clinic closure, see Jane E. Brody, "Benefits of Transsexual Surgery Disputed as Leading Hospital Halts the Procedure," *New York Times*, October 2, 1979.

60. Money and Schwartz, "Public Opinion and Social Issues," 255. Jules Gill-Peterson discusses G. L.'s case at length to argue that the part trans children played in the establishment of these clinics has been overlooked; see Jules Gill-Peterson, *Histories of the Transgender Child* (Minneapolis: University of Minnesota Press, 2018), 130–33.

61. Daniel St. Albin Greene, "What Makes a Person Want to Switch Sexes?," *National Observer* (USA), October 16, 1976.

62. *Dog Day Afternoon* (1975) was directed by Sidney Lumet. In the film, the main character, Sonny Wortzik, played by Al Pacino, robs a bank to help his transgender partner pay for her surgery. *The Rocky Horror Picture Show* (1975) was directed by Jim Sharman. Tim Curry plays Dr. Frank N. Furter, a self-proclaimed "sweet transvestite from Transsexual, Transylvania." The 1970 film *Myra Breckinridge*, based on a 1968 novel of the same name by Gore Vidal, tells the story of Myra, a transgender woman who undergoes a "sex change operation." The main character was played by Raquel Welch.

63. See J. P. Scott, "Obituary: William C. Young 1899–1965," *Anim Behav* 15, no. 1 (1967): 205.

64. See Moore and Price, "Gonad Hormone Functions."

65. See Edward W. Dempsey, Roy Hertz, and William C. Young, "The Experimental Induction of Oestrus (Sexual Receptivity) in the Normal and Ovariectomized Guinea Pig," *Am J Physiol* 116 (1936): 201–9; Hugh I. Myers, William C. Young, and Edward W. Dempsey, "Graafian Follicle Development throughout the Reproductive Cycle in the Guinea Pig, with Especial Reference to Changes during Oestrus (Sexual Receptivity)," *Anat Rec* 65, no. 4 (1936): 381–401; Vincent J. Collins et al., "Quantitative Studies of Experimentally Induced Sexual Receptivity in the Spayed Guinea-Pig," *Endocrinology* 23, no. 2 (1938): 188–96. On Young, see Robert W. Goy, "Biography: William Caldwell Young," *Anat Rec* 157, no. 1 (1967): 3–11. On his approach to behavior, see Frank Ambrose Beach, "Historical Origins of Modern Research on Hormones and Behavior," *Horm Behav* 15, no. 4 (1981): 325–76, esp. 337.

66. Phoenix et al., "Organizing Action of Prenatally Administered Testosterone Propionate."

67. Researchers used animal experiments to prove this hypothesis. They measured gendered behavior by observing the sexual behavior of guinea pigs that had been prenatally masculinized. There are a lot of problems with this assumption of sexual behavior as an indicator of gender, not least of which is its disregard of the complexity of animal mating behavior (not to mention that of humans). For an analysis of the acceptance and extensions of OT, see Marianne van den Wijngaard, *Reinventing the Sexes: Feminism and Biomedical Construction of Femininity and Masculinity, 1959–1985* (Amsterdam: Uitgeverij Eburon, 1991); Jordan-Young, *Brain Storm*.

68. Hampson, "Human Hermaphroditism."

69. John L. Hampson and Joan G. Hampson, "The Ontogenesis of Sexual Behavior in Man," in *Sex and Internal Secretions*, ed. Edgar Allen and William C. Young (Baltimore: Williams and Wilkins, 1961), 1401–32.

70. See Jordan-Young, *Brain Storm*, 28–29. See also Karkazis, *Fixing Sex*, 67–68.

71. Jordan-Young, *Brain Storm*, 30.

72. John Money, "Influence of Hormones on Sexual Behavior," *Annu Rev Med* 16, no. 1 (1965): 67–82; quotation is from p. 69. See also Jordan-Young, *Brain Storm*, 30–31.

73. Money, "Influence of Hormones," 69.

74. See for example John Money, Anke A. Ehrhardt, and D. N. Masica, "Fetal Feminization Induced by Androgen Insensitivity in the Testicular Feminizing Syndrome: Effect on Marriage and Maternalism," *Johns Hopkins Med Jl* 123, no. 3 (1968): 105–14.

75. Money, "Influence of Hormones," 69–70.

76. Money, 70. See also Jordan-Young, *Brain Storm*, 31.

77. Later renamed androgen insensitivity syndrome.

78. Money, "Influence of Hormones," 70.

79. Jordan-Young, *Brain Storm*, 32ff. The acceptance and extension of the OT to human behavior also faced opposition, most famously by the psychologist Frank A. Beach, chair of the Psychology Department at the University of California, Berkeley, from 1958 to 1978. Beach studied the effects of hormones on animal behavior, and in 1971 he penned a critical (and humorous) article on the methodological faults and assumptions of OT experiments; see Frank Ambrose Beach, "Hormonal Factors Controlling the Differentiation, Development and Display of Copulatory Behavior in the Ramstergig and Related Species," in *Biopsychology of Development*, ed. Edith Tobach and Matthew H. Adamson (New York: Academic Press, 1971), 249–96.

80. Jordan-Young, *Brain Storm*, 32.

81. See Ehrhardt, Evers, and Money, "Influence of Androgen."

82. Jordan-Young, *Brain Storm*, 33. See Anke A. Ehrhardt and John Money, "Progestin Induced Hermaphroditism: IQ and Psychosexual Identity in a Study of Ten Girls," *J Sex Res* 3, no. 1 (1967): 83–100.

83. Money, Ehrhardt, and Masica, "Fetal Feminization."

84. Jordan-Young, *Brain Storm*, 33.

85. Money and Ehrhardt, *Man and Woman, Boy and Girl*, back cover.

86. See John Money, "This Week's Citation Classic," in *Current Contents*, no. 11 (March 16, 1987), 12.

87. Money and Ehrhardt, *Man and Woman, Boy and Girl*, back cover.

88. See Milam, *Creatures of Cain*; Wijngaard, *Reinventing the Sexes*.

89. Money and Ehrhardt, *Man and Woman, Boy and Girl*, 98–101.

90. On OT and masculine and feminine sexuality, see Jordan-Young, *Brain Storm*, 114–18.

91. Money and Ehrhardt, *Man and Woman, Boy and Girl*, 102.

92. Money and Ehrhardt, 103. See also Jordan-Young, *Brain Storm*, 34–35.

93. Money and Ehrhardt, *Man and Woman, Boy and Girl*, 118. See also John Money, "Ablatio Penis: Normal Male Infant Sex-Reassigned as a Girl," *Arch Sex Behav* 4, no. 1 (1975): 65–71.

94. The sexologist Milton Diamond, who had long been critical of John Money's work, published an article with Keith Sigmundson to expose that the child's reassignment from male to female had failed; Milton Diamond and H. Keith Sigmundson, "Sex Reassignment at Birth: Long-Term Review and Clinical Implications," *Arch Pediatr Adolesc Med* 151, no. 3 (1997): 298–304.

95. Bernice L. Hausman, "Do Boys Have to Be Boys? Gender, Narrativity, and the John/Joan Case," *NWSA Journal* 12, no. 3 (2000): 114–38, esp. 121.

96. Money and Ehrhardt, *Man and Woman, Boy and Girl*, 118. Further citations of this work are given in the text.

97. Money, "Ablatio Penis," 66. A great part of his case description was simply adapted from Money and Ehrhardt, *Man and Woman, Boy and Girl*.

98. Money, "Ablatio Penis," 71.

99. See Diamond and Sigmundson, "Sex Reassignment at Birth."

100. In 1997, *Rolling Stone* published the journalist John Colapinto's article on David Reimer and John Money, "The True Story of John/Joan," which Colapinto followed with a book-length account two years later. His narrative privileged the idea of a true biological sex that could not be overwritten by Money's experimentations; see John Colapinto, "The True Story of John/Joan," *Rolling Stone*, December 11, 1997; Colapinto, *As Nature Made Him*. Jeffrey Eugenides also modeled the psychologist in his novel *Middlesex* after John Money; see Eugenides, *Middlesex*.

101. See Hausman, "Do Boys Have to Be Boys?"; Judith Butler, "Doing Justice to Someone: Sex Reassignment and Allegories of Transsexuality," *GLQ: A Journal of Lesbian and Gay Studies* 7, no. 4 (2001): 621–36; Sharon E. Preves, "Sexing the Intersexed: An Analysis of Sociocultural Responses to Intersexuality," *Signs* 27, no. 2 (2002): 523–56.

102. News reports often claimed that this was an important case for feminists in the nurture-over-nature debate. I have yet to find much published feminist discussion of this case before 1983. Most notable is a critical evaluation of the gendered double standard applied; see Margrit Eichler, "Sex Change Operations: The Last Bulwark of the Double Standard," in *Feminist Frontiers: Rethinking Sex, Gender, and Society*, ed. Verta A. Taylor and Laurel Richardson (Reading, MA: Addison-Wesley, 1983), 106–15.

103. For Money's stance against a supposedly antisex feminist movement, see John Money, *The Destroying Angel: Sex, Fitness and Food in the Legacy of Degeneracy Theory; Graham Crackers, Kellogg's Corn Flakes and American Health History* (Buffalo, NY: Prometheus Books, 1985).

104. Jordan-Young, *Brain Storm*, 35–36.

105. Money and Ehrhardt, *Man and Woman, Boy and Girl*, 121.

106. Money and Ehrhardt, 122.

107. See for example Money's talk at the 1963 symposium "The Potential of Woman" at the University of California, San Francisco, Medical Center: John Money, "Developmental Differentiation of Femininity and Masculinity Compared," in *Man and Civilization: The Potential of Woman—a Symposium*, ed. Seymour M. Farber and Roger H. L. Wilson (New York: McGraw-Hill, 1963), 51–65.

108. "The Central Program of the 1972 AAAS Annual Meeting," *Science* 178, no. 4063 (1972): 886–914.

109. "Biological Imperatives," *Time*, January 8, 1973, 34.

110. "Biological Imperatives," 34.

111. By the end of the 1960s, the *Berkeley Barb* had a circulation of between seventy thousand and ninety thousand copies per week; see Sinead McEneaney, "Sex and the Radical Imagination in the *Berkeley Barb* and the *San Francisco Oracle*," *Radical Americas* 3, no. 16 (2018): 1–19.

112. Jean Baker Miller, "Psychoanalysis, Patriarchy, and Power: One Viewpoint on Women's Goals and Needs," *Chrysalis, a Magazine of Women's Culture*, no. 2 (February 1, 1977): 19–25; quotations are from p. 20. As references, Miller listed Stoller and Money and Ehrhardt. Germon discusses the relatively belated uptake of gender by feminist psychologists in the late 1970s. For a discussion of the work of Nancy Chodorow, Dorothy Dinnerstein, Dorothy Ullian, and Rhoda Unger, see Germon, *Gender*, 97–101.

113. See Judy Tzu-Chun Wu, "US Feminisms and Their Global Connections," in *The Oxford Handbook of American Women's and Gender History*, ed. Ellen Hartigan-O'Connor and Lisa G. Materson (New York: Oxford University Press, 2018), 488; Becky Thompson, "Multiracial Feminism: Recasting the Chronology of Second Wave Feminism," *Feminist Studies* 28, no. 2 (2002): 337–60; Estelle B. Freedman, *No Turning Back: The History of Feminism and the Future of Women* (New York: Ballantine Books, 2002).

114. By the 1990s, feminists had increasingly realized that the sex/gender split had relegated "sex" to biology and nature, making it an ahistorical and essential category. Yet, as historians and feminist scholars have shown, sex is as much made/constructed as gender is. For early challenges to the naturalness of "sex," see Catherine Gallagher and Thomas Walter Laqueur, eds., *The Making of the Modern Body: Sexuality and Society in the Nineteenth Century* (Berkeley: University of California Press, 1987); Laqueur, *Making Sex*; Schiebinger, *Nature's Body*; Judith Butler, *Bodies That Matter: On the Discursive Limits of "Sex"* (New York: Routledge, 1993); Oudshoorn, *Beyond the Natural Body*.

115. Kate Millett, *Sexual Politics* (Garden City, NY: Doubleday, 1970), 29.

116. On the shift from *sex* to *gender* in titles of academic publications, see David Haig, "The Inexorable Rise of Gender and the Decline of Sex: Social Change in Academic Titles, 1945–2001," *Arch Sex Behav* 33, no. 2 (2004): 87–96. On the slow uptake of gender as an idea in the 1970s, see chap. 3 in Germon, *Gender*.

117. Jessie Bernard, *Women and the Public Interest* (Piscataway, NJ: Transaction, 1971), 16. Further citations of this work are given in the text.
118. Bernard also cites Mead as one of the thinkers who pointed out the cultural contents of gender in her work.
119. Germon, *Gender*, 95.
120. Ann Oakley, *Sex, Gender and Society*, Towards a New Society (London: Maurice Temple Smith, 1972), 95.
121. Oakley, 50.
122. Germon, *Gender*, 95. See also David A. Rubin, "'An Unnamed Blank That Craved a Name': A Genealogy of Intersex as Gender," *Signs* 37, no. 4 (2012): 883–908.
123. Robin Morgan, ed., *Sisterhood Is Powerful: An Anthology of Writings from the Women's Liberation Movement* (New York: Random House, 1970), xvii.
124. Jo Freeman, ed., *Women: A Feminist Perspective* (Palo Alto, CA: Mayfield, 1975).
125. Lenore J. Weitzman, "Sex-Role Socialization," in *Women: A Feminist Perspective*, ed. Jo Freeman (Palo Alto, CA: Mayfield, 1975), 105–44; quotation is from p. 107. Weitzman noted that the article had originally been written between 1970 and 1971.
126. Mead, *Coming of Age in Samoa*; Mead, *Sex and Temperament*.
127. Mead was assistant curator of ethnology at the American Museum of Natural History from 1926 to 1942, promoted in 1942 to the rank of associate curator, and in 1964 to curator until she retired in 1969; see David Hurst Thomas, "Margaret Mead as a Museum Anthropologist," *American Anthropologist* 82, no. 2 (1980): 354–61, esp. 354.
128. The anthropologist Paul Shankman provides an in-depth analysis of Mead's shifting position as a *Redbook* columnist in Paul Shankman, "The Public Anthropology of Margaret Mead: *Redbook*, Women's Issues, and the 1960s," *Current Anthropology* 59, no. 1 (2018): 55–73. Further citations of this work are given in the text.
129. Margaret Mead, "What Shall We Tell Our Children?," *Redbook*, June 1970, 35.
130. Margaret Mead, "Women: A Time for Change," *Redbook*, March 1970, 62. Further citations of this work are given in the text.
131. Through the 1970s, Stoller and the psychiatrist Richard Greene studied "feminine boys" or "sissies" and used behavior modification tactics to transform them into gender-conforming men. See Phyllis Burke, *Gender Shock: Exploding the Myths of Male and Female* (New York: Anchor Books, 1996).
132. Meyerowitz, "History of 'Gender,'" 1354.
133. "Biological Imperatives," 34.
134. Edward T. Adelson, MD, and Society of Medical Psychoanalysts, eds., *Sexuality and Psychoanalysis* (New York: Brunner / Mazel, 1975).
135. John Money, "Nativism versus Culturalism in Gender-Identity Differentiation," in *Society of Medical Psychoanalysts*, ed. Edward T. Adelson, MD, and Society of Medical Psychoanalysts (New York: Brunner / Mazel, 1975), 61.

136. Money, 62.

137. Janice G. Raymond, "Transsexualism: The Ultimate Homage to Sex-Role Power," *Chrysalis, a Magazine of Women's Culture*, no. 3 (March 1, 1977): 11–24.

138. Another early critique of Money came from the British anthropologist Marilyn Strathern; see Barbara Bloom Lloyd and John Archer, *Exploring Sex Differences* (London: Academic Press, 1976). Barbara Fried also criticized Money in Barbara R. Fried, Mary Sue Henifin, and Ruth Hubbard, *Women Look at Biology Looking at Women: A Collection of Feminist Critiques* (Boston: Hall, 1979). See Germon, *Gender*, 112–13.

139. Raymond, "Transsexualism," 14. Raymond referred to Money's earlier work in her footnotes but cited Money and Ehrhardt, *Man and Woman, Boy and Girl*. In addition, she lambasted Robert Stoller for describing mothers as the main source of problems in gender identity development in his writings about transsexuality.

140. Raymond deepened her feminist critique of the conception of transsexuality as a tool for reinforcing gender stereotypes in her 1979 book; see Janice G. Raymond, *The Transsexual Empire: The Making of the She-Male* (Boston: Beacon Press, 1979). At the time, it was positively reviewed, for example by the psychiatrist Thomas Szasz, author of *The Myth of Mental Illness: Foundations of a Theory of Personal Conduct* (1961); see Thomas Szasz, "Male and Female Created He Them: Transsexual," *New York Times*, June 10, 1979. As Susan Stryker argues, Raymond's book played an important role in the political history of transgender; see Stryker, *Transgender History*, 106.

141. Finn Enke, "Collective Memory and the Transfeminist 1970s: Toward a Less Plausible History," *TSQ: Transgender Studies Quarterly* 5, no. 1 (2018): 9–29; quotation is from p. 12. See also Cristan Williams, "Radical Inclusion: Recounting the Trans Inclusive History of Radical Feminism," *Transgender Studies Quarterly* 3, nos. 1–2 (2016): 254–58. For an account of trans-positive second-wave feminisms, see Stryker, *Transgender History*, 108–9. The feminist Andrea Dworkin, for example, took a different stance from Raymond on trans women; see Andrea Dworkin, *Woman Hating* (New York: Dutton, 1974), 186. Stryker also described how, when the feminist Robin Morgan gave the keynote speech at the West Coast Lesbian Conference in 1973 in which she criticized Beth Elliott, a trans lesbian performer who was on the organizing committee, the *Lesbian Tide* publisher Jeanne Cordova and the lesbian activist the Reverend Freda Smith of Sacramento spoke out in support of Elliott. Another critic of Morgan was the socialist feminist Shulamite Firestone. See Stryker, *Transgender History*, 103–5.

142. Laud Humphreys, *Out of the Closets: The Sociology of Homosexual Liberation*, A Spectrum Book, S-288 (Englewood Cliffs, NJ: Prentice-Hall, 1972), 164.

143. Jim Green, "Gender-Fuck Is the Name of the Game," *Berkeley (California) Barb*, May 25–31, 1973, 6.

144. Moon, "Crazy Ladies," *Lavender Woman*, March 1, 1973, 12.

145. Robbie, "Cosmic Light in 'Lanta,'" *Great Speckled Bird* (Atlanta), November 5, 1973, 23.
146. "Freaking Them Out in the Windy City," *Philadelphia Gay News*, March 1, 1976, B2.
147. Ruth Batchelor, "The Reigning Queens of the Sunset Strip," *Los Angeles Free Press*, October 24–30, 1975, 12.
148. Gayle Rubin, "The Traffic in Women: Notes on the 'Political Economy' of Sex," in *Toward an Anthropology of Women* (New York: Monthly Review Press, 1975), 159. Rubin started working on the essay in 1969 and first published it in 1974. Gayle Rubin and Judith Butler, "Sexual Traffic," *A Journal of Feminist Cultural Studies* 6, no. 2 (1994), 62–99; Gayle S. Rubin, *Deviations: A Gayle Rubin Reader* (Durham, NC: Duke University Press, 2011).
149. Rubin, "Traffic in Women," 167–68.
150. Rubin and Butler, "Sexual Traffic," 72.
151. Personal communication with Gayle Rubin, July 31, 2020.

EPILOGUE

Epigraphs: Denise Riley, *"Am I That Name?": Feminism and the Category of "Women" in History, Language, Discourse, Society* (Houndmills, UK: Macmillan Press, 1988), 6; Joan Wallach Scott, "Gender: Still a Useful Category of Analysis?," *Diogenes* 57, no. 1 (2010): 7–14; quotation is from p. 12.

1. The only dissent came from geneticists such as Milton Diamond, who objected to Money's culturalist approach and focus on genitals as signifier of sex and who argued that a child with XY chromosomes should never be assigned as female, even if he did not have a penis. Money and his supporters would have argued that a child would find it hard to develop a convincing male gender role without a penis.
2. Suzanne J. Kessler, "The Medical Construction of Gender: Case Management of Intersexed Infants," *Signs* 16, no. 1 (1990): 3–26; quotations are from p. 7n9. See also Kessler's book *Lessons from the Intersexed*.
3. See Jordan-Young, *Brain Storm*.
4. Fausto-Sterling, "The Five Sexes"; Fausto-Sterling, "How Many Sexes Are There?"
5. Cheryl Chase, "Letters from Readers," *Sciences*, July/August 1993, 3.
6. Dreger, *Hermaphrodites*. Alice Domurat Dreger, *Intersex in the Age of Ethics* (Hagerstown, MD: University Publishing Group, 1999); Alice D. Dreger, "Intersex and Human Rights: The Long View," in *Ethics and Intersex*, ed. Sharon E. Sytsma (Dordrecht: Springer Science, 2006), 73–86. On the ethics of intersex case management, see also Feder, *Making Sense of Intersex*.
7. Dreger was also a member and chair of the Intersex Society of North America for nine years, where she served as chair and president of the board for six years, chair of the Fundraising Committee for one year, and

the first Director of Medical Education. On this alliance, see for example Alice Domurat Dreger and M. April Herndon, "Progress and Politics in the Intersex Rights Movement: Feminist Theory in Action," *GLQ: A Journal of Lesbian and Gay Studies* 15, no. 2 (2009): 199–224.

8. In 2019, the European Parliament passed a resolution calling on all member states to end genital surgeries. Elizabeth Reis notes that congenital adrenal hyperplasia has become a notable exception in this rejection of surgery. The CARES Foundation, a large parent organization dedicated to the treatment and support of children with CAH, considers it a separate condition and rejects subsuming it under the differences of sex development/intersex umbrella. CARES also opposes a ban on early nonconsensual genital surgery, maintaining that these interventions are "medically necessary" or, if not necessary in the strictest sense, then at least beneficial and desirable. This definition of medical necessity includes psychological health. See Elizabeth Reis, *Bodies in Doubt*, 2nd ed. (Baltimore: Johns Hopkins University Press, 2021).

9. As of this writing, two institutions have decided to stop medically unnecessary surgeries on children born with intersex traits: the Ann and Robert H. Lurie Children's Hospital, Chicago (2018), and the Boston Children's Hospital (2020).

10. Betty Friedan, *The Feminine Mystique* (New York: W. W. Norton, 1963).

11. This idea of a relatively uniform female gender in opposition to a male gender and its underlying bias was criticized by Elizabeth Spelman among others in the late 1980s; see Elizabeth V. Spelman, *Inessential Woman: Problems of Exclusion in Feminist Thought* (Boston: Beacon Press, 1988).

12. Since the 1980s, feminist science scholars have analyzed how the concept of gendered hormonal and chromosomal body was shaped by the material conditions and practices of the scientific work as well as cultural assumptions; see for example Oudshoorn, *Beyond the Natural Body*; Richardson, *Sex Itself*. Thomas Laqueur, for example, shows that until the late eighteenth century, female and male sexes were not considered to be distinct categories with specific traits; see Laqueur, *Making Sex*. For a feminist critique of biological sex, see also Fausto-Sterling, *Myths of Gender*; Ruth Hubbard, *The Politics of Women's Biology* (New Brunswick, NJ: Rutgers University Press, 1990); Janice M. Irvine, *Disorders of Desire: Sex and Gender in Modern American Sexology*, Health, Society, and Policy (Philadelphia: Temple University Press, 1990); Janice M. Irvine, "From Difference to Sameness: Gender Ideology in Sexual Science," *J Sex Res* 27, no. 1 (1990): 7–24.

13. Judith Butler, *Gender Trouble: Feminism and the Subversion of Identity*, Thinking Gender (New York: Routledge, 1990), 9–10. Elizabeth Grosz, who differentiates her gender theories from Butler's, also argues that sex is neither fixed nor given; see Elizabeth A. Grosz, *Volatile Bodies: Toward a Corporeal Feminism* (Bloomington: Indiana University Press, 1994).

14. Butler elaborates on this in Butler, *Bodies That Matter*.

NOTES TO PAGES 229–230

15. Fausto-Sterling describes how osteoporosis is related to expectations about gender, women's diet, and their exercise; see Anne Fausto-Sterling, "The Bare Bones of Sex: Part 1—Sex and Gender," *Signs* 30, no. 2 (2005): 1491–1527. For menopause and local biologies, see Margaret Lock and Patricia Kaufert, "Menopause, Local Biologies, and Cultures of Aging," *Am J Hum Biol* 13, no. 4 (2001): 494–504.

16. See C. Riley Snorton, *Black on Both Sides: A Racial History of Trans Identity* (Minneapolis: University of Minnesota Press, 2017); Enke, "Collective Memory and the Transfeminist 1970s"; Gill-Peterson, *Histories of the Transgender Child*; Jesse Bayker, "Before Transsexuality: Transgender Lives and Practices in Nineteenth-Century America" (PhD diss., Rutgers University, 2019); Emily Skidmore, *True Sex: The Lives of Trans Men at the Turn of the Twentieth Century* (New York: New York University Press, 2019); Jen Manion, *Female Husbands: A Trans History* (Cambridge: Cambridge University Press, 2020).

17. In 2010 Scott, revisited her famous question from 1986; see Scott, "Gender: A Useful Category of Historical Analysis"; Scott, "Gender: Still a Useful Category of Analysis?" For a critique of the postmodern shift from women to gender, see for example Laura Lee Downs, "If 'Woman' Is Just an Empty Category, Then Why Am I Afraid to Walk Alone at Night? Identity Politics Meets the Postmodern Subject," *Comparative Studies in Society And History* 35, no. 2 (1993): 414–37.

18. Ellen Hartigan-O'Connor and Lisa G. Materson, eds., *The Oxford Handbook of American Women's and Gender History*, Oxford Handbooks Online (Oxford: Oxford University Press, 2018), 3. Since the 1970s, women's and gender historians have built a field that is more than simply another subfield of history. Rather, as historians Ellen Hartigan-O'Connor and Lisa Materson argue in the case of US gender historians, a focus on women and gender challenges the conventional chronology and national focus of US history.

19. Scott, "Gender: A Useful Category of Historical Analysis."

Bibliography

Abraham, Tara H. "Transcending Disciplines: Scientific Styles in Studies of the Brain in Mid-Twentieth Century America." *Studies in History and Philosophy of Science Part C: Studies in History and Philosophy of Biological and Biomedical Sciences* 43, no. 2 (2012): 552–68.

Adelson, Edward T., MD, ed., and Society of Medical Psychoanalysts. *Sexuality and Psychoanalysis*. [Conference papers.] New York: Brunner / Mazel, 1975.

Allport, Gordon W. *Personality: A Psychological Interpretation*. New York: Henry Holt, 1937.

Allport, Gordon W., and Edwin G. Boring. "Psychology and Social Relations at Harvard University." *Am Psychol* 1, no. 4 (1946): 119.

Armstrong, D. "The Patient's View." *Soc Sci Med* 18, no. 9 (1984): 737–44.

Barnett, Henry L., and L. Emmett Holt. *Pediatrics*. 15th ed. New York: Appleton-Century-Crofts, 1972.

———. *Pediatrics*. 14th ed. New York: Appleton-Century-Crofts, 1968.

Barr, Murray L., and Ewart G. Bertram. "A Morphological Distinction between Neurones of the Male and Female, and the Behaviour of the Nucleolar Satellite during Accelerated Nucleoprotein Synthesis." *Nature* 163, no. 4148 (1949): 676–77.

Bartter, F. C., F. Albright, A. P. Forbes, A. Leaf, E. Dempsey, and E. Carroll. "The Effects of Adrenocorticotropic Hormone and Cortisone in the Adrenogenital Syndrome Associated with Congenital Adrenal Hyperplasia: An Attempt to Explain and Correct Its Disordered Hormonal Pattern." *J Clin Investig* 30, no. 3 (March 1951): 237–51.

Bauer, Raymond Augustine. *How the Soviet System Works: Cultural, Psychological, and Social Themes*. Russian Research Center Studies. Cambridge, MA: Harvard University Press, 1956.

Bayer, Ronald. *Homosexuality and American Psychiatry: The Politics of Diagnosis*. New York: Basic Books, 1981.

Bayker, Jesse. "Before Transsexuality: Transgender Lives and Practices in Nineteenth-Century America." PhD diss., Rutgers University, 2019.

Beach, Frank Ambrose. "Historical Origins of Modern Research on Hormones and Behavior." *Horm Behav* 15, no. 4 (1981): 325–76.

———. "Hormonal Factors Controlling the Differentiation, Development and Display of Copulatory Behavior in the Ramstergig and Related Species." In *Biopsychology of Development*, edited by Edith Tobach and Matthew H. Adamson, 249–96. New York: Academic Press, 1971.

Beatty, Barbara, Emily D. Cahan, and Julia Grant. *When Science Encounters the Child: Education, Parenting, and Child Welfare in 20th-Century America*. Reflective History Series. New York: Teachers College Press, 2006.

Beauvoir, Simone de. *The Second Sex*: Translated and Edited by H. M. Parshley. London: J. Cape, 1953.

Beecher, Henry K. "Ethics and Clinical Research." In *Biomedical Ethics and the Law*, edited by James M. Humber, 215–27. Boston: Springer, 1966.

Benedict, Ruth. "Anthropology and the Abnormal." *J Gen Psychology* 10, no. 1 (January 1, 1934): 59–82.

———. *The Chrysanthemum and the Sword: Patterns of Japanese Culture*. Boston: Houghton Mifflin, 1946.

Benjamin, Harry. "Clinical Aspects of Transsexualism in the Male and Female." *Am J Psychother* 18, no. 3 (1964): 458–69.

———. *The Transsexual Phenomenon*. New York: Julian Press, 1966.

———. "Transsexualism and Transvestism—a Symposium: Transsexualism and Transvestism as Psychosomatic and Somato-Psychic Syndromes." *Am J Psychother* 8, no. 2 (1954): 219–30.

Berg, Marc, and Paul Harterink. "Embodying the Patient: Records and Bodies in Early 20th-Century US Medical Practice." *Body and Society* 10, nos. 2–3 (2004): 13–41.

Bernard, Claude, A. Dastre, and Muséum national d'Histoire naturelle. *Leçons sur les phenomenes de la vie, communs aux animaux et aux vegetaux*. Paris: J.-B. Bailliere, 1878.

Bernard, Jessie. *Women and the Public Interest*. Piscataway, NJ: Transaction, 1971.

Berube, Allan. *Coming Out under Fire: The History of Gay Men and Women in World War Two*. New York: Free Press, 1990.

"Biological Imperatives." *Time*, January 8, 1973, 34.

Blackless, Melanie, Anthony Charuvastra, Amanda Derryck, Anne Fausto-Sterling, Karl Lauzanne, and Ellen Lee. "How Sexually Dimorphic Are We? Review and Synthesis." *Am J Hum Biol* 12, no. 2 (2000): 151–66.

Blizzard, Robert M. "Pediatric Profiles: Lawson Wilkins (1894–1963)." *J Pediatr* 133, no. 4 (1998): 577–80.

Boake, Corwin. "From the Binet-Simon to the Wechsler-Bellevue: Tracing the History of Intelligence Testing." *J Clin Exp Neuropsychol* 24, no. 3 (2002): 383–405.

Boas, Franz. *The Mind of Primitive Man: A Course of Lectures Delivered before the Lowell Institute, Boston, Mass., and the National University of Mexico, 1910–1911*. New York: Macmillan, 1911.

"A Body to Match the Mind." *Time*, December 2, 1966, 52–57.

Borst, Charlotte G. *Catching Babies: The Professionalization of Childbirth, 1870–1920*. Cambridge, MA: Harvard University Press, 1995.

Bourne, Geoffrey H. *An Introduction to Medical History and Case Taking*. Edinburgh: E. and S. Livingstone, 1931. Cited in D. Armstrong, "The Patient's View," 738.

Brandt, Allan M., and Martha Gardner. "The Golden Age of Medicine?" In *Medicine in the Twentieth Century*, edited by Roger Cooter and John V. Pickstone, 21–38. Amsterdam: Harwood Academic, 2000.

Brattain, Michelle. "Race, Racism, and Antiracism: UNESCO and the Politics of Presenting Science to the Postwar Public." *American Historical Review* 112, no. 5 (2007): 1386–1413.

Brody, Eugene B. "Jacob E. Finesinger, M.D." *Am J Psychiatry* 116, no. 4 (1959): 383–84.

Brown-Séquard, Charles-Edouard. "Recherches expérimentales sur la physiologie des capsules surrénales." *Comptes rendus de l'Académie des Sciences* 43 (1856): 422.

Bulloch, W., and J. H. Sequeira. "On the Relation of the Suprarenal Capsules to the Sexual Organs." *Transactions of the Pathological Society of London* 56 (1905): 189–208.

Bullough, Vern L. *Before Stonewall: Activists for Gay and Lesbian Rights in Historical Context*. Haworth Gay and Lesbian Studies. New York: Harrington Park Press, 2002.

Burke, Phyllis. *Gender Shock: Exploding the Myths of Male and Female*. New York: Anchor Books, 1996.

Burnham, John C. "American Medicine's Golden Age: What Happened to It?" *Science* 215, no. 4539 (1982): 1474–79.

Burns, Charles Louis Crawford. *Maladjusted Children*. London: Hollis and Carter, 1955.

Butler, Judith. *Bodies That Matter: On the Discursive Limits of "Sex."* New York: Routledge, 1993.

———. "Doing Justice to Someone: Sex Reassignment and Allegories of Transsexuality." *GLQ: A Journal of Lesbian and Gay Studies* 7, no. 4 (2001): 621–36.

———. *Gender Trouble: Feminism and the Subversion of Identity*. Thinking Gender. New York: Routledge, 1990.

Canaday, Margot. *The Straight State: Sexuality and Citizenship in Twentieth-Century America*. Politics and Society in Twentieth-Century America. Princeton, NJ: Princeton University Press, 2009.

Canguilhem, Georges. *On the Normal and the Pathological*. Translated by Carolyn R. Fawcett. Studies in the History of Modern Science, vol. 3. Dordrecht, Holland: D. Reidel, 1978.

Cantor, David. "Cortisone and the Politics of Drama, 1949–55." In *John V. Pickstone, Hg., Medical Innovations in Historical Perspective*, 165–84. London: Macmillan, 1992.

Cappon, Daniel, Calvin Ezrin, and Patrick Lynes. "Psychosexual Identification (Psychogender) in the Intersexed." *Can Psychiatr Assoc J* 4, no. 2 (1959): 90–106.

Cauldwell, David O. "Psychopathia Transexualis." *Sexology* 16 (1949): 274–80.

"The Central Program of the 1972 AAAS Annual Meeting." *Science* 178, no. 4063 (1972): 886–914.

Chauncey, George. "From Sexual Inversion to Homosexuality: Medicine and the Changing Conceptualization of Female Deviance." *Salmagundi* (1982): 114–46.

Chesser, Eustace, and Zoe Dawe. *The Practice of Sex Education: A Plain Guide for Parents and Teachers*. New York: Roy, 1946.

Childs, B. "Park, Edwards A." *J Pediatr* 125, no. 6 (December 1994): 1009–13.

Clarke, Adele E. "Research Material and Reproductive Science in the United States, 1910–1940." In *Physiology in the American Context, 1850–1940*, 323–50. Baltimore: American Physiological Society, 1987. Distributed by Williams and Wilkins.

Cobb, Stanley. *Borderlands of Psychiatry*. Harvard University Monographs in Medicine and Public Health. Cambridge, MA: Harvard University Press, 1943.

Cohen-Cole, Jamie. *The Open Mind: Cold War Politics and the Sciences of Human Nature*. Chicago: University of Chicago Press, 2014.

Colapinto, John. *As Nature Made Him: The Boy Who Was Raised as a Girl*. New York: HarperCollins, 2000.

———. "The True Story of John/Joan." *Rolling Stone*, December 11, 1997, 54–73+.

Collins, Vincent J., John L. Boiling, Edward W. Dempsey, and William C. Young. "Quantitative Studies of Experimentally Induced Sexual Receptivity in the Spayed Guinea-Pig." *Endocrinology* 23, no. 2 (1938): 188–96.

Comfort, Nathaniel C. *The Science of Human Perfection: How Genes Became the Heart of American Medicine*. New Haven, CT: Yale University Press, 2012.

Comptes-rendus du Sixième congrès international de pédiatrie/Transactions of the Sixth International Congress of Pediatrics (Zurich, July 24–28, 1950).

Condrau, Flurin. "The Patient's View Meets the Clinical Gaze." *Soc Hist Med* 20, no. 3 (2007): 525–40.

Corber, Robert J. *Homosexuality in Cold War America: Resistance and the Crisis of Masculinity*. New Americanists. Durham, NC: Duke University Press, 1997.

Cory, Donald Webster. *The Homosexual in America: A Subjective Approach*. New York: Greenberg, 1951.

Creighton, Sarah M., Julie A. Greenberg, Roen Katrina, and Volcano Del LaGrace. "Intersex Practice, Theory, and Activism: A Roundtable Discussion." *GLQ: A Journal of Lesbian and Gay Studies* 15, no. 2 (2009): 249–60.

Daston, Lorraine, and Peter Galison. *Objectivity*. New York: Zone Books, 2007. Distributed by MIT Press.

De Crecchio, L. "Sopra un caso di apparenze virili in una donna." *Morgagni* 7 (1865): 151–89.

Degler, Carl N. *In Search of Human Nature: The Decline and Revival of Darwinism in American Social Thought*. New York: Oxford University Press, 1991.

D'Emilio, John. *Sexual Politics, Sexual Communities: The Making of a Homosexual Minority in the United States, 1940–1970*. Chicago: University of Chicago Press, 1983.

D'Emilio, John, and Estelle B. Freedman. *Intimate Matters: A History of Sexuality in America*. New York: Harper and Row, 1988.

Dempsey, Edward W., Roy Hertz, and William C. Young. "The Experimental Induction of Oestrus (Sexual Receptivity) in the Normal and Ovariectomized Guinea Pig." *Am J Physiol* 116 (1936): 201–9.

Diamond, Milton. "A Critical Evaluation of the Ontogeny of Human Sexual Behavior." *Q Rev Biol* 40, no. 2 (1965): 147–75.

———. "Genetic-Endocrine Interactions and Human Psychosexuality." *Perspectives in Reproduction and Sexual Behavior* (1968): 417–43.

Diamond, Milton, and H. Keith Sigmundson. "Sex Reassignment at Birth: Long-Term Review and Clinical Implications." *Arch Pediatr Adolesc Med* 151, no. 3 (1997): 298–304.

Dodds, E. C., L. Goldberg, W. Lawson, and R. Robinson. "Oestrogenic Activity of Certain Synthetic Compounds." *Nature* 141, no. 3562 (February 1, 1938): 247–48.

Dorcus, Roy M., and G. Wilson Shaffer. *Textbook of Abnormal Psychology*. 4th ed. Baltimore: Williams and Wilkins, 1950.

Downing, Lisa, Iain Morland, and Nikki Sullivan. *Fuckology: Critical Essays on John Money's Diagnostic Concepts*. Chicago: University of Chicago Press, 2015.

Downs, Laura Lee. "If 'Woman' Is Just an Empty Category, Then Why Am I Afraid to Walk Alone at Night? Identity Politics Meets the Postmodern Subject." *Comparative Studies in Society and History* 35, no. 2 (1993): 414–37.

Dreger, Alice Domurat. *Hermaphrodites and the Medical Invention of Sex*. Cambridge, MA: Harvard University Press, 1998.

———. *Intersex in the Age of Ethics*. Hagerstown, MD: University Publishing Group, 1999.

———. "Intersex and Human Rights: The Long View." In *Ethics and Intersex*, edited by Sharon E. Sytsma, 73–86. Dordrecht: Springer Science, 2006.

Dreger, Alice Domurat, and M. April Herndon. "Progress and Politics in the Intersex Rights Movement: Feminist Theory in Action." *GLQ: A Journal of Lesbian and Gay Studies* 15, no. 2 (2009): 199–224.

Drucker, Donna J. *The Classification of Sex: Alfred Kinsey and the Organization of Knowledge*. Pittsburgh: University of Pittsburgh Press, 2014.

———. "Keying Desire: Alfred Kinsey's Use of Punched-Card Machines for Sex Research." *Journal of the History of Sexuality* 22, no. 1 (2013): 105–25.

———. "The Machines of Sex Research." In *The Machines of Sex Research*, 1–18: Heidelberg: Springer, 2014.

———. "Male Sexuality and Alfred Kinsey's 0–6 Scale: Toward 'a Sound Understanding of the Realities of Sex.'" *J Homosex* 57, no. 9 (2010): 1105–23.

———. "'A Noble Experiment': The Marriage Course at Indiana University, 1938–1940." *Indiana Magazine of History* (2007): 231–64.

Dworkin, Andrea. *Woman Hating*. New York: Dutton, 1974.

Eder, Sandra. "From 'Following the Push of Nature' to 'Restoring One's Proper Sex'—Cortisone and Sex at Johns Hopkins's Pediatric Endocrinology Clinic." *Endeavour* 36, no. 2 (2012): 69–76.

———. "Gender and Cortisone: Clinical Practice and Transatlantic Exchange in the Medical Management of Intersex in the 1950s." *Bull Hist Med* 92, no. 4 (2018): 604–33.

———. "The Volatility of Sex: Intersexuality, Gender and Clinical Practice in the 1950s." *Gender and History* 22, no. 3 (November 2010): 692–707.

Ehrhardt, Anke A., Ralph Epstein, and John Money. "Fetal Androgens and Female Gender Identity in the Early-Treated Adrenogenital Syndrome." *Johns Hopkins Med J* 122, no. 3 (1968): 160.

Ehrhardt, Anke A., Kathryn Evers, and John Money. "Influence of Androgen and Some Aspects of Sexually Dimorphic Behavior in Women with the Late-Treated Andrenogenital Syndrome." *Johns Hopkins Med J* 123, no. 3 (1967): 115–22.

Ehrhardt, Anke A., and John Money. "Progestin-Induced Hermaphroditism: IQ and Psychosexual Identity in a Study of Ten Girls." *J Sex Res* 3, no. 1 (1967): 83–100.

Eichler, Margrit. "Sex Change Operations: The Last Bulwark of the Double Standard." In *Feminist Frontiers: Rethinking Sex, Gender, and Society*, edited by Verta A. Taylor and Laurel Richardson, 106–15. Reading, MA: Addison-Wesley, 1983.

Elliott, T. R. "The Sidney Ringer Memorial Lecture on the Adrenal Glands: Delivered at University College Hospital Medical School, June, 1914." *Br Med J* 1, no. 2791 (June 27, 1914): 1393–97.

Ellis, Albert. *Homosexuality: Its Causes and Cure*. New York: Lyle Stuart, 1965.

———. "Reviews, Abstracts, Notes, and Correspondence: The Sexual Psychology of Human Hermaphrodites." *Psychosom Med* 7, no. 2 (1945): 108–25.

Ellis, Albert, and Shawn Blau. *The Albert Ellis Reader: A Guide to Well-Being Using Rational Emotive Behavior Therapy*. New York: Citadel Press, 1998.

Ellis, Havelock. *Studies in the Psychology of Sex*. Vol. 7, *Eonism and Other Supplementary Studies*. Philadelphia: F. A. Davis, 1928.

Ellis, Havelock, and John Addington Symonds. *Sexual Inversion*. Studies of the Psychology of Sex. London: Wilson and Macmillan, 1897.

Engerman, David C. "Social Science in the Cold War." *Isis* 101, no. 2 (June 1, 2010): 393–400.

Enke, Finn. "Collective Memory and the Transfeminist 1970s: Toward a Less Plausible History." *TSQ: Transgender Studies Quarterly* 5, no. 1 (2018): 9–29.

Epstein, Julia. "Either/Or-Neither/Both: Sexual Ambiguity and the Ideology of Gender." *Genders* 7 (1990): 99–142.

Eugenides, Jeffrey. *Middlesex*. New York: Picador / Farrar, Straus and Giroux, 2003.

Farber, Seymour M., and Roger H. L. Wilson, eds. *Man and Civilization: The Potential of Woman; A Symposium*. New York: McGraw-Hill, 1963.

Fass, Paula S. *The End of American Childhood: A History of Parenting from Life on the Frontier to the Managed Child*. Princeton, NJ: Princeton University Press, 2016.

Fausto-Sterling, Anne. "The Bare Bones of Sex: Part 1—Sex and Gender." *Signs* 30, no. 2 (2005): 1491–1527.

———. "The Five Sexes: Why Male and Female Are Not Enough." *Sciences*, 33, no. 2 (March–April 1993): 20–24.

———. *Myths of Gender: Biological Theories about Women and Men*. New York: Basic Books, 1985.

———. *Sexing the Body: Gender Politics and the Construction of Sexuality*. New York: Basic Books, 2000.

Feder, Ellen K. *Making Sense of Intersex: Changing Ethical Perspectives in Biomedicine*. Bloomington: Indiana University Press, 2014.

Feder, Ellen K., and Katrina Karkazis. "What's in a Name?: The Controversy over 'Disorders of Sex Development.'" *Hastings Cent Rep* 38, no. 5 (September–October 2008): 33–36.

Ferguson-Smith, M. A. "Cytogenetics in Man." *Arch Intern Med* 105, no. 4 (1960): 627–39.

Feudtner, John Christopher. *Bittersweet: Diabetes, Insulin, and the Transformation of Illness*. Studies in Social Medicine. Chapel Hill: University of North Carolina Press, 2003.

Finesinger, Jacob E., Joe V. Meigs, and Hirsh W. Sulkowitch. "Clinical, Psychiatric and Psychoanalytic Study of a Case of Male Pseudohermaphroditism." *Am J Obstet Gynecol* 44, no. 2 (1942): 310–17.

Fisher, Delbert A. "A Short History of Pediatric Endocrinology in North America." *Pediatr Res* 55, no. 4 (2004): 716–26.

Fleck, Ludwik. *Genesis and Development of a Scientific Fact*. Translated by Fred Bradley and Thaddeus J. Trenn. Chicago: University of Chicago Press, 1979.

Ford, C. E., K. W. Jones, P. E. Polani, J. C. De Almeida, and J. H. Briggs. "A Sex-Chromosome Anomaly in a Case of Gonadal Dysgenesis (Turner's Syndrome)." *Lancet* 273, no. 7075 (April 4, 1959): 711–13.

Fraser, R. W., A. P. Forbes, F. Albright, H. Sulkowitch, and E. C. Reifenstein. "Colorimetric Assay of 17-Ketosteroids in Urine—a Survey of the Use of This Test in Endocrine Investigation, Diagnosis and Therapy." *J Clin Endocrinol* 1, no. 3 (March 1941): 234–56.

Freedman, Estelle B. *No Turning Back: The History of Feminism and the Future of Women*. New York: Ballantine Books, 2002.

Freeman, Jo, ed. *Women: A Feminist Perspective*. Palo Alto, CA: Mayfield, 1975.

Freud, Anna. "Sex in Childhood." *Health Educ J* 2, no. 1 (1944): 2–6.

Freud, Sigmund. "Three Essays on the Theory of Sexuality (1905)." In *A Case of Hysteria, Three Essays on Sexuality and Other Works*, translated from the German under the general editorship of James Strachey, in collaboration with Anna Freud and with the assistance of Alix Strachey and Alan Tyson: 123–246. Vol. 7 (1901-1905) of *The Standard Edition of the Complete Psychological Works of Sigmund Freud*. London: Hogarth Press and the Institute of Psychoanalysis, 1953.

Fried, Barbara R., Mary Sue Henifin, and Ruth Hubbard. *Women Look at Biology Looking at Women: A Collection of Feminist Critiques*. Boston: Hall, 1979.

Friedan, Betty. *The Feminine Mystique*. New York: W. W. Norton, 1963.

Gallagher, Catherine, and Thomas Walter Laqueur, eds. *The Making of the Modern Body: Sexuality and Society in the Nineteenth Century*. Berkeley: University of California Press, 1987.

Gardetto, Darlaine Claire. "Engendered Sensations: Social Construction of the Clitoris and Female Orgasm, 1650–1975." PhD diss., University of California, Davis, 1992.

Gardner, Lytt I., ed. *Adrenal Function in Infants and Children: A Symposium*. Syracuse: Public Relations Office, Upstate Medical Center, State University of New York, 1954. Conference abstracts.

———, ed. *Adrenal Function in Infants and Children: A Symposium*. New York: Grune and Stratton, 1956.

———. *Endocrine and Genetic Diseases of Childhood*. Philadelphia: Saunders, 1969.

———. *Endocrine and Genetic Diseases of Childhood and Adolescence*. 2nd ed. Philadelphia: Saunders, 1975.

Garfinkel, Harold. "Passing and the Managed Achievement of Sex Status in an 'Intersexed' Person." In *The Transgender Studies Reader*, edited by Susan Stryker and Stephen Whittle, 58–93. New York: Routledge, 2006.

Gathorne-Hardy, Jonathan. *Alfred C. Kinsey: Sex the Measure of All Things; A Biography*. London: Chatto and Windus, 1998.

Gaudillière, Jean-Paul. "Paris–New York Roundtrip: Transatlantic Crossings and the Reconstruction of the Biological Sciences in Post-War France." *Stud Hist Philos Sci C* 33, no. 3 (2002): 389–417.

Germon, Jennifer. *Gender: A Genealogy of an Idea*. New York: Palgrave Macmillan, 2009.

Gibson, Campbell, and Kay Jung. *Historical Census Statistics on Population Totals by Race, 1790 to 1990, and by Hispanic Origin, 1790 to 1990, for the United States, Regions, Divisions, and States*. Washington, DC: US Census Bureau, 2002.

Gill-Peterson, Jules. *Histories of the Transgender Child*. Minneapolis: University of Minnesota Press, 2018.

Gillis, Jonathan. "Taking a Medical History in Childhood Illness: Representations of Parents in Pediatric Texts since 1850." *Bull Hist Med* 79 (2005): 393–429.

Gleason, Philip. "Americans All: World War II and the Shaping of American Identity." *Review of Politics* 43, no. 4 (1981): 483–518.

Golden, Janet, Richard A. Meckel, and Heather Munro Prescott. *Children and Youth in Sickness and in Health: A Historical Handbook and Guide*. Children and Youth: History and Culture. Westport, CT: Greenwood Press, 2004.

Goldie, Terry. *The Man Who Invented Gender: Engaging the Ideas of John Money*. Sexuality Studies Series. Vancouver: UBC Press, 2014.

Goldschmidt, Richard. *Mechanismus und Physiologie der Geschlechtsbestimmung*. Berlin: Gebr. Borntraeger, 1920.

Goldschmidt, Richard, and William J. Dakin. *The Mechanism and Physiology of Sex Determination*. London: Methuen, 1923.

Goodenough, Florence Laura. *Measurement of Intelligence by Drawings*. New York: World Book, 1926.

Goy, Robert W. "Biography: William Caldwell Young." *Anat Rec* 157, no. 1 (1967): 3–11.

Grant, Julia. *Raising Baby by the Book: The Education of American Mothers*. New Haven, CT: Yale University Press, 1998.

———. "A 'Real Boy' and Not a Sissy: Gender, Childhood, and Masculinity, 1890–1940." *Journal of Social History* 37, no. 4 (2004): 829–51.

Green, Richard. "The Three Kings: Harry Benjamin, John Money, Robert Stoller." *Arch Sex Behav* 38, no. 4 (2009): 610–13.

Grob, Gerald N. "Presidential Address: Psychiatry's Holy Grail; The Search for the Mechanisms of Mental Diseases." *Bull Hist Med* 72, no. 2 (1998): 189–219.

Grollman, Arthur. *The Adrenals*. Baltimore: Williams and Wilkins, 1936.

Grosz, Elizabeth A. *Volatile Bodies: Toward a Corporeal Feminism*. Bloomington: Indiana University Press, 1994.

Grumbach, M. M. "Further Studies on the Treatment of Congenital Adrenal Hyperplasia with Cortisone: IV. Effect of Cortisone and Compound B in Infants with Disturbed Electrolyte Metabolism, by John F. Crigler Jr, MD, Samuel H. Silverman, MD, and Lawson Wilkins, MD, *Pediatrics*, 1952; 10: 397–413." Pt. 2. *Pediatrics* 102, no. 1 (July 1998): 215–21.

György, P., J. Stokes, W. Rashkind, A. Michie, P. Brown, M. Dratman Wishner, et al. "Inter-University Round Table Conference by the Medical Faculties of the University of Pennsylvania and Johns Hopkins University: Psychological Aspects of the Sexual Orientation of the Child with Particular Reference to the Problem of Intersexuality." *J Pediatr* 47, no. 6 (1955): 771–90.

Ha, Nathan Q. "The Riddle of Sex: Biological Theories of Sexual Difference in the Early Twentieth-Century." *J Hist Biol* 44, no. 3 (2011): 505–46.

Haig, David. "The Inexorable Rise of Gender and the Decline of Sex: Social Change in Academic Titles, 1945–2001." *Arch Sex Behav* 33, no. 2 (2004): 87–96.

Hall, Lesley A. "Hauling down the Double Standard: Feminism, Social Purity and Sexual Science in Late Nineteenth-Century Britain." *Gender and History* 16, no. 1 (April 2004): 36–56.

———. *Sex, Gender and Social Change in Britain since 1880*. Gender and History. New York: Palgrave Macmillan, 2012.

Haller, Lea. *Cortison: Geschichte eines Hormons, 1900–1955*. Zurich: Chronos, 2012.

Halpern, Sydney A. *American Pediatrics: The Social Dynamics of Professionalism, 1880–1980*. Berkeley: University of California Press, 1988.

———. "Medicalization as Professional Process: Postwar Trends in Pediatrics." *J Health Soc Behav* 31 (March 1990): 28–42.

Hampson, Joan G. "Hermaphroditic Genital Appearance, Rearing and Eroticism in Hyperadrenocorticism: Psychologic Findings." In *Adrenal Function in Infants and Children: A Symposium*, edited by Lytt I. Gardner, 17–19. Syracuse: Public Relations Office, Upstate Medical Center, State University of New York, 1954.

———. "Hermaphroditic Genital Appearance, Rearing and Eroticism in Hyperadrenocorticism." *Bulletin of the Johns Hopkins Hospital* 96, no. 6 (June 1955): 265–73.

———. "Hermaphroditic Genital Appearance, Rearing and Eroticism in Hyperadrenocorticism." In *Adrenal Function in Infants and Children: A Symposium*, edited by Lytt I. Gardner, 11936. New York: Grune and Stratton, 1956.

———. "Human Hermaphroditism: Establishment of Gender Role and Erotic Practices." In *Symposium: Genetic, Psychological and Hormonal Factors in the Establishment and Maintenance of Patterns of Sexual Behavior in Mammals; November 17–19, 1954*, comp. William C. Young, 292–315. Held at the Lord Jeffrey, Amherst, Massachusetts. Lawrence, KS, 1954. Unpublished conference report bound and held at the University of Kansas.

Hampson, John L., and Joan G. Hampson. "The Ontogenesis of Sexual Behavior in Man." In *Sex and Internal Secretions*, edited by Edgar Allen and William C. Young, 1401–32. Baltimore: Williams and Wilkins, 1961.

Hampson, John L., Joan G. Hampson, and John Money. "The Syndrome of Gonadal Agenesis (Ovarian Agenesis) and Male Chromosomal Pattern in Girls and Women: Psychologic Studies." *Bulletin of the Johns Hopkins Hospital* 97, no. 3 (September 1955): 207–26.

Handler, Richard. "Boasian Anthropology and the Critique of American Culture." *AQ* 42, no. 2 (1990): 252–73.

Haraway, Donna. "Situated Knowledges: The Science Question in Feminism and the Privilege of Partial Perspective." *Feminist Studies* 14, no. 3 (1988): 575–99.

Hartigan-O'Connor, Ellen, and Lisa G. Materson, eds. *The Oxford Handbook of American Women's and Gender History*. Oxford Handbooks Online. Oxford: Oxford University Press, 2018.

Hartman, Saidiya. *Wayward Lives, Beautiful Experiments: Intimate Histories of Social Upheaval*. New York: W. W. Norton, 2019.

Hausman, Bernice L. *Changing Sex: Transsexualism, Technology, and the Idea of Gender*. Durham, NC: Duke University Press, 1995.

———. "Do Boys Have to Be Boys? Gender, Narrativity, and the John/Joan Case." *NWSA Journal* 12, no. 3 (Fall 2000): 114–38.

Heape, Walter. *Sex Antagonism*. New York: G. P. Putnam's Sons, 1913.

Heiman, Marcel. "Comment on Dr Stoller's Paper." *Int J Psychoanal* 49 (1968): 368.

Hench, P. S. "Potential Reversibility of Rheumatoid Arthritis." *Ann Rheum Dis* 8, no. 2 (June 1949): 90–96.

Henderson, John. "Ernest Starling and 'Hormones': An Historical Commentary." *J Endocrinol* 184, no. 1 (2005): 5–10.

Hinman Jr., Frank. "Advisability of Surgical Reversal of Sex in Female Pseudohermaphroditism." *JAMA* 146, no. 5 (1951): 423–29.

———. "Sexual Trends in Female Pseudohermaphrodism." *J Clin Endocrinol Metab* 11, no. 5 (1951): 477–86.

Hoberman, John M. *Testosterone Dreams: Rejuvenation, Aphrodisia, Doping*. Berkeley: University of California Press, 2005.

Hollinger, David A. *Cosmopolitanism and Solidarity: Studies in Ethnoracial, Religious, and Professional Affiliation in the United States*. Madison: University of Wisconsin Press, 2006.

———. "Science as a Weapon in Kulturkampfe in the United States during and after World War II." *Isis* 86, no. 3 (1995): 440–54.

Holmes, Morgan, ed. *Critical Intersex*. London: Routledge, 2016.

———. *Intersex: A Perilous Difference*. Selinsgrove, PA: Susquehanna University Press, 2008.

Holt, L. Emmett Jr., Rustin MacIntosh, Henry L. Barnett, and L. Emmett Holt. *Pediatrics*. 13th ed. New York: Appleton-Century-Crofts, 1962.

Holt, L. Emmett Jr., Rustin MacIntosh, and L. Emmett Holt. *Holt Pediatrics*. 12th ed. New York: Appleton-Century-Crofts, 1953.

hooks, bell. *Feminist Theory: From Margin to Center*. London: Pluto Press, 2000.

Howard, William Lee. "Effeminate Men and Masculine Women." *New York Medical Journal* 71, no. 5 (May 5, 1900): 686–87. Cited in Terry, "'Momism' and the Making of Treasonous Homosexuals," 169.

Hubbard, Ruth. *The Politics of Women's Biology*. New Brunswick, NJ: Rutgers University Press, 1990.

Hughes, Arthur F. "A History of Endocrinology." *J Hist Med Allied Sci* 32, no. 3 (1977): 292–313.

Humphreys, Laud. *Out of the Closets: The Sociology of Homosexual Liberation*. A Spectrum Book, S-288. Englewood Cliffs, NJ: Prentice-Hall, 1972.

Ingersoll, F. M., and J. E. Finesinger. "A Case of Male Pseudohermaphroditism, the Importance of Psychiatry in the Surgery of This Condition." *Surg Clin North Am* 27 (October 1947): 1218–25.

Institute for Sex Research and Alfred C. Kinsey. *Sexual Behavior in the Human Female*. Philadelphia: Saunders, 1953.

Irvine, Janice M. *Disorders of Desire: Sex and Gender in Modern American Sexology*. Health, Society, and Policy. Philadelphia: Temple University Press, 1990.

———. "From Difference to Sameness: Gender Ideology in Sexual Science." *J Sex Res* 27, no. 1 (1990): 7–24.

Isaac, Joel. *Working Knowledge: Making the Human Sciences from Parsons to Kuhn*. Cambridge, MA: Harvard University Press, 2012.

Jacobs, Patricia A., and John Anderson Strong. "A Case of Human Intersexuality Having a Possible XXY Sex-Determining Mechanism." *Nature* 183, no. 4657 (1959): 302–3.

Jacobsen, A. W., et al. "The Adrenal Gland in Health and Disease." *Pediatrics* 3, no. 4 (April 1949): 515–48.

Jewson, N. D. "The Disappearance of the Sick-Man from Medical Cosmology, 1770–1870." *Sociology* 10, no. 2 (1976): 225–44.

Johns Hopkins Hospital. *Administrative and Statistical Report: Sixth Report of the Superintendent of the Johns Hopkins Hospital*. Baltimore: Johns Hopkins Hospital, 1894–1900.

———. *Administrative and Statistical Report: Thirty-Fourth Report of the Director of the Johns Hopkins Hospital*. Baltimore: Johns Hopkins Hospital, 1921–24.

Johnson, David K. *The Lavender Scare: The Cold War Persecution of Gays and Lesbians in the Federal Government*. Chicago: University of Chicago Press, 2004.

Jones, Howard Wilbur. "Female Hermaphroditism without Virilization." *Obstet Gynecol Surv* 12, no. 4 (1957): 433–60.

Jones, Howard Wilbur, and Georgeanna Seegar Jones. "The Gynecological Aspects of Adrenal Hyperplasia and Allied Disorders." *Am J Obstet Gynecol* 68, no. 5 (November 1954): 1330–65.

Jones, Howard Wilbur, Georgeanna Seegar Jones, and William E. Ticknor. *Richard Wesley TeLinde*. Baltimore: Williams and Wilkins, 1986.

Jones, Howard Wilbur, and William Wallace Scott. *Hermaphroditism, Genital Anomalies and Related Endocrine Disorders*. Baltimore: Williams and Wilkins, 1958.

Jones, James H. *Alfred C. Kinsey: A Public/Private Life*. New York: W. W. Norton, 1997.

Jordan-Young, Rebecca M. *Brain Storm: The Flaws in the Science of Sex Differences*. Cambridge, MA: Harvard University Press, 2010.

Jordan-Young, Rebecca M., and Katrina Karkazis. *Testosterone: An Unauthorized Biography*. Cambridge, MA: Harvard University Press, 2019.

Karkazis, Katrina Alicia. *Fixing Sex: Intersex, Medical Authority, and Lived Experience*. Durham, NC: Duke University Press, 2008.

Katz, Jonathan. *Gay American History: Lesbians and Gay Men in the U.S.A.; A Documentary History*. Rev. ed. New York: Meridian, 1992.

Kendall, Edward C. "The Development of Cortisone as a Therapeutic Agent." Nobel Lecture, December 11, 1950. NobelPrize.org., https://www.nobelprize .org/prizes/medicine/1950/kendall/lecture/.

———. "The Development of Cortisone as a Therapeutic Agent." *Indian Med J* 45, no. 10 (October 1951): 239–41.

Kenen, Stephanie Hope. "Scientific Studies of Human Sexual Difference in Interwar America." PhD diss.,University of California, Berkeley, 1998.

———. "Who Counts When You're Counting Homosexuals? Hormones and Homosexuality in Mid-Twentieth Century America." In *Science and Homosexualities*, edited by Vernon A. Rosario, 197–218. New York: Routledge, 1997.

Kessler, Suzanne J. "The Medical Construction of Gender: Case Management of Intersexed Infants." *Signs* 16, no. 1 (1990): 3–26.

———. *Lessons from the Intersexed*. New Brunswick, NJ: Rutgers University Press, 1998.

Kevles, Daniel J. *In the Name of Eugenics: Genetics and the Uses of Human Heredity*. Berkeley: University of California Press, 1986.

———. "Testing the Army's Intelligence: Psychologists and the Military in World War I." *Journal of American History* 55, no. 3 (1968): 565–81.

King, Michael, and Eastern Southland Gallery, Gore, NZ. *Splendours of Civilisation: The John Money Collection at the Eastern Southland Gallery*. Dunedin, NZ: Eastern Southland Gallery in association with Longacre Press, 2006.

Kinsey, Alfred C. "Homosexuality: Criteria for a Hormonal Explanation of the Homosexual." *J Clin Endocrinol* 1, no. 5 (May 1941): 424–28.

Kinsey, Alfred C., Wardell Baxter Pomeroy, and Clyde Eugene Martin. *Sexual Behavior in the Human Male*. Philadelphia: W. B. Saunders, 1948.

Klebs, E. *Handbuch der pathologischen Anatomie*. Berlin: Hirschwald, 1876.

Kleinman, Arthur. *Writing at the Margin: Discourse between Anthropology and Medicine*. Berkeley: University of California Press, 1995.

Kline, Wendy. *Bodies of Knowledge: Sexuality, Reproduction, and Women's Health in the Second Wave*. Chicago: University of Chicago Press, 2010.

———. *Building a Better Race: Gender, Sexuality, and Eugenics from the Turn of the Century to the Baby Boom*. Berkeley: University of California Press, 2001.

Klöppel, Ulrike. *XX0XY Ungelöst: Hermaphroditismus, Sex und Gender in der deutschen Medizin; Eine historische Studie zur Intersexualität*. Vol. 12. Bielefeld: Transcript 2010.

Kluckhohn, Clyde. *Mirror for Man: The Relation of Anthropology to Modern Life*. New York: Whittlesey House, 1949.

Kluckhohn, Clyde, and Henry A. Murray. *Personality in Nature, Society, and Culture*. New York: A. A. Knopf, 1948.

Krabbe, Knud H. "The Relation between the Adrenal Cortex and Sexual Development." *New York Medical Journal* 114 (1921): 4–8.

Kuhn, Thomas S. *The Structure of Scientific Revolutions*. Chicago: University of Chicago Press, 1962.

Kuriyama, Shigehisa. *The Expressiveness of the Body and the Divergence of Greek and Chinese Medicine*. 1st pbk. ed. New York: Zone Books, 2002.

Lamb, S. D. *Pathologist of the Mind: Adolf Meyer and the Origins of American Psychiatry*. Baltimore: Johns Hopkins University Press, 2014.

Laqueur, Thomas Walter. *Making Sex: Body and Gender from the Greeks to Freud*. Cambridge, MA: Harvard University Press, 1990.

———. *Solitary Sex: A Cultural History of Masturbation*. New York: Zone Books, 2003.

Lemov, Rebecca M. *World as Laboratory: Experiments with Mice, Mazes, and Men*. New York: Hill and Wang, 2005.

Lewis, Roger A., and Lawson Wilkins. "The Effect of Adrenocorticotrophic Hormone in Congenital Adrenal Hyperplasia with Virilism and in Cushing's Syndrome Treated with Methyl Testosterone." *J Clin Investig* 28, no. 2 (March 1949): 394–400.

Leys, Ruth. "Types of One: Adolf Meyer's Life Chart and the Representation of Individuality." *Representations*, no. 34 (1991): 1–28.

Leys Stepan, Nancy. "Race, Gender, Science and Citizenship." *Gender and History* 10, no. 1 (1998): 26–52.

Lillie, Frank R. "The Free-Martin: A Study of the Action of Sex Hormones in the Foetal Life of Cattle." *J Exp Zool* 308, no. 3 (1917): 371–452.

Lisser, Hans. "The Endocrine Society—the First 40 Years (1917–1957)." *Endocrinology* 80, no. 7 (1967): 5–28.

Lloyd, Barbara Bloom, and John Archer. *Exploring Sex Differences*. London: Academic Press, 1976.

Lock, Margaret, and Patricia Kaufert. "Menopause, Local Biologies, and Cultures of Aging." *Am J Hum Biol* 13, no. 4 (2001): 494–504.

Long Hall, Diana. "Biology, Sex Hormones and Sexism in the 1920s." *Philosophical Forum* 5, nos. 1–2 (1974): 81–96.

Long Hall, Diana, and Thomas F. Glick. "Endocrinology: A Brief Introduction." *J Hist Biol* 9, no. 2 (Autumn 1976): 229–33.

Lorenz, Konrad Z. "The Companion in the Bird's World." *Auk* 54, no. 3 (1937): 245–73.

———. *King Solomon's Ring: New Light on Animal Ways*. New York: Crowell, 1952.

———. *Man Meets Dog*. London: Methuen, 1954.

———. *On Aggression*. London: Methuen, 1966.

Magubane, Zine. "Spectacles and Scholarship: Caster Semenya, Intersex Studies, and the Problem of Race in Feminist Theory." *Signs* 39, no. 3 (2014): 761–85.

Mak, Geertje. *Doubting Sex: Inscriptions, Bodies and Selves in Nineteenth-Century Hermaphrodite Case Histories*. Manchester: Manchester University Press, 2012.

———. "Doubting Sex from Within: A Praxiographic Approach to a Late Nineteenth Century Case of Hermaphroditism." *Gender and History* 18, no. 2 (2006): 332–56.

Mandler, Peter. "One World, Many Cultures: Margaret Mead and the Limits to Cold War Anthropology." *History Workshop Journal*, no. 68 (2009): 149–72.

Manion, Jen. *Female Husbands: A Trans History*. Cambridge: Cambridge University Press, 2020.

———. "Transgender Representations, Identities, and Communities." In *The Oxford Handbook of American Women's and Gender History*, edited by Ellen Hartigan-O'Connor and Lisa G. Materson, 311–31. New York: Oxford University Press, 2018.

Marks, Harry M. "Cortisone, 1949: A Year in the Political Life of a Drug." *Bull Hist Med* 66, no. 3 (Fall 1992): 419–39.

Martucci, Jessica. "'A Habit That Worries Me Very Much': Raising Good Boys and Girls in the Postwar Era." In *Pink and Blue: Gender, Culture, and the Health of Children*, edited by Elena Conis, Sandra Eder, and Aimee Madeiros, 31–50. New Brunswick, NJ: Rutgers University Press, 2021.

Masters, William H., Virginia E. Johnson, and Reproductive Biology Research Foundation (USA). *Human Sexual Response*. Boston: Little, Brown, 1966.

Matta, Christina. "Ambiguous Bodies and Deviant Sexualities: Hermaphrodites, Homosexuality, and Surgery in the United States, 1850–1904." *Perspect Biol Med* 48, no. 1 (Winter 2005): 74–83.

May, Elaine Tyler. *Homeward Bound: American Families in the Cold War Era*. New York: Basic Books, 1988.

McEneaney, Sinead. "Sex and the Radical Imagination in the *Berkeley Barb* and the *San Francisco Oracle*." *Radical Americas* 3, no. 16 (2018): 1–19.

McMaster, Elizabeth Wilkins. "Lawson Wilkins: Recollections by His Daughter." *Int J Pediatr Endocrinol*, suppl. 1 (May 2014): S1.

Mead, Margaret. *And Keep Your Powder Dry: An Anthropologist Looks at America*. New York: William Morrow, 1942.

———. *Coming of Age in Samoa: A Psychological Study of Primitive Youth for Western Civilisation*. New York: William Morrow, 1928.

———. *Male and Female: A Study of the Sexes in a Changing World*. New York: William Morrow, 1949.

———. *Sex and Temperament in Three Primitive Societies*. New York: William Morrow, 1935.

———. "What Shall We Tell Our Children?" *Redbook*, June 1970, 35, 37, 39, 41.

———. "Women: A Time for Change." *Redbook*, March 1970, 60, 62, 64, 67.

Mead, Margaret, and Rhoda Métraux. *The Study of Culture at a Distance*. Chicago: University of Chicago Press, 1953.

Medvei, Victor Cornelius. *The History of Clinical Endocrinology: A Comprehensive Account of Endocrinology from Earliest Times to the Present Day*. Carnforth, UK: Parthenon, 1993.

———. *A History of Endocrinology*. Lancaster, UK: MTP Press, 1982.

Meyerowitz, Joanne J. "Beyond the Feminine Mystique: A Reassessment of Postwar Mass Culture, 1946–1958." *Journal of American History* 79, no. 4 (1993): 1455–82.

———. "A History of 'Gender.'" *Am Hist Rev* 113, no. 5 (2008): 1346–56.

———. "'How Common Culture Shapes the Separate Lives': Sexuality, Race, and Mid-Twentieth-Century Social Constructionist Thought." *Journal of American History* 96, no. 4 (2010): 1057–84.

———. *How Sex Changed: A History of Transsexuality in the United States*. Cambridge, MA: Harvard University Press, 2002.

———. "Sex Change and the Popular Press: Historical Notes on Transsexuality in the United States, 1930–1955." *GLQ: A Journal of Lesbian and Gay Studies* 4, no. 2 (1998): 159–87.

———. "Transforming Sex: Christine Jorgensen in the Postwar US." *OAH Magazine of History* 20, no. 2 (2006): 16–20.

Migeon, C. J. "Lawson Wilkins and My Life: Part 3." *Int J Pediatr Endocrinol* (2014): suppl. 1, "Remembering Doctor Lawson Wilkins: A Pioneer of Pediatric Endocrinology," S4.

Mikesell, William Henry. *Psychology of Adjustment*. The Van Nostrand Series in Psychology. New York: Van Nostrand, 1952.

Milam, Erika Lorraine. *Creatures of Cain: The Hunt for Human Nature in Cold War America*. Princeton, NJ: Princeton University Press, 2019.

Miller, Arthur. *Death of a Salesman*. New York: Viking. 1949.

Miller, Fiona Alice. "'Your True and Proper Gender': The Barr Body as a *Good Enough* Science of Sex." *Stud Hist Philos Biol Biomed Sci* 37 (2006): 449–83.

Miller, Jean Baker. "Psychoanalysis, Patriarchy, and Power: One Viewpoint on Women's Goals and Needs." *Chrysalis, a Magazine of Women's Culture*, no. 2 (February 1, 1977): 19–25.

Millett, Kate. *Sexual Politics*. Garden City, NY: Doubleday, 1970.

Mol, Annemarie. *The Body Multiple: Ontology in Medical Practice*. Science and Cultural Theory. Durham, NC: Duke University Press, 2002.

Money, John. "Ablatio Penis: Normal Male Infant Sex-Reassigned as a Girl." *Arch Sex Behav* 4, no. 1 (1975): 65–71.

———. *The Adam Principle: Genes, Genitals, Hormones and Gender; Selected Readings in Sexology*. Buffalo, NY: Prometheus Books, 1993.

———. "Critique of 'Gender Role Determination: A Critical Review of the Evidence from Hermaphroditism,' by B. Zuger." *Psychosom Med* 32 (1970): 463–65.

———. "Delusion, Belief and Fact." *Psychiatry* 11 (1948): 33–38.

———. *The Destroying Angel: Sex, Fitness and Food in the Legacy of Degeneracy Theory; Graham Crackers, Kellogg's Corn Flakes and American Health History*. Buffalo, NY: Prometheus Books, 1985.

———. "Developmental Differentiation of Femininity and Masculinity Compared." In *Man and Civilization: The Potential of Woman—a Symposium*, edited by Seymour M. Farber and Roger H. L. Wilson, 51–65. New York: McGraw-Hill, 1963.

———. "An Examination of the Concept of Psychodynamics." *Psychiatry* 17 (1954): 325–30.

———. "Explorations in Human Behavior." In *The History of Clinical Psychology in Autobiography*, edited by C. Eugene Walker, 2:231–71. Pace Grove, CA: Thomson Brooks / Cole, 1991.

———. *A First Person History of Pediatric Psychoendocrinology, 1951–2000*. New York: Kluwer Academic / Plenum, 2002.

———. "Hermaphroditism." In *The Encyclopedia of Sexual Behavior*, edited by Albert Ellis and Albert Abarbanel, 472–84. New York: Hawthorn Books, 1961.

———. "Hermaphroditism, Gender and Precocity in Hyperadrenocorticism: Psychological Findings." In *Adrenal Function in Infants and Children: A Symposium*, ed. Lytt I. Gardner, 15–16. Syracuse: Public Relations Office, Upstate Medical Center, State University of New York, 1954.

———. "Hermaphroditism, Gender and Precocity in Hyperadrenocorticism: Psychological Findings." *Bulletin of the Johns Hopkins Hospital* 96, no. 6 (June 1955): 253–64.

———. "Hermaphroditism: An Inquiry into the Nature of a Human Paradox." PhD diss., Harvard University, 1952.

———. "Influence of Hormones on Sexual Behavior." *Annu Rev Med* 16, no. 1 (1965): 67–82.

———. "Nativism versus Culturalism in Gender-Identity Differentiation." In *Society of Medical Psychoanalysts*, edited by Edward T. Adelson and Society of Medical Psychoanalysts, 48–66. New York: Brunner / Mazel, 1975.

————. "Once upon a Time I Met Alfred C. Kinsey." *Arch Sex Behav* 31, no. 4 (August 2002): 319–22.

————. *The Psychologic Study of Man.* Springfield, IL: Charles C. Thomas, 1957.

————. "This Week's Citation Classic." In *Current Contents*, no. 11 (March 16, 1987): 12.

————. "Unanimity in the Social Sciences with Reference to Epistemology, Ontology and Scientific Method." *Psychiatry* 12 (1949): 211–21.

————. *Venuses Penuses: Sexology, Sexosophy, and Exigency Theory.* Buffalo, NY: Prometheus Books, 1986.

Money, John, and Anke A. Ehrhardt. *Man and Woman, Boy and Girl: Differentiation and Dimorphism of Gender Identity from Conception to Maturity.* (Baltimore: Johns Hopkins University Press, 1972).

Money, John, Anke A. Ehrhardt, and D. N. Masica. "Fetal Feminization Induced by Androgen Insensitivity in the Testicular Feminizing Syndrome: Effect on Marriage and Maternalism." *Johns Hopkins Medical Journal* 123, no. 3 (1968): 105–14.

Money, John, Joan G. Hampson, and John L. Hampson. "An Examination of Some Basic Sexual Concepts: The Evidence of Human Hermaphroditism." *Bulletin of the Johns Hopkins Hospital* 97, no. 4 (October 1955): 301–19.

————. "Hermaphroditism: Recommendations concerning Assignment of Sex, Change of Sex and Psychological Management." *Bulletin of the Johns Hopkins Hospital* 97, no. 4 (October 1955): 284–300.

————. "Imprinting and the Establishment of Gender Role." *Arch Neurol Psychiatry* 77 (1957): 333–36.

————. "Sexual Incongruities and Psychopathology: The Evidence of Human Hermaphroditism." *Bulletin of the Johns Hopkins Hospital* 98, no. 1 (January 1956): 43–57.

Money, John, John L. Hampson, and Joan G. Hampson. "Hermaphroditism: Psychology and Case Management." *Can Psychiatr Assoc J* 5, no. 2 (1960): 131–33.

Money, John, and Florence Schwartz. "Public Opinion and Social Issues in Transsexualism: A Case Study in Medical Sociology." In *Transsexualism and Sex Reassignment*, edited by Richard Green and John Money, 253–66. Baltimore: Johns Hopkins University Press, 1969.

Moon. "Crazy Ladies." *Lavender Woman*, March 1, 1973, 12.

Moore, Carl R., and Dorothy Price. "Gonad Hormone Functions, and the Reciprocal Influence between Gonads and Hypophysis with Its Bearing on the Problem of Sex Hormone Antagonism." *Am J Anat* 50, no. 1 (March 1932): 13–71.

Moore, K. L., M. A. Graham, and M. L. Barr. "The Detection of Chromosomal Sex in Hermaphrodites from a Skin Biopsy." *Surg Gynecol Obstet* 96, no. 6 (1953): 641–48.

Moore, Lisa Jean, and Adele E. Clarke. "Clitoral Conventions and Transgressions: Graphic Representations in Anatomy Texts, c1900–1991." *Feminist Studies* 21, no. 2 (Summer 1995): 255–301.

Morgan, Christiana D., and Henry A. Murray. "A Method for Investigating Fantasies: The Thematic Apperception Test." *Arch Neurol Psychiatry* 34, no. 2 (1935): 289–306.

Morgan, Clifford Thomas. *Introduction to Psychology*. New York: McGraw-Hill, 1956.

Morgan, Robin, ed. *Sisterhood Is Powerful: An Anthology of Writings from the Women's Liberation Movement*. New York: Random House, 1970.

Morland, Iain. "What Can Queer Theory Do for Intersex?" *GLQ: A Journal of Lesbian and Gay Studies* 15, no. 2 (2009): 285–312.

Murray, Henry A., and Harvard Psychological Clinic, Harvard University. *Explorations in Personality: A Clinical and Experimental Study of Fifty Men of College Age*. New York: Oxford University Press, 1938.

Myers, Hugh I., William C. Young, and Edward W. Dempsey. "Graafian Follicle Development throughout the Reproductive Cycle in the Guinea Pig, with Especial Reference to Changes during Oestrus (Sexual Receptivity)." *Anat Rec* 65, no. 4 (1936): 381–401.

Nelson, Waldo E., ed. *Textbook of Pediatrics*. 7th ed. Philadelphia: W. B. Saunders, 1959.

———. *Textbook of Pediatrics*. 8th ed. Philadelphia: W. B. Saunders, 1964.

Neugebauer, Franz Ludwig von. *Hermaphroditismus beim Menschen*. Vol. 2. Leipzig: Klinkhardt, 1908.

Oakley, Ann. *Sex, Gender and Society*. Towards a New Society. London: Maurice Temple Smith, 1972.

Oever, Roel van den. *Mama's Boy: Momism and Homophobia in Postwar American Culture*. New York: Palgrave Macmillan, 2012.

Oudshoorn, Nelly. *Beyond the Natural Body: An Archaeology of Sex Hormones*. New York: Routledge, 1994.

———. "On the Making of Sex Hormones: Research Material and the Production of Knowledge." *Social Studies of Science* 20 (1990): 5–33.

Owens, Deirdre Cooper. *Medical Bondage: Race, Gender, and the Origins of American Gynecology*. Athens, GA: University of Georgia Press, 2017.

Park, Edwards A. *The Harriet Lane Home: A Model and a Gem*. Baltimore: Department of Pediatrics, School of Medicine, Johns Hopkins University, 2006.

———. "Lawson Wilkins." *J Pediatr* 57, no. 3 (September 1960): 317–22.

Parsons, Talcott. *The Social System*. Glencoe, IL: Free Press, 1951.

Parsons, Talcott, and Edward Shils. *Toward a General Theory of Action*. Cambridge, MA: Harvard University Press, 1951.

Pernick, Martin S. *A Calculus of Suffering: Pain, Professionalism, and Anesthesia in Nineteenth-Century America*. New York: Columbia University Press, 1985.

Phoenix, Charles H., Robert W. Goy, Arnold A. Gerall, et al. "Organizing Action of Prenatally Administered Testosterone Propionate on the Tissues Mediating Mating Behavior in the Female Guinea Pig." *Endocrinology* 65 (1959): 369–82.

Pietila, Antero. *The Ghosts of Johns Hopkins: The Life and Legacy That Shaped an American City*. Lanham, MD: Rowman and Littlefield, 2018.

Plant, Rebecca Jo. *Mom: The Transformation of Motherhood in Modern America*. Chicago: University of Chicago Press, 2010.

———. "The Repeal of Mother Love: Momism and the Reconstruction of Mother-hood in Philip Wylie's America." PhD diss., Johns Hopkins University, 2001.

Porter, Roy. "The Patient's View: Doing Medical History from Below." *Theory and Society* 4 (1985): 175–98.

Prader, Andrea. "Cortison Dauerbehandlung des kongenitalen adrenogenitalen Syndroms." *Helv Paediatr Acta* 5 (1953): 368–423.

———. "Gonadendysgenesie und testikuläre Feminisierung." *Schweiz Med Wochen-schr* 87 (1957): 278–85.

———. *Intersexualität: Habilitationsschrift*. Labhart, Klinik der inneren Sekretion. Berlin: Springer, 1957.

———. "Pseudohermaphroditismus Femininus mit kongenitaler Nebennierenrinden-Insuffizienz: Günstige Wirkung von Cortison, Desoxycorticosteronacetat und Kochsalz." *Helv Paediatr Acta* 5 (1950): 426–33.

Pressman, Jack David. *Last Resort: Psychosurgery and the Limits of Medicine*. Cambridge: Cambridge University Press, 1998.

———. "Psychiatry and Its Origins." *Bull Hist Med* 71, no. 1 (1997): 129–39.

Preves, Sharon E. "Sexing the Intersexed: An Analysis of Sociocultural Responses to Intersexuality." *Signs* 27, no. 2 (2002): 523–56.

Quirke, Viviane. "Making British Cortisone: Glaxo and the Development of Corticosteroids in Britain in the 1950s–1960s." *Stud Hist Philos Sci C* 36, no. 4 (2005): 645–74.

Rasmussen, Nicolas. "Steroids in Arms: Science, Government, Industry, and the Hormones of the Adrenal Cortex in the United States, 1930–1950." *Med Hist* 46, no. 3 (2002): 299–324.

Raymond, Janice G. *The Transsexual Empire: The Making of the She-Male*. Boston: Beacon Press, 1979.

———. "Transsexualism: The Ultimate Homage to Sex-Role Power." *Chrysalis, a Magazine of Women's Culture*, no. 3 (March 1, 1977): 11–24.

Redick, Alison. "American History XY: The Medical Treatment of Intersex, 1916–1955." PhD diss., New York University, 2004.

Reed, Matt T. "Historicizing Inversion: Or, How to Make a Homosexual." *History of the Human Sciences* 14, no. 4 (2001): 1–29.

Reis, Elizabeth. *Bodies in Doubt: An American History of Intersex*. Baltimore: Johns Hopkins University Press, 2009.

———. *Bodies in Doubt: An American History of Intersex*. 2nd ed. Baltimore: Johns Hopkins University Press, 2021.

Reumann, Miriam G. *American Sexual Character: Sex, Gender, and National Identity in the Kinsey Reports*. Berkeley: University of California Press, 2005.

Reynolds, Thelma. "A Metabolism Bed." *American Journal of Nursing* 43, no. 2 (February 1943): 183–85.

Richardson, Sarah S. *Sex Itself: The Search for Male and Female in the Human Genome*. Chicago: University of Chicago Press, 2013.

Richardson, Theresa R. *The Century of the Child: The Mental Hygiene Movement and Social Policy in the United States and Canada*. Albany: SUNY Press, 1989.

Riley, Denise. *"Am I That Name?": Feminism and the Category of "Women" in History*. Language, Discourse, Society. Houndmills, UK: Macmillan Press, 1988.

Risse, Guenter B., and John Harley Warner. "Reconstructing Clinical Activities: Patient Records in Medical History." *Soc Hist Med* 5, no. 2 (1992): 183–205.

Ritchie, James, and Jane Ritchie. "Beaglehole, Ernest." Orig. pub. 2000 in *The Dictionary of New Zealand Biography*, which is now online as part of *Te Ara—the Encyclopedia of New Zealand*, accessed September 13, 2021, https://teara.govt.nz/en/biographies/5b15/beaglehole-ernest.

Riviere, Joan. "Womanliness as a Masquerade." In *Female Experience: Three Generations of British Women Psychoanalysts on Work with Women*, edited by Joan Raphael-Leff and Rosine Jozef Perelberg, 228–36. London: Routledge, 1997.

Robinson, Paul A. *The Modernization of Sex: Havelock Ellis, Alfred Kinsey, William Masters, and Virginia Johnson*. New York: Harper and Row, 1976.

Rockefeller Foundation. *The Rockefeller Foundation Annual Report 1950*. N.p.: Rockefeller Foundation, 1950.

Rodriguez, Sarah B. *Female Circumcision and Clitoridectomy in the United States: A History of a Medical Treatment*. Rochester Studies in Medical History. Rochester, NY: University of Rochester Press, 2014.

Rose, N. "Beyond Medicalisation." *Lancet* 369, no. 9562 (February 24, 2007): 700–702.

Rosenberg, Charles E. "Disease in History: Frames and Framers." *Milbank Quarterly* 67 (1989): 1–15.

Rosenberg, Charles E., and Janet Lynne Golden. *Framing Disease: The Creation and Negotiation of Explanatory Schemes*. The Milbank Quarterly. New York: Published for the Milbank Memorial Fund by Cambridge University Press, 1989.

Rosenberg, Charles E., Janet Lynne Golden, and Francis Clark Wood Institute for the History of Medicine. *Framing Disease: Studies in Cultural History*. Health and Medicine in American Society. New Brunswick, NJ: Rutgers University Press, 1992.

Rothman, David J. *Strangers at the Bedside: A History of How Law and Bioethics Transformed Medical Decision Making*. New York: Basic Books, 1991.

Rothman, Sheila M. *Living in the Shadow of Death: Tuberculosis and the Social Experience of Illness in America*. New York: Basic Books, 1994.

Rubin, David A. "'An Unnamed Blank That Craved a Name': A Genealogy of Intersex as Gender." *Signs* 37, no. 4 (2012): 883–908.

Rubin, Gayle S. *Deviations: A Gayle Rubin Reader*. Durham, NC: Duke University Press, 2011. doi:10.2307/j.ctv11smmmj.

———. *The Traffic in Women: Notes on the "Political Economy" of Sex*. Toward an Anthropology of Women, edited by Rayna R. Reiter. New York: Monthly Review Press, 1975.

Rubin, Gayle S., and Judith Butler. "Sexual Traffic." *A Journal of Feminist Cultural Studies* 6, no. 2 (1994), 62–99.

Russett, Cynthia Eagle. *Sexual Science: The Victorian Construction of Womanhood*. Cambridge, MA: Harvard University Press, 1989.

Sappol, Michael. *A Traffic of Dead Bodies: Anatomy and Embodied Social Identity in Nineteenth-Century America*. Princeton, NJ: Princeton University Press, 2002.

Savitt, Todd Lee. *Race and Medicine in Nineteenth- and Early-Twentieth-Century America*. Kent, OH: Kent State University Press, 2007.

Schaefer, Leah Cahan, and Connie Christine Wheeler. "Harry Benjamin's First Ten Cases (1938–1953): A Clinical Historical Note." *Arch Sex Behav* 24, no. 1 (1995): 73–93.

Schiebinger, Londa. *Nature's Body: Gender in the Making of Modern Science*. Boston: Beacon Press, 1993.

Schoen, Johanna. *Choice and Coercion: Birth Control, Sterilization, and Abortion in Public Health and Welfare*. Chapel Hill: University of North Carolina Press, 2005.

Scott, J. P. "Obituary: William C. Young 1899–1965." *Anim Behav* 15, no. 1 (1967): 205.

Scott, Joan Wallach. "Gender: A Useful Category of Historical Analysis." *American Historical Review* 91, no. 5 (1986): 1053–75.

———. "Gender: Still a Useful Category of Analysis?" *Diogenes* 57, no. 1 (2010): 7–14.

Sengoopta, Chandak. *The Most Secret Quintessence of Life: Sex, Glands, and Hormones, 1850–1950*. Chicago: University of Chicago Press, 2006.

Shankman, Paul. "The Public Anthropology of Margaret Mead: *Redbook*, Women's Issues, and the 1960s." *Current Anthropology* 59, no. 1 (2018): 55–73.

Siotos, C., P. M. Neira, B. D. Lau, J. P. Stone, J. Page, G. D. Rosson, and D. Coon. "Origins of Gender Affirmation Surgery: The History of the First Gender Identity Clinic in the United States at Johns Hopkins." *Ann Plast Surg* 83, no. 2 (August 2019): 132–36.

Sippell, Wolfgang G., ed. *ESPE—the First 50 Years: A History of the European Society for Paediatric Endocrinology*. Basel: S. Karger, 2011.

Skidmore, Emily. *True Sex: The Lives of Trans Men at the Turn of the Twentieth Century*. New York: New York University Press, 2019.

Skloot, Rebecca. *The Immortal Life of Henrietta Lacks*. New York: Crown, 2010.

Smith-Rosenberg, Carroll, and Charles Rosenberg. "The Female Animal: Medical and Biological Views of Woman and Her Role in Nineteenth-Century America." *Journal of American History* (1973): 332–56.

Snodgrass, S. Robert. "Stanley Cobb, the Rockefeller Foundation and the Evolution of American Psychiatry." *History of Psychiatry* 29, no. 4 (2018): 438–55.

Snorton, C. Riley. *Black on Both Sides: A Racial History of Trans Identity*. Minneapolis: University of Minnesota Press, 2017.

Solovey, Mark, and Hamilton Cravens, eds. *Cold War Social Science: Knowledge Production, Liberal Democracy, and Human Nature*. New York: Palgrave Macmillan, 2012.

Spelman, Elizabeth V. *Inessential Woman: Problems of Exclusion in Feminist Thought*. Boston: Beacon Press, 1988.

Stein, Melissa N. *Measuring Manhood: Race and the Science of Masculinity, 1830–1934*. Minneapolis: University of Minnesota Press, 2015.

Stern, Alexandra Minna. *Eugenic Nation: Faults and Frontiers of Better Breeding in Modern America*. 2nd ed. American Crossroads 17. Oakland: University of California Press, 2016.

———. "Sterilized in the Name of Public Health." *Am J Public Health* 95, no. 7 (July 1, 2005): 1128–38.

Stern, Alexandra Minna, and Howard Markel. *Formative Years: Children's Health in the United States, 1880–2000*. Ann Arbor: University of Michigan Press, 2009.

Stoller, Robert J. "A Contribution to the Study of Gender Identity." *Int J Psychoanal* 45 (April–July 1964): 220–26.

———. "A Further Contribution to the Study of Gender Identity." *Int J Psychoanal* 49 (1968): 364.

———. "Gender-Role Change in Intersexed Patients." *JAMA* 188 (May 18, 1964): 684–85.

———. *Sex and Gender: On the Development of Masculinity and Femininity*. New York: Science House, 1968.

Stone, Sandy. "The Empire Strikes Back: A Posttranssexual Manifesto." In *The Transgender Studies Reader*, edited by Susan Stryker and Stephen Whittle, 221–35. New York: Routledge, 2006.

Stryker, Susan. *Transgender History*. Seal Studies. Berkeley, CA: Seal Press, 2008. Distributed by Publishers Group West.

Swift, Edith Hale. *Step by Step in Sex Education*. New York: Macmillan, 1948.

Talbot, Nathan B. *Functional Endocrinology, from Birth through Adolescence*. Cambridge, MA: Harvard University Press, 1952.

Talbot, Nathan B., A. M. Butler, and R. A. Berman. "Adrenal Cortical Hyperplasia with Virilism: Diagnosis, Course and Treatment." *J Clin Invest* 21 (1942): 559–70.

Terman, Lewis Madison. *The Measurement of Intelligence: An Explanation of and a Complete Guide for the Use of the Stanford Revision and Extension of the Binet-Simon Intelligence Scale*. Boston: Houghton Mifflin, 1916.

Terry, Jennifer. *An American Obsession: Science, Medicine, and Homosexuality in Modern Society*. Chicago: University of Chicago Press, 1999.

———. "'Momism' and the Making of Treasonous Homosexuals." In *"Bad" Mothers: The Politics of Blame in Twentieth-Century America*, edited by Molly Ladd-Taylor and Lauri Umansky, 169–90. New York: New York University Press, 1998.

Thomas, David Hurst. "Margaret Mead as a Museum Anthropologist." *Am Anthropol* 82, no. 2 (1980): 354–61.

Thompson, Becky. "Multiracial Feminism: Recasting the Chronology of Second Wave Feminism." *Feminist Studies* 28, no. 2 (2002): 337–60.

Timmons, Stuart. *The Trouble with Harry Hay: Founder of the Modern Gay Movement*. Boston: Alyson, 1990.

Tinbergen, Niko. *The Study of Instinct*. Oxford: Clarendon Press, 1951.

Tjio, Joe Hin, and Albert Levan. "The Chromosome Number of Man." *Hereditas* 42, nos. 1–2 (1956): 1–6.

Tomes, Nancy. *The Gospel of Germs: Men, Women, and the Microbe in American Life*. Cambridge, MA: Harvard University Press, 1998.

Triplet, Rodney G. "Henry A. Murray: The Making of a Psychologist?" *Am Psychol* 47, no. 2 (1992): 299–307.

Tudico, Christopher. *The History of the Josiah Macy Jr. Foundation*. New York: Josiah Macy Jr. Foundation; September 2012.

United States. Children's Bureau. *The Story of the White House Conferences on Children and Youth*. Washington, DC: US Department of Health, Education, and Welfare, Social Rehabilitation Service, Children's Bureau, 1967.

Vicedo, Marga. "Cold War Emotions: Mother Love and the War over Human Nature." In *Cold War Social Science: Knowledge Production, Liberal Democracy, and Human Nature*, edited by Mark Solovey and Hamilton Cravens, 233–50. New York: Palgrave Macmillan, 2012.

———. *The Nature and Nurture of Love: From Imprinting to Attachment in Cold War America*. Chicago: University of Chicago Press, 2013.

Vidich, Arthur J. "The Department of Social Relations and 'Systems Theory' at Harvard: 1948–50." *International Journal of Politics, Culture, and Society* 13, no. 4 (2000): 607–48.

Wailoo, Keith. *Dying in the City of the Blues: Sickle Cell Anemia and the Politics of Race and Health*. Studies in Social Medicine. Chapel Hill: University of North Carolina Press, 2001.

———. "Historical Aspects of Race and Medicine: The Case of J. Marion Sims." *JAMA* 320, no. 15 (2018): 1529–30.

Warner, John Harley. "The Uses of Patient Records by Historians—Patterns, Possibilities, and Perplexities." *Health History* 1 (1999): 101–11.

Washington, Harriet A. *Medical Apartheid: The Dark History of Medical Experimentation on Black Americans from Colonial Times to the Present*. New York: Doubleday, 2006.

Wechsler, David, and Psychological Corporation. *Wechsler Intelligence Scale for Children: Manual*. New York: Psychological Corporation, 1949.

Weinstein, Deborah. *The Pathological Family: Postwar America and the Rise of Family Therapy*. Ithaca, NY: Cornell University Press, 2013.

Weissmann, G. "Cortisone and the Burning Cross: The Story of Percy Julian." *Pharos Alpha Omega Alpha Honor Med Soc* 68, no. 1 (Winter 2005): 13–16.

Weisz, George. *Divide and Conquer: A Comparative History of Medical Specialization*. Oxford: Oxford University Press, 2006.

———. "The Emergence of Medical Specialization in the Nineteenth Century." *Bull Hist Med* 77, no. 3 (Fall 2003): 536–75.

———. "Medical Directories and Medical Specialization in France, Britain, and the United States." *Bull Hist Med* 71, no. 1 (Spring 1997): 23–68.

Weitzman, Lenore J. "Sex-Role Socialization." In *Women: A Feminist Perspective*, edited by Jo Freeman, 105–44. Palo Alto, CA: Mayfield, 1975.

Wijngaard, Marianne van den. *Reinventing the Sexes: Feminism and Biomedical Construction of Femininity and Masculinity, 1959–1985*. Amsterdam: Uitgeverij Eburon, 1991.

Wilkins, L., W. Fleischmann, and J. E. Howard. "Macrogenitosomia Precox Associated with Hyperplasia of the Androgenic Tissue of the Adrenal and Death from Corticoadrenal Insufficiency." *Endocrinology* 26 (March 1940): 385–95.

Wilkins, L., R. Klein, and R. A. Lewis. "The Response to ACTH in Various Types of Adrenal Hyperplasia." In *Proceedings of the First Clinical ACTH Conference*, edited by John R. Mote, 184–92. Philadelphia: Blakiston, 1950.

Wilkins, L., R. A. Lewis, R. Klein, L. I. Gardner, J. F. Crigler Jr., E. Rosemberg, and C. J. Migeon. "Treatment of Congenital Adrenal Hyperplasia with Cortisone." *J Clin Endocrinol* 11 (1951): 1–25.

Wilkins, Lawson. "Acceptance of the Howland Award." Pt. 2. *J Pediatr* 63, no. 4 (October 1963): 808–11.

———. *The Diagnosis and Treatment of Endocrine Disorders in Childhood and Adolescence.* Springfield, IL: Thomas, 1950.

———. *The Diagnosis and Treatment of Endocrine Disorders in Childhood and Adolescence.* 2nd ed. Springfield, IL: Thomas, 1957.

———. *The Diagnosis and Treatment of Endocrine Disorders in Childhood and Adolescence.* With the assistance of Robert M. Blizzard and Claude J. Migeon. 3rd ed. Springfield, IL: Thomas, 1965.

———. "The Diagnosis of the Adrenogenital Syndrome and Its Treatment with Cortisone." *J Pediatr* 41, no. 6 (1952): 860–74.

———. "Epilepsy in Childhood: I. A Statistical Study of Clinical Types." *J Pediatr* 10, no. 3 (March 1937): 317–28.

———. "Epilepsy in Childhood: II. The Incidence of Remissions." *J Pediatr* 10, no. 3 (March 1937): 329–40.

———. "Epilepsy in Childhood: III. Results with the Ketogenic Diet." *J Pediatr* 10, no. 3 (March 1937): 341–57.

Wilkins, Lawson, Alfred M. Bongiovanni, George W. Clayton, Melvin M. Grumbach, and Judson J. Van Wyk. "Virilizing Adrenal Hyperplasia: Its Treatment with Cortisone and the Nature of the Steroid Abnormalities." *Ciba Foundation Colloquia on Endocrinology* 8 (1955): 460–86.

Wilkins, Lawson, and Jose Cara. "Further Studies on the Treatment of Congenital Adrenal Hyperplasia with Cortisone: V. Effects of Cortisone Therapy on Testicular Development." *J Clin Endocrinol Metab* 14, no. 3 (1954): 287–96.

Wilkins, Lawson, John F. Crigler, Samuel H. Silvermann, Lytt I. Gardner, and Claude J Migeon. "Further Studies on the Treatment of Congenital Adrenal Hyperplasia with Cortisone: II. The Effects of Cortisone on Sexual and Somatic Development, with an Hypothesis concerning the Mechanism of Feminization." *J Clin Endocrinol Metab* 12 (1952): 277–307.

Wilkins, Lawson, Melvin M. Grumbach, Judson J. Van Wyk, Thomas H. Shepard, and Constantine Papadatos. "Hermaphroditism: Classification, Diagnosis, Selection of Sex and Treatment." *Pediatrics* 16 (1955): 287–302.

Wilkins, Lawson, R. A. Lewis, R. Klein, and E. Rosemberg. "The Suppression of Androgen Secretion by Cortisone in a Case of Congenital Adrenal Hyperplasia." *Bulletin of the Johns Hopkins Hospital* 86 (1950): 249–52.

Wilkins, Lawson, and Curt P. Richter. "A Great Craving for Salt by a Child with Cortico-Adrenal Insufficiency." *JAMA* 114, no. 10 (March 9, 1940): 866–68.

Williams, Cristan. "Radical Inclusion: Recounting the Trans Inclusive History of Radical Feminism." *Transgender Studies Quarterly* 3, nos. 1–2 (2016): 254–58.

Wu, Judy Tzu-Chun. "US Feminisms and Their Global Connections." In *The Oxford Handbook of American Women's and Gender History*, edited by Ellen Hartigan-O'Connor and Lisa G. Materson, 487–510. New York: Oxford University Press, 2018.

Wylie, Philip. *Generation of Vipers*. New York: Rinehart, 1942.

Young, Hugh Hampton. *Genital Abnormalities: Hermaphroditism and Related Adrenal Diseases*. Baltimore: Williams and Wilkins, 1937.

Young, William C., and Edgar Allen, eds. *Sex and Internal Secretions*. 3rd ed. Baltimore: Williams and Wilkins, 1961.

Yudell, Michael. *Race Unmasked: Biology and Race in the Twentieth Century*. New York: Columbia University Press, 2014.

Zachmann, Milo. "Andrea Prader 1919–2001." *Horm Res Paediatr* 56, nos. 5–6 (2001): 205–7.

Zondek, Bernhard. "Mass Excretion of Oestrogenic Hormones in the Urine of the Stallion." *Nature* 133 (February 10, 1934): 209–10.

Züblin, W. "Zur Psychiatrie des adrenogenitalen Syndroms bei kongenitaler Nebennierenrinden-Hyperplasie." *Helv Paediatr Acta* 8 (1953): 117–35.

Zuger, Bernard. "Gender Role Determination: A Critical Review of the Evidence from Hermaphroditism." *Psychosom Med* 32, no. 5 (1970): 449–63.

———. "Rebuttal." *Psychosom Med* 32, no. 5 (1970): 465–67.

Index

Page numbers in italics refer to figures.

ACTH. *See* adrenocorticotrophic hormone (ACTH)
adaptations: and behavior, 43, 55; and clinical data, 168; and gender, 16, 33, 43, 168, 171, 175, 179, 195–224; and ICM, 170
Addison's disease, 38, 191
adrenal androgens, 37, 153. *See also* congenital adrenal hyperplasia (CAH)
adrenalectomies, 18, 28, 31, 38, 73
"Adrenal Function in Infants and Children" (Money and Hampson symposium), 120–21
"Adrenal Gland in Health and Disease, The" (Wilkins panel discussion), 31–32
adrenal glands: and AGS, 28; as ambisexual, 28; and compound E, isolated, 38; conference about, 120; and deoxycorticosterone production, 243n4; and hormonal treatments, 42; and hormones, 27; physiology of, 25; research on, early years of, 244–45n25; and sex, 24–28; and sex glands, 27; surgical removal of, 18; as vital for survival, 25. *See also* adrenalectomies; adrenogenital syndrome (AGS); congenital adrenal hyperplasia (CAH)
adrenal hyperplasia. *See* congenital adrenal hyperplasia (CAH)

adrenocorticotrophic hormone (ACTH), 31, 39
adrenogenital syndrome (AGS), 25, 27–28, 45, 171–74, 180, 274n43, 276n75, 277n77. *See also* congenital adrenal hyperplasia (CAH); hermaphroditism
"Advisability of Surgical Reversal of Sex in Female Pseudohermaphroditism" (Hinman), 65
Afro-American (Baltimore newspaper), 204–5
AGS. *See* adrenogenital syndrome (AGS)
Albert Einstein College of Medicine (Bronx, NY), 122
Albright, Fuller, 97, 272n12
aldosterone, 243n4
Allport, Gordon W., 94–95, 257n46
AMA. *See* American Medical Association (AMA)
ambisexual, 27–28, 221
amenorrhea, 79
American Academy of Pediatrics, 31–32, 97
American Association for the Advancement of Science, 215
American Cancer Society, 42
American Journal of Obstetrics and Gynecology, 57
American Medical Association (AMA), 64–66
American People, The (Gorer), 104

American Society of Clinical Investigation, 272n12

anatomical sex, 15, 54, 75. *See also* biological sex

anatomy: and behavior, 29; clitoral, 270n26; and gender identity, 197; hermaphroditic, 177; and homosexuality, 63–64; and physiology, 29, 197, 202; and psychology, 59, 113–14; and psychosexuality, 61, 67–68, 75, 113; and somatic sexuality, 181–82. *See also* reproductive organs

And Keep Your Powder Dry (Mead), 104

androgen, overproduction of. *See* congenital adrenal hyperplasia (CAH)

anesthesia, 36, 54, 56–57, 120, 126, 151, 251n23

animal behavior, 88, 132–33, 195, 268n68, 282n79. *See also* behavior

Ann and Robert H. Lurie Children's Hospital (Chicago), 288n9

anthropology, 285n128, 286n138; and adaptation, 219; and child rearing, 88; cultural, 55, 93; and culture, 258–59n64; and culture vs. biology, 85–87, 100, 103–4, 256n26; and psychiatry, 55; and psychology, 91, 94–95; and race, 85–87; and scientific racism, 86; and sex/gender system, 223–24; and sex roles, 3; social, 93; and social relations, 257n46; and sociology, 3; and war efforts, 93, 104, 258–59n64; and women's biological destiny, 245n31

anti-adrenal drug, 37–38

antiseptics, 36

antisex feminist movement, 283n103

antisexualism, hysteria of Victorianism, 100

Appel, Kenneth, 118

Archives of Sexual Behavior, 213

asepsis, 56

Association for the Advancement of Psychotherapy, 279n27

Baltimore Sun, 166, 249n97

Barnett, Henry L., 122, 124, 179–80

Barr, Murray Llewellyn, 130, 148, 238n5, 267n52

Barr body test, 13, 37, 111, 129–30, 143, 148–50, 183, 238n5, 267nn52–53, 270n14

Bartter, Frederic C., 97, 169, 272n12

Bateson, George, 104, 262n97

Beach, Frank Ambrose, 207–8, 281n65, 282n79

Beaglehole, Ernest, 91

Beauvoir, Simone de, 6

Beecher, Henry K., 264n23

behavior: and adaptation, 43, 55; and adjustment, 55; and anatomy, 29; and biology, 5, 15, 86, 108, 119, 239n14; and character, 119; and cultural patterns, 85–90; and culture, 5, 15, 85–86, 119, 139, 142, 256n26; and desire, 59, 116; and environment, 15, 55, 85–86, 119; and experience, 55; female/feminine, 58–59, 160; and gender, 58–59, 119, 215–16, 230; gender inversion in, 116; and gender roles, 3, 109; and habitus, 35; and hormones, 6, 119, 210; and human nature, 86; and ideology, 12–13; and instinct, 6, 239n14; learned, 10–11, 86, 88, 134, 139; measurement of, 75; and norms, 96; and nurture, 55; and personality, 4–5, 8, 15, 85–86, 119, 128–29, 139, 142, 184; and physiology, 208; and play, observations of, 116, 210; and psychiatry, 21; and psychology, 174–75; and psychosexuality, 106; and race, 86; science of, 239n12; and self-identification, 215; and sex assignment/reassignment, 4, 43, 119; and sex changes, 116; and sex determination, 5; and sex roles, 6, 85; and sexual orientation, 107; and sexual traits, 210; social, 89; stereotypical (gender), 220; and trans people, 220; and women, 218. *See also* animal behavior; sexual behavior

behavioral endocrinology, 208

behavioral sciences, 15, 85, 93; and social sciences, 85

Bellevue Hospital (New York), 171

Benedict, Ruth, 89, 91, 95, 104, 256nn26–27

Benjamin, Harry, 202–5, 279n27, 279n29

Berkeley Barb (underground newspaper), 216, 223, 284n111

Bernard, Jessie, 218

Bernreuter Personality Inventory, 60

better sex: determining/finding for CAH patients, 38, 146, 152; and true sex, 14–15, 18–44, 148. *See also* biological sex; proper sex; true sex

Binet, Alfred, 259–60n77

bioethics, 227
biological determinism, 6, 55, 89, 139–40, 216–17, 224. *See also* environmental determinism; social determinism
"Biological Imperatives" (*Time* magazine), 215
biological norms, 7, 33; and social norms, 21, 116, 164, 216. *See also* gender norms; sexual norms; social norms
biological sex, 2–3, 10, 32–33, 36–37, 43, 56–57, 74–75, 102–3, 117–18, 125–26, 130, 137–38, 142, 184–85, 201, 206, 221–24, 228, 283n100; and feminism, 26, 288n12. *See also* anatomical sex; better sex; proper sex; true sex
biology: and behavior, 5, 15, 86, 108, 119, 239n14; and culture, 5, 85–86, 113–20, 218, 228; and environment, 134, 222; and gender, 4, 10; of hormones, 26; and instinct, 239n14; and personality, 88, 95, 218; and psychiatry, 55; psycho-, 55, 111, 131; and psychology, 97–98, 118; and race, 85; reproductive, 125; and sex, 10; and sex determination, 5; and social causes, 26–27; and socialization, 222; and social sciences, 8. *See also* reproductive biology
biomedicine, 13–14, 19, 23, 143, 156, 207
biopolitics, of childbearing/child rearing, 89–90
bisexuality, 8, 27–28, 34, 63–64, 118, 200, 202; and heterosexuality, 63; and homosexuality, 63
Bleuler, Manfred, 173–75
Blizzard, Robert, 177
Boas, Franz, 86–87
body morphology: and intersexuality, 98; and physiology, 96
Borderlands of Psychiatry (Cobb), 97
Borst, Charlotte G., 251n25
Boston Children's Hospital, 96–97, 288n9
Boston City Hospital, 58
Boston Psychopathic Hospital, 58
Brady Urological Institute (Johns Hopkins), 28, 32, 58, 73, 153
brain: and gender/sex, 207–16, 221–22; and hormones, 210–11
British Journal of Medical Psychology, 131
Bulletin of the Johns Hopkins Hospital, 39–40, 127, 266n40

Butler, Judith, 228, 288nn13–14

CAH. *See* congenital adrenal hyperplasia (CAH)
CAH patients, 45–52, 76–83; better/proper sex, determining/finding for, 38, 146, 152; and diagnoses, 118; and drugs for virilization, 31; and happiness, 68–73; intersex psychosexuality of, 175; intersex studies of, 175; as intersexuality, 237n3; medical management of, 76, 158; medical practices for, 143–44; physical examination of, 149; and postcortisone, chromosomally female children, 270n22; and precortisone treatments, 129; psychiatric study of, 173–74; psychological findings on, 121; psychological health of, 15, 109; psychological sex of, evaluation, 173–75; and sex assignment/reassignment, 14–15; steroid hormones for, 39; studies of, 127–28; and sweeping changes in American culture and biomedicine, 19; therapeutic success for, 192; treatment, 97, 151–56
Canadian Psychiatric Association Journal, 181, 272n7
Canguilhem, Georges, 142
Cantor, David, 248n80, 248n83
Cappon, Daniel, 181–84, 275n63, 275n66
CARES Foundation, 288n8
case histories/studies, 8–9, 13, 15, 18–19, 25, 28, 54, 68, 75, 95–97, 99, 102–3, 105–6, 112, 114, 116, 128, 138, 142–44, 152, 168, 170, 173, 197–200, 209, 212–16, 263n6, 272n16
case management, 6–7, 16, 44, 156–64, 166–86. *See also* intersex case management (ICM); treatment plans
Cauldwell, David O., 201–2
Chase, Cheryl, 227
childhood science, 256n32
children: adrenal function in, 120–21; with CAH, 19–20; clinical encounters with, 46; and history of childhood, 262n96; hormones in, 24, 210; and intersexuality, 1, 4, 9–10; normalizing procedures inflicted on, 10; protection of by mothers/parents, 46, 70; and their development, 56
Children's Hospital of Philadelphia, 114, 117

chromosomes. *See* sex chromosomes
Chrysalis: A Magazine of Women's Culture,
 216–17, 221
civil rights, and homosexuality, 261n90
clinic: and gender, 4, 12, 16–17, 141–65,
 224, 226; and gender roles, 5, 16; and
 medical approaches to sex, 43–44;
 patient-physician relationship, 243n48;
 patient records, 13–14, 16; and sex,
 75, 97; sex/gender binary in, 14; social
 relations in, 99–106. *See also* gender
 identity: clinics for; medicine
"Clinical Aspects of Transsexualism in the
 Male and Female" (Benjamin), 202
clinical endocrinology, 97, 245n25
clinical research, and ethics, 264n23
clitoral anatomy, history of, 270n26
clitoral stimulation, 274n51
clitoridectomies, 270n27, 274n51; and
 consequences for women's eroticism,
 123–24; consequences of, 66, 123–24,
 178; delayed/deferred, 57, 66, 122, 161;
 as drastic surgical intervention, 155;
 at early age, 66, 122, 155, 161–62; for
 enlarged clitoris, 35–36, 152, 164; and
 eroticism, 123–24; and feminization, 66,
 121, 123; history of, 35, 152–53, 155–
 56; and homosexuality, to combat, 35;
 and hypersexuality, to combat, 35; and
 masturbation, to curb, 35; and normalization, 158, 164; post-surgery evaluation, 154; and preservation of erotic
 sensation, 123–24; and psychological
 difficulties, 123; and psychologization,
 61, 155–56; raison d'être, 155; and sex
 assignment/reassignment, 35; as treatment to restore patient health, 153
clitoris: cosmetic, 155, 271n37; as sexually
 important organ, 178–79; size of, 35–36,
 61, 77, 122, 147, 152–53, 155, 157–58,
 164
Cobb, Stanley, 96–97
Colapinto, John, 254n5, 283n100
Columbia University, 62, 179
Coming of Age in Samoa (Mead), 219
compound E. *See* cortisone
congenital adrenal hyperplasia (CAH), 1–2,
 288n8; and clinical options, 32; diagnosing, 16, 144–51; and gender roles,
 16; as inborn hyperplasia of adrenal
 glands, 1; as life-threatening adrenal

pathology, 19; maintenance, 16; and
 metabolic problems, 1; and normalization, 164–65; and push of nature,
 31–37; as rare condition, initially, 126;
 and restoration of proper sex, 39–42;
 results in lack of cortisol and overproduction of androgen, 1; and salt loss,
 1, 16, 30, 110–11, 152, 156; treatment
 and management, 16; and true sex, 19,
 30–38. *See also* adrenogenital syndrome
 (AGS); CAH patients
Conn, Jacob H., 69–71
contrasexism, 201, 203, 278n23
Cordova, Jeanne, 286n141
Cornell University Medical College, 122
Corner, George, 126
cortisol, lack of. *See* congenital adrenal
 hyperplasia (CAH)
cortisone: compound E as, 38–39, 79; dramatic effects, 38; lower costs, 39; mass
 production of, 39; politics of drama in
 introduction of, 248n83; synthesized
 from soybeans, 39
"Cortisone Helps to Restore Sex Balance"
 (*Washington Post*), 42
cortisone treatments: for CAH patients, 2,
 30–31, 37–45, 66, 71–72, 81, 109–11,
 115, 121, 141, 152, 156–57, 159–60,
 164, 168–73, 186, 270n22, 272nn12–13;
 for disease, 39; and feminization, 41; as
 lifelong management strategy, 42; and
 pediatric endocrinology, 172–73; for
 rheumatoid arthritis, 38–39, 248n80;
 success and therapeutic achievements,
 249n97
Cory, Donald Webster (Edward Sagarin),
 261n90, 268n90
Crigler, John, 151
cultural patterns, 257n46; and behavior,
 85–90; and environment, 85–86; and
 gender, 15, 84–109; and heterosexuality, 63–64; and personality, 85–86; and
 psychological sex, 15, 54; and social relations, 99–106; and social sciences, 86–90
cultural relativism, 6, 85–90, 258n64
culture: and anthropology, 258–59n64; and
 behavior, 5, 15, 85–86, 119, 139, 142,
 256n26; and biology, 5, 85–86, 113–20,
 218, 228; and environment, 15, 54, 85,
 87, 119, 132, 139; and gender, 15, 84–
 109, 228–29; holistic view of, 256n26;

and homosexuality, 63–64, 252n45; and
personality, 15, 43, 54, 84–109, 139,
252n45, 256n26, 256n30, 262n97; and
race, 89–90; and sex roles, 97; and social
sciences, 139, 259n64
Cushing syndrome, 41–42, 160
cybernetics, 258n52

Darwinism, and adaptation, 55
Death of a Salesman (A. Miller), 55
De Crecchio, Luigi, 25
Degler, Carl, 86
deoxycorticosterone, 243n4
despair, 45, 48, 187–94
determinism. *See* biological determinism;
environmental determinism; social
determinism
Diamond, Milton, 184–85, 212, 276n75,
283n94, 287n1
discrimination. *See* gender discrimination;
sex/sexual discrimination
disease: as biological pathology, 188; and
clinical practice, 13; cortisone as
therapeutic for, 39; endocrine, 19; and
germs, 143; and heredity, 73; meanings of, 143; prevention, 24; rare, 24;
understandings/study of, 11, 24, 143.
See also health
Diseases of Infancy and Childhood (Holt), 179
disorders of sex development (DSD), 1–2,
9, 237n3
Dog Day Afternoon (film), 207, 281n62
drag queens, 223
Dreger, Alice Domurat, 227, 232, 249n100,
287–88n7
DSD. *See* disorders of sex development (DSD)
Dworkin, Andrea, 286n141

Eder, Sandra, 269, 272n16
Edgerton, Milton T., 206, 279n38
effeminacy/effeminate behavior, 253n64,
285n131; and homosexuality, 105, 184
Ehrhardt, Anke, 210–14, 217, 221, 224,
286n139
electrolytes: abnormality, control of, 151;
defects, 41, 157; loss of, 243n4
Elkes, Joel, 203
Elliott, Beth, 286n141
Ellis, Albert, 62–64, 67, 102, 274n37,
279n26
Ellis, Havelock, 8, 251n31, 278n23

endocrinology, 125; behavioral, 208; clinical, 97, 245n25; and disease, 19; golden
age of, 24; medical technologies in, 10;
and natural experiments, 197; psychosyndrome, 174–75. *See also* pediatric
endocrinology
environment: and behavior, 15, 55, 85–86,
119; and biology, 134, 222; and cultural
patterns, 85–86; and culture, 15, 54, 85,
87, 119, 132, 139; and heredity, 211;
and nurture, 55; and personality, 15,
54, 95, 139; and psychology, 66–67; and
psychosexuality, 59, 67–68; scientific,
85; and sex, 116; and sex roles, 216;
social, 55, 87
environmental determinism, 6, 125.
See also biological determinism; social
determinism
eonism, 201, 278n23
erections, frequent: and masturbation, 153;
as sexual difficulty, 74
Erickson, Reed, 203
Erickson Educational Foundation, 203
Erikson, Erik, 88
eroticism, 7, 85, 123–24, 128
ethics: bio-, 227; and clinical research,
264n23; of ICM, 10–11, 287n6; and
medicine, 45–52, 120
ethnography, 89, 103
ethnology, 285n127
eugenics, 89–90, 255n25
Eustachius, Bartolomeo, 25, 244n22
"Examination of Some Basic Sexual Concepts, An" (Money), 133
exhibitionism, as sexual difficulty, 74
Ezrin, Calvin, 181, 183–84

facies, 49, 250n7
Fanconi, Guido, 171, 173–74
fatherhood, 73, 88, 200
Fausto-Sterling, Anne, 11, 227, 238n4,
238n8, 265n30, 288n12, 289n15
Feminine Mystique, The (Friedan), 227–28,
264n16
femininity, and homosexuality, 60
feminism, 283nn102–3, 284n114; and
biological sex, 26, 288n12; and gender,
3–4, 16–17, 195–96, 215–24, 227–28,
288nn11–12; trans-, 222, 229, 286n141;
and transsexuality, 286n140. *See also*
women's emancipation/liberation

feminization: and CAH, 199; and clitoridectomies, 66, 121, 123; and cortisone
treatments, 41; early surgical, 121; in
female patients, 41; and hormone replacement therapy, 212; parents' role in
sons', 200; and puberty, 212; signs of,
41; and start of sex-specific adolescence,
41; surgical, 121, 123; testicular, 172;
and virilization, 41, 74
Finesinger, Jacob E., 57–61, 65, 75, 252n51
Firestone, Shulamite, 286n141
Five Colleges (Amherst, MA), 221
Flexner Report, 120, 264n22
Frame, Janet, 257n36
Fremont-Smith, Frank, 111, 119, 264n20
Freud, Anna, 252n41, 270n32, 297
Freud, Sigmund, 58, 63, 88, 94, 154, 224,
252n41
Friedan, Betty, 227–28, 264n16
Frisch, Karl von, 133
Fromm, Erich, 88
*Functional Endocrinology, from Birth through
Adolescence* (Talbot), 272n13

Gardner, George, 96, 107–8
Gardner, Lytt I., 179, 265n31, 275n54
Garfinkel, Harold, 253n72, 278n6
gays: and group identity, 261–62n90; as
oppressed minority, 102. *See also* homosexuality; lesbianism/lesbians
gender: at birth, 218, 226; and child
rearing, 166, 168, 174, 177, 179, 226;
conformity, 264n16; cross-, 8; differences, 216; discomfort, 203; as dynamic
category, 5–6; as expression of human
behavior, potential, and creativity, 230;
feeling, 203; formative conversations
about, 113; formulated, 3, 4–10, 16,
208; genealogy of (1940s to 1970s), 14,
17, 225; history of, 17, 289nn17–18;
inequalities, 3, 230; invented and
transformed within US medicine, 3–10;
as language of power, 230; learned,
98, 202, 217, 228; life of, 16, 195–224;
matters, 225; medical history/origin of,
10–14, 17, 216; as normative concept,
226; opposite, 216; orientation, 158,
202–3; psycho-, 181–82; as real, 228; as
reformulation of sex, 6; and research,
196, 211; and self-identification, 215; as
self-regulating system, 258n52; and sex,

3–6, 13, 16–17, 70, 140, 210, 216–17,
224, 228, 284n116; and sexual behavior,
281n67; and sexual difference, 195–96;
social, 228–30; spectrum, 3; term, as
ubiquitous, 3, 223; term, defined, 3;
term, usage, 3, 16–17, 110, 128, 195–96,
216–19, 222–25, 227, 284n116; transformations, 186; trap, 216; unicorn, 3.
See also gender roles
gender discrimination, 3, 16–17, 216–17,
229–30. *See also* sex: discrimination
gender-fuck, 17, 222–23
gender identity, 8, 196–201, 216–17,
240n20; and child rearing, 213; clinics for, 3, 16, 202–7, 216, 220, 229,
280n59; core, 198–201; and gender
roles, 195–201; and imprinting, 201;
and intersexuality, 187; normal, 42; and
psychological sex, 16, 195; and psychology, 16, 125; and sex chromosomes,
185; term, usage, 3, 203, 216. *See also*
transsexuality
gender inequality index, 3
gender inversion: in behavior, 116; and
homosexuality, 103, 116; term, usage,
251n31. *See also* sexual inversion
gender nonbinary individuals, 10, 229–30,
253n72
gender norms, 3, 220–22. *See also* biological norms; sexual norms; social
norms
gender roles, 127–31; assessment, 144; at
birth, 132; and CAH, 16; and child
rearing, 177; clinical formulation of, 5;
as cultural process, 228; emergence and
formulation of, 138; empirical origin,
110; flexibility and rigidity, 135–38;
formulated, 4–10, 138–39; as indelibly
imprinted, 133–34; learned, 2–3, 5–6,
15–17, 84, 110, 116, 134–35, 138–39,
168, 174, 181, 195, 209–11, 213, 217–
18, 220–21, 226–28; legacy of, 226; in
medical practices, 16; normative, 226–
27; as real, 226; term, defined, 3; term,
usage, 3, 125, 128, 177, 203, 216; theory
of, 120–21. *See also* sex roles
Generation of Vipers (Wylie), 70
"Genetic, Psychological and Hormonal
Factors in the Establishment and Maintenance of Patterns of Sexual Behavior
in Mammals" (conference), 125, 208

genetics, 177, 245n30; and hormones, 245n30. *See also* heredity
Genital Abnormalities, Hermaphroditism, and Related Adrenal Diseases (H. H. Young), 28, 30
genitals, 1–4, 7, 20, 61, 76–77, 98, 110–11, 113, 118, 147, 180, 208, 270n30; as determining sex variable/as signifier of sex, 185–86, 265n29, 266n51, 287n1; and hermaphroditism, 28, 177; and hormones, 125; and surgeries, 2–3, 57, 61, 74, 78, 85, 121–22, 169–70, 175–78, 189, 191, 227, 288n8
Gerall, Arnold A., 208
Germon, Jennifer, 258n52, 284n112
Gillis, Jonathan, 46, 242n47
Gill-Peterson, Jules, 281n60
gonadal sex/gonads, 26–29, 33, 35, 37, 54, 56–57, 65, 68, 75, 111, 113–16, 118–20, 129, 135–36, 178, 180, 184, 237n2, 240n22, 252n38
gonads, and hormones, 56
Goodenough, Florence Laura, 100
Gorer, Geoffrey, 95, 104
Goy, Robert W., 208
Great Speckled Bird (underground newspaper), 223
Greene, Richard, 279n29, 285n131
Greenson, Ralph, 277–78n2
Grosz, Elizabeth, 288n13
Grumbach, Melvin M., 180, 265n24, 272n11, 275n56
György, Paul, 113, 117, 119

habitus, 34–35, 37
Hampson, Joan, 2, 4–6, 15–16, 110–13, *112*, 115, 122–23, 125–27, 130, 136–38, 140, 141, 156, 166–69, 172–73, 177–78, 182, 196, 208, 214, 218, 253n49, 264–65n24, 265–66n38, 266n45, 272n7, 275–76n67; and theory of human gender role, 120–21
Hampson, John, 2, 4–6, 15–16, 110, 112, *112*, 130, 138, 140, 166–69, 172–73, 177, 182, 196, 208, 214, 218, 272n7, 275–76n67, 280n58
Harriet Lane Home for Invalid Children (HLH), 2, 3–4, 9, 18–19, *22*, *23*, 30, 47, 68, 111, *112*, 141, 145, 147–48, 169; as first children's hospital in the US associated with a medical school, 21; specialty clinics, 21

Harry Benjamin Foundation, 203
Hartigan-O'Connor, Ellen, 289n18
Hartman, Saidiya, 9
Harvard Medical School (Boston), 58, 96
Harvard Psychological Clinic, 92, 94
Harvard University: Dept. of Neurology, 96–97; Dept. of Psychiatry, 96–97; Dept. of Psychology, 94; Dept. of Social Relations, 84, 90–96, 108, 111, 128, 257n46
health: and adjustment, 16, 68; and case management, 44; and clinical practice, 13; information shared with patients and families, 120; meanings of, 143; and treatment plans, 44; understandings of, 143. *See also* disease; medicine; psychological health
Heape, Walter, 245n31, 245n33
hegemony, in ICM, 226
Hench, Philip, 38–39, 248n76
Henry Phipps Psychiatric Clinic (Johns Hopkins), 55, 107, 111, 167
heredity: and child rearing, 89; and disease, 73; and environment, 211; same sex, 218. *See also* genetics
hermaphroditism, 8–9, 77, 113–15, 119, 121, 123–28, 135–36, 203; and bisexuality, 64; and experimentation, 62–64, 97, 125, 131; first recorded case of, 25; and genitals, 28, 177; and happiness, 64–68, 73–75; and heterosexuality, 62, 67; and homosexuality, 56, 62, 64, 138; and ICM, 173–74, 177–82, 186; as living paradox, 96; management and treatment of, 131; and masculine psychosexuality, 105; medicalized, 123; as naturally occurring sexual variation, 8; and personality, 108; and physiology, 64; and psychoanalysis, 56–59; psychoanalytic perspective of, 56–59; and psychological health, 127–28, 136; psychologic pertinence of, 131; and psychology, 56, 131; and psychosexuality, 56, 58–59, 62–65, 96, 105–6, 125, 127; as rare condition, 126; and sex assignment/reassignment, 215–16, 275n66; and sex chromosomes, 267n52; and sexed body, 29; and sexual orientation, 62–63; and sibling neurosis, 124; studying of, 28–30, 96–99; surgery for, 28–30, 36, 56, 177; and transforming sex, 131–32; and

hermaphroditism (*cont.*)
  transsexuality, 203; and true sex, 27,
  113. *See also* adrenogenital syndrome
  (AGS); pseudo-hermaphroditism
"Hermaphroditism, Gender and Precocity
  in Hyperadrenocorticism" (Money), 131
"Hermaphroditism: An Inquiry into the Nature of a Human Paradox" (Money), 97
Hermaphroditism monograph (H. H. Young),
  178
heteronormativity, 10–11
heterosexual–homosexual rating scale
  (Kinsey), 7
heterosexuality: and bisexuality, 63; and
  cultural patterns, 63–64; and cultural
  tropes of gender, 160; as gender orientation by default, 210; and hermaphroditism, 62, 67; and homosexuality, 116;
  and masculine role, 105; as normal,
  42, 63; and psychosexuality, 63; and
  social norms, 10, 29, 43, 119; in wedlock, 7
Hinman, Frank, Jr., 64–69, 72–73, 75,
  252n51, 253n59, 274n37
Hirschfeld, Magnus, 8, 240n22
HLH. *See* Harriet Lane Home for Invalid
  Children (HLH)
Holt, L. E. (Luther Emmett), Jr., 171, 176,
  179–80
Holt Pediatrics (Holt), 275n55
homeostasis, 258n52
homophile groups/movements, 7, 63,
  239n16, 261n88, 261n90
Homosexual in America, The (Cory),
  261–62n90
homosexuality, 252n38; and anatomy,
  63–64; anxiety about, 116, 137–38;
  avoidance of, 116; to be avoided, 116;
  and bisexuality, 63; causes of, 63;
  chromosomal setup of, 130; and civil
  rights, 261n90; and clitoral surgeries to
  combat, 35; and clitoris, size of, 36, 153;
  and culture, 63–64, 252n45; degeneration as cause of, challenged, 63; and ef-
  feminacy/effeminate behavior, in boys,
  105, 184; and environmental theory of
  sex, 116; exclusive, 63; and exposure
  to wrong hormone in utero, 210; as
  failed adjustment to sex of rearing, 102;
  fantasies as pathological, 58; fear of,
  116, 137; and femininity, to avoid con-

notations of, 60; as form of crossgender
  identification, 8; and fragile status as
  males or females, 103; and gender,
  261n88; and gender inversion, 103, 116;
  and gender roles, 116, 137–38, 210; and
  hermaphroditism, 56, 62, 64, 138; and
  heterosexuality, 116; inability to speak
  freely about, 102; as inborn or acquired,
  62; inclusion of in repertoire of normal
  human sexuality, 102; instrumental
  in development of treatment standards, 116; intensification of anxiety
  about, 116; laws against, 219; linked
  to psychological unhealthiness, 137;
  and maladjustment, 102–3, 105, 116,
  137; male, 63, 115, 184; medical and
  scientific engagement with, 252n43;
  as minority group, 261n90, 268n90; as
  naturally occurring sexual variation, 8;
  and normalization, 102, 116; as normal
  sexual behavior, 7; and oppressed minority of gays and lesbians, 102; perceived threat from, 116; persecution of,
  261n88; and personality, 105, 252n45;
  practice of relating shape of genitals
  to, 251n21; problems in boys, 124;
  psychologically, 118; and psychology,
  118; and psychosexuality, 60, 63–64, 96,
  102–3; scientific study of, 148, 261n88,
  267n53; and sex assignment/reassign-
  ment, 115–16; and sex changes, 116,
  138; as sexual deviance, 137; as sexual
  inversion, 8, 103; and sexual orientation, 137; as sexual outlet, 137; speaking about, 102; stigma of, 138; study
  of, 85; as unrecognized minority group,
  deserving of civil rights, 261n90; widely
  debated, 102. *See also* gays; lesbianism/
  lesbians
Hoopes, John E., 203–6
hope, 45–52, 99, 144
Hopkins Gender Identity Clinic, 16, 280n59
hormone replacement therapy, and puberty
  and feminization, regulated by, 212
hormones: adrenal cortical, 79, 248n76;
  and adrenal glands, 27; and behavior,
  6, 119, 210; and brain, 210–11; and chromosomes, 56, 209, 245n30; and genetics,
  245n30; and genitals, 125; and gonads,
  56; quantity vs. quality, 8; role of, 24;
  sex, 8, 26–27, 34, 54, 56, 58–59, 62, 98,

106, 148, 244n18; and sex glands, 27; steroid, 19, 39, 243n4; and transsexuality, 239n14; in utero, 210. *See also specific hormone(s)*

Horney, Karen, 88

human behavior. *See* behavior

"Human Hermaphroditism" (Money and Hampson), 125

human nature, 85–86

hyperadrenocorticism, 121–22, 127, 156, 181, 266n41; and masturbation, 156

hypersexuality: and clitoridectomies, to combat, 35; and clitoris, size of, 36

hypospadias, 105, 113–14

Icahn School of Medicine at Mount Sinai (New York), 200

ICM. *See* intersex case management (ICM)

ideology, 12–13, 26, 69–70, 264n16

illness, as an experience, 188

imprinting, 132–36, 138, 165, 174–75, 181–85, 201, 204, 226, 228, 267n63

Ingersoll, Francis M., 59–61, 252n51

instinct: and behavior, 6, 239n14; and biology, 239n14; and psychosexual development, 63; and psychosexuality, 63; reformulations of, 133–34; and sex determination, 107; and sexual determination, 107

intelligence tests, 60, 99–100, 116, 128, 259n77, 260n78; and race, 259n77

International Journal of Psychoanalysis, 196, 277–78n2

International Psychoanalytic Congress (Sweden), 277–78n2

intersex case management (ICM), 166–86, 226–27; and adaptations, 170; and afterlife of gender, 16; clinical practices of, 108; ethics of, 10–11, 287n6; and gender roles, 9; hegemony in, 226; Hopkins history of, 15–16, 110–40, 204; Hopkins protocols, 143, 168–76, 182, 186; model of, 9, 166, 168, 179; normalizing approach to, 85; recommendations about, 16; and social sciences, 108; standardized, 11–12, 186, 195; success of, 186

intersex research/studies, 2, 8, 85, 130, 148, 175, 196–97, 267n53

Intersex Society of North America, 227, 240–41n27, 287n7

intersexuality, 237n3; and body morphology, 98; and children, 1, 4, 9–10; and diagnoses, 118; and experimentation, 197; and gender, 3–4; and gender identity, 187; and gender roles, 2, 5, 218, 220; habilitation thesis on, 174; and happiness, 6–7, 269n94; history of, 9; management protocols, 84; and psychological health, 98; and psychological sex, 75; and psychosexuality, 65–66, 173–75, 274n43; and race, 8–10, 262n104; and sex assignment/reassignment, 5; and sex determination, 4–5; and surgeries, 288n9; and true sex, 34

Isaac, Joel, 93

James Buchanan Brady Urological Institute. *See* Brady Urological Institute (Johns Hopkins)

Jewett, Hugh, 32

Johns Hopkins Hospital and University (Baltimore), 2, 3–5, 12, 15–16, 57–58, 69, 77, 110–40, 187, 203–6, 219; Dept. of Child Psychiatry, 207; Dept. of Pediatrics, 21, 110, *112*; Dept. of Psychiatry, 110; Moore Clinic, 203; Phipps Clinic, 55, 107, 111, 167; and surrounding Black neighborhoods, 241n28

Johns Hopkins Medical Institutions (Baltimore), 206

Johns Hopkins School of Medicine, 21, 23, 57–58, 65, 111

Johnson, Virginia E., 178–79, 274n51

Jones, Georgeanna E. S., 160–61

Jones, Howard Wilbur, 4, 115, 149–50, 160–63, 177–79, 180, 270n26

Jordan-Young, Rebecca, 209–10, 232

Jorgensen, Christine, 7, 201, 204, 240n19

Josiah Macy Jr. Foundation, 111, 119, 264n20

Journal of Pediatrics, 180

Judge Baker Child Guidance Clinic (Boston), 96

Julian, Percy, 39, 248–49n87

Jung, Carl, 94

Kanner, Leo, 48–49, 52, 111, *112*

Kardiner, Abram, 256n30

Karel, Frank, 205

Karkazis, Katrina Alicia, 247n62

Kendall, Edward C., 38, 248n76

Kessler, Suzanne J., 226–27, 269n94
Kinsey, Alfred C., 7, 100–102, 137, 203, 206–8, 239n17, 239–40n18, 260n83, 265–66n38, 268–69n90
Kinsey Reports, 7, 137, 211
Klebs, Theodor Albrecht, 129, 237n2
Kleinman, Arthur, 188
Klinefelter's syndrome, 275n67
Kluckhohn, Clyde, 94–96, 258–59n64
Knorr, Norman J., 206, 279n38

laparotomies, 36–37, 48, 53, 58–59, 69, 73, 77, 147–49, 189
Laqueur, Thomas, 288n12
Lavender Scare, 102, 137–38
Lavender Woman (lesbian periodical), 223
lesbianism/lesbians, 222–23; and clitoris, size of, 36; and group identity, 261–62n90; as oppressed minority, 102; and trans women, 222, 286n141. *See also* gays; homosexuality
Lesbian Tide (lesbian periodical), 286n141
Lévi-Strauss, Claude, 224
LGBTQ community, 217, 222–23
loneliness, as medical prognosis, 73
Look (magazine), 71
Lorenz, Konrad, 132–34, 181, 267n66, 268n68, 268n71, 268n73, 275n63
Lumet, Sidney, 281n62
Lynes, Patrick, 181, 183–84

MacCollum, Donald W., 97
macrogenitosomia precox, 146, 149
Magubane, Zine, 9, 262n104
Mak, Geertje, 57, 242n43
maladjustment: and adjustment, 15, 54–56, 64–65, 73–75, 109; and homosexuality, 102–3, 105, 116, 137; and masturbation, 154; and parental influence, 70; and psychiatry, 55; and psychosexuality, 103; and transsexuality, 239n14
Male and Female (Mead), 88
Man and Woman, Boy and Girl (Money and Ehrhardt), 211–15, 217, 221, 224
Mandler, Peter, 262n97
Manion, Jen, 204
Marx, Karl, 224
Marzo, Giuseppe, 25
Massachusetts General Hospital (Boston), 24, 53, 58, 96, 169
Masters, William H., 178–79, 274n51

masturbation: anti-, hysteria of Victorianism, 100; by children, 154–55; and clitoral surgeries to curb, 35; and clitoris, size of, 36, 153, 155; conservative religious attitudes toward, 101; and erections, frequent, 153; and estrogen therapy, 48; fears about, 153; history of, 260n85; and hyperadrenocorticism, 156; and maladjustment, 154; as normal sexual behavior, 7; as one stage of normal sexual development, 271n32; parental concerns/perceptions, 154, 271n32; and psychological maladjustments, 154; and psychology, 154; and psychosexuality, 60; as sexual difficulty, 74; sporadic practice by children, 154–55
Materson, Lisa, 289n18
Mayo Clinic (Rochester, MN), 38
Mead, Margaret, 87–91, 95, 104, 217–20, 222, 255nn16–17, 256n26, 259n64, 261n87, 262nn97–98, 285n118, 285nn127–28
medicine, 125; confidence in, 120; and ethics, 45–52, 120; golden age of, 47, 250n5; and hope, 45–52, 99, 144; praxiographic approach to, 242n43; psychosomatic, 96–97; public trust in, 47. *See also* clinic; health
Medvei, Victor Cornelius, 244n17, 245n25
Meigs, Joe V., 57
mental health, 55–56, 98. *See also* psychological health
Meyer, Adolf, 55, 96–97, 107, 111
Meyerowitz, Joanne, 10, 89–90, 220, 238n8, 239n14, 240n19, 256n30, 264n16
Midcentury White House Conference on Children and Youth (1950), 90
midwives, 127, 251n25
Migeon, Claude J., *112*, 177, 264–65n24
Milam, Erika Lorraine, 268n68
Miller, Arthur, 55
Miller, Fiona Alice, 148, 267n53
Miller, Jean Baker, 217, 284n112
Millett, Kate, 217–18
mind-body unit, 64, 96–97, 131–35, 139, 228
Minnesota Multiphasic Personality Inventory (MMPI), 60
MMPI. *See* Minnesota Multiphasic Personality Inventory (MMPI)
Mol, Annemarie, 242n43

Momism, 70, 253n65, 261n88
Money, Grace, 167
Money, John, 19, 52, 90–91, 110–41, *112*, 194, 195–98, 201–3, 205, 208–22, *211*, 228–29, 233, 235, 240n18, 257n36, 263nn5–6, 264–65n24, 266nn40–41, 266nn44–45, 272n7, 274n36, 274n43, 275n54, 275n63, 275n66, 279n26, 279n29, 283n97, 284n107, 284n112; on adaptation, 175; on assigned (biological) sex vs. reassignment, 116; and behavioral sciences, 15–16; on boyhood, 104; on CAH, 266n41; and case management, 166–68, 170, 172–77, 179–86, 195; as clinician, 4, 15, 99–106, 131, 196, 218; critics of, 286n138; and culturalist approach, 85–86, 90–92, 95–109, 134, 221, 287n1; and Diamond, 276n75, 283n94, 287n1; and economic constraints, 91; and ego function, 102; and Ehrhardt, 210–12; experimentations, 283n100; and feminism/liberated women, 216, 218–21, 283n103; focus on genitals as signifier of sex, 287n1; on gender open to manipulation, 139; on gender roles, 2–10, 15–16, 43, 84–86, 98, 109, 111, 120–21, 125, 127–29, 133–38, 179, 181–84, 196–97, 209–11, 214, 216–22, 226, 258n52; and the Hampsons, 16, 112, 115, 118, 120–23, 126–30, 136, 138, 140, 166–70, 172–77, 180–85, 201, 208, 214, 218, 263n2, 265–66n38, 266n40, 266n45, 275n67; on hermaphroditism, 179; on his own sex life, 262n91; and homosexuality, 102–3, 115–16; on hormone effects, 210, 221–22; and ICM, 226; on imprinting, 133–34, 267n63; and intersex cases, 84, 108, 172–73, 186, 195–97, 218; and Lorenz, 268n71; on male gender role and penis, 287n1; on mind-body unit, 97; and Murray, 95; and normalization, 148, 150, 161, 163–65; and objectivity of science, 109; and patient data as human studies, 195; and psychoanalytic theories, 107; and psychological appraisals, 99–100, 103, 179; and psychology, 131, 163, 175, 214; and psychosexuality, 102, 107; on race, 105–6; as ruthless experimenter on children, 213–14; and science, 91; and scientific authority,

15–16; and sex assignment/reassignment, 122, 184, 215–16, 218, 276n75, 283n94; on sex changes, 277n77; and sexual determination, 107; and sexual orientation, 107, 266n45; and social determination, 85–86; and social learning, 103, 222; and social sciences, 15–16, 108; and sociology, 258n52; on syndromes, 275–76n67; textbook, 131; and transformation of sex, 4; and transsexuality, 203, 221–22, 224, 286n139; and true biological sex, 283n100; and Wilkins, 84, 96–98, 109, 111–12, 131, 177, 263n6; and W. C. Young, 208; and Zuger, 184
Moore, Carl, 27
Moore Clinic (Johns Hopkins), 203
Morgan, Christiana, 95
Morgan, Murray, 95
Morgan, Robin, 218–19, 286n141
Morland, Iain, 258n52
motherhood, 37, 46, 70–71, 81, 90, 109, 132–33, 200, 210, 212, 215, 253n66, 256n32, 276n75, 286n139
Mount Sinai School of Medicine (New York), 200
Murray, Henry A., 92, 94–96, 100, 107, 258n55
Myra Breckinridge (film), 207, 281n62

National Observer, 207
National Research Council (US), 38–39
"Nativism and Culturalism in Gender Identity Differentiation" (Money), 215
Nelson, Waldo E., 176
Neugebauer, Franz von, 177–78, 259n76
neurology, 96, 191
New Directions for Women (newsletter), 216
New York Daily News, 205
New York Medical Journal, 253n64
New York Times, 38, 55, 205–6, 211, 227, 249n97
New York Times Book Review, 211
New York University School of Medicine, 184, 202
normalization: gender in clinic/process of, 16, 141–65; and gender roles, 159–60; and homosexuality, 102, 116; and social functionality, 164
norms. *See* biological norms; gender norms; sexual norms; social norms

Northwestern University Medical School, Gender Study and Research Program (Evanston, IL), 207
nurture: and behavior, 55; and environment, 55; and nature, 5, 55, 75, 89–90, 125, 195, 201–2, 214, 225–26, 228, 283n102, 284n114
NYU Grossman School of Medicine, 184

Oakley, Ann, 218
ontogeny, and sex roles, 265n31
Organization Theory (OT), 208–9, 211, 226, 276n75, 281n67, 282n79
osteoporosis, 288–89n15
ostracism, social, 174
OT. See Organization Theory (OT)

Park, Edwards A., 21–24, 241n29
Parsons, Talcott, 93–95, 128–29, 257n46, 258n52
patient-physician relationship, 243n48
patriarchy, 85, 214–15, 217, 224, 227
Pavlov, Ivan, 58
pediatric endocrinology: and cortisone treatment, 172–73; and genital surgery, 176; as new perspective, 21–24; and personality, 97; and research, 169; as subspecialty, 21–24; and transformation of sex, 4
Pediatric Endocrinology Clinic (Johns Hopkins), 2, 4–5, 9, 12–15, 17, 19–21, 24, 30, 32, 43–45, 47, 68, 78–79, 98, 107, 109, 110–12, 122, 127, 130, 141, 148, 150–53, 155–57, 164, 168–69, 174, 177–79, 190, 195; as nation's first medical center devoted to hormonal problems in children, 19; and standardized recommendations for diagnosing sex, 68. See also Wilkins, Lawson
pediatricians, and gender, 120–25
Pediatrics (Holt), 275n55
penis size, 247n62
personality: and behavior, 4–5, 8, 15, 85–86, 119, 128–29, 139, 142, 184; and biology, 88, 95, 218; and child rearing, 88; and cultural patterns, 85–86; and culture, 15, 43, 54, 84–109, 139, 252n45, 256n26, 256n30, 262n97; and environment, 15, 54, 95, 139; and families, 71; and gender, 15, 84–109; and homosexuality, 105, 252n45; and normative social

roles, 103; and psychology, 90–92, 95; and psychopathology, 201; and sex assignment/reassignment, 4; and social determinants, 88; and social sciences, 15, 93; term, usage, 95; and women, 218
Personality in Nature, Society, and Culture (anthology), 95
petting, as normal sexual behavior, 7
phallic standard, 34, 122, 247n62, 265n30
Phipps Psychiatric Clinic (Johns Hopkins), 55, 107, 111, 167
Phoenix, Charles H., 208
physiology: of adrenal glands, 25; and anatomy, 29, 197, 202; and behavior, 208; and body morphology, 96; and hermaphroditism, 64; and psychiatry, 55; reformulations of, 27; sexual, 27
Plant, Rebecca Jo, 70–71
plastic surgery, 10, 72, 97, 189, 203, 212
"Potential of Woman, The" (Money), 284n107
Prader, Andrea, 171–76, 274n43
pragmatism, 3, 5, 21, 34–35, 43, 67, 115, 119, 121–22, 131, 139
praxiographic approach, to medical practice, 242n43
premarital sex, as normal sexual behavior, 7
Price, Dorothy, 27
proper sex, 36, 38–44, 71–72, 169–70. See also better sex; biological sex; true sex
pseudo-hermaphroditism: female, 1–2, 31–32, 35, 40–41, 53–54, 63, 65, 73–75, 78–79, 103, 106, 147–51, 157, 171, 177, 181, 185, 237n3; gonads as determiner of sex in, 75, 129, 237n2; and heterosexuality, 67; male, 1–2, 53–54, 63, 65, 75, 105–6, 124, 149–50, 181, 185; masculinity or femininity of, 63; ovaries as determiner of sex in, 129; and psychosexuality, 74–75, 106; sibling neurosis, 124; surgery for, 36; testes as determiner of sex in, 129. See also hermaphroditism
psychiatry, 125; and anthropology, 55; and behavior, 21; and biology, 55; and child rearing, 88; and maladjustment, 55; and neurology, 96; and physiology, 55; and psychoanalysis, 54, 58–59, 75, 97; and psychogenics, 63; and psychol-

ogy, 5, 62, 64, 66–67, 74–75, 142; and
psychosexuality, 61; and social sciences,
71; and transformation of sex, 4
Psychiatry, 131
psychoanalysis, 139, 217, 221; and child
rearing, 88; and hermaphroditism,
56–59; and psychiatry, 54, 58–59, 75,
97; and psychology, 56, 59, 94; and
psychosexuality, 107; studies, 58, 75;
theories, 94, 107
"Psychoanalysis, Patriarchy, and Power"
(J. B. Miller), 217
psychoanalytic perspective, 56–61, 63; of
hermaphroditism, 56–59
psychobiology, 55, 111, 131
psychological health, 2, 13, 15, 34, 44, 68,
84, 98–100, 103–4, 108–9, 127–28, 136,
139–40, 158, 165, 169, 172, 178–79,
288n8. *See also* mental health; psychological sex
psychological sex, 33, 56, 59, 61–64, 67–68,
71–75, 139, 195–97, 226; of CAH patients, evaluation of, 173–75; children's,
67; and cultural patterns, 15, 54; and
gender identity, 16, 195; and gender
roles, 110, 195; and intersexuality, 75;
and normalization, 142, 149–50; and
personality, 97–98, 109; and sex assign-
ment/reassignment, 69, 73–75. *See also*
psychological health; psychosexuality
Psychological Study of Man, The (Money),
131
psychologic sex, and gender roles, 110
psychologization: and adjustment/malad-
justment paradigm, 15, 64–65, 74–75;
of American society, 15, 74–75; and
clinical engagement with sex assignment, 54; and clitoridectomies, 155–56;
of everyday life, 69; and medical evaluation of sex, 15, 54, 69, 74–75; of sex,
in 1930s and 1940s, 15, 53–75; and sex
assignment/reassignment, 57, 73; and
true sex, 57
psychology: and anatomy, 59, 113–14; and
anthropology, 91, 94–95; applied, 56;
and behavior, 174–75; and biology, 97–
98, 118; and child's behavior, 174–75;
clinical, 86; and environment, 66–67;
and gender identity, 16, 125; and hermaphroditism, 56, 131; and homosexuality, 118; and masturbation, 154; and

personality, 90–92, 95; and psychiatry,
5, 62, 64, 66–67, 74–75, 142; and
psychoanalysis, 56, 59, 94; psychosomatic, 131; and sex roles, 97; and
social adjustment, 42; and social relations, 94–96; and social sciences, 5; and
sociology, 118; and transformation of
sex, 4
"Psychopathia Transexualis" (Cauldwell),
201–2
psychopathology, 98, 181, 201; and psychosexuality, 98
psychophysiology, 95
"Psychosexual Development and Behavior
Problems in Human Hermaphrodites"
(Money and Hampson), 125
"Psychosexual Development in Relation to
Homosexuality" (Money), 96
"Psychosexual Identification (Psychogender) in the Intersexed" (Cappon, Ezrin,
and Lynes), 181
psychosexuality: and anatomy, 61, 67–68,
75, 113; and behavior, 106; of CAH patients, 175; cause-and-effect mechanism
of, 62; of children, 118; and conflict, 98,
107–8; development of, 59, 62–63; and
ego function, 102; and environment,
59, 67–68; and gender roles, 180; and
hermaphroditism, 56, 58–59, 62–65,
96, 105–6, 125, 127; and heterosexuality, 63; and homosexuality, 60, 63–64,
96, 102–3; and immaturity, 64; and
instinct, 63; and intersexuality, 65–66,
173–75, 274n43; and maladjustment,
103; and masturbation, 60; and orientation, 96, 98, 108, 118, 177, 180; and
perceived as male or female, 64; and
pseudo-hermaphroditism, 74–75, 106;
and psychiatry, 61; and psychoanalysis,
107; and psychopathology, 98; and
psychoses, 107; and racial stereotypes,
106; and sexual and social orientation,
61; and sexual desire, 58; and sexual
orientation, 67; and true sex, 28–29, 60,
74–75, 97. *See also* psychological sex
psychosomatic medicine, 96–97
Psychosomatic Medicine, 62, 184
psychosomatic psychology, 131
puberty, and feminization, regulated by
hormone replacement therapy, 212
puritanism, 87, 100–101

queer, 64
queer community, and gender, 16–17, 195–
    96, 216, 222–23
Quirke, Viviane, 39

race: and anthropology, 85–87; and behav-
    ior, 86; and biology, 85; and culture,
    89–90; and gender, 9, 105–6; and intel-
    ligence tests, 259–60n77; and inter-
    sexuality, 8–10, 262n104; and mistrust,
    241n30; and sex/gender binary, 8–10
racialization, of bodies, 240n24
racism, 8, 86–87, 254n11
Rado, Sandor, 63
Rashkind, W., 114, 117
Raymond, Janice G., 221–22, 286nn139–41
Redbook (magazine), 219–20, 285n128
reformulations: of gender, 16, 168, 195–
    224; of instinct, 133–34; of physiology,
    27; of sex, 6, 43
Reimer, David/Brenda (né Bruce), 212–14,
    220, 283n100
Reimer twins, 214–16, 220
Reis, Elizabeth, 37, 232, 250n5, 288n8
reproductive biology, 125
reproductive organs, 3, 20, 29, 33–37, 69,
    73, 111, 129, 147, 150, 208–9. See also
    anatomy; specific organ(s)
Richardson, Sarah, 228, 245n30
Rockefeller Foundation, 55, 96–97, 111, 173
Rocky Horror Picture Show, The (film), 207,
    281n62
Rodriguez, Sarah B., 35, 152–53, 178–79
Rolling Stone, 283n100
Rorschach test, 60, 92, 100
Rosenberg, Charles, 11, 143
Rosenzweig, Saul, 84, 92, 95
Rubin, Gayle, 223–24, 287n148

Sagarin, Edward, 261–62n90. See also Cory,
    Donald Webster (Edward Sagarin)
same-sex desire/practice, 99, 102–3, 137,
    218, 251n31
San Francisco General Hospital, 65
Sapir, Edward, 91
schizophrenia, 39, 173
Sciences, 227
scientific authority, 15, 131
Scott, Joan Wallach, 229, 289n17
Scott, William W., 4, 149, 177–79, 270n26,
    274n44

self-identification, 215
Sengoopta, Chandak, 244n18, 247n59
sex, 240n20; and adrenal glands, 24–28;
    as ahistorical and essential category,
    284n114; as anatomy and physiology,
    202; biological definition of, 99; and bi-
    ology, 284n114; and brain, 207–16; and
    child rearing, 180–81; contradictions,
    53, 135; diagnosing, 146–51, 164–65;
    discrimination, 229–30; divergence
    of development, 237n3; and gender,
    3–6, 13, 16–17, 70, 140, 210, 216–17,
    224, 228, 284n116; and gender, terms,
    usage, 284n116; medical approaches to,
    43–44; pragmatic reformulation of, 43;
    quantification of, 260n82; reformula-
    tions of, 6, 43; and sexuality, 4; term,
    usage, 3; transformation of, 4, 10, 43–
    44, 131–32. See also sex roles
Sex, Gender and Society (Oakley), 218
Sex and Gender (Stoller), 196, 201, 220
Sex and Internal Secretions (W. C. Young),
    168, 208
Sex and Temperament in Three Primitive Soci-
    eties (Mead), 87–88, 219
sex antagonism, 26–28, 245n31, 245n33,
    247n59
Sex Antagonism (Heape), 245n31
sex assignment/reassignment, 9, 283n94;
    and behavior, 4, 43, 119; at birth, 2–3,
    72, 113–15, 118, 121, 129, 146, 150,
    155, 181, 197, 212, 215–16, 218; and
    clinical setting, 126; and consequent
    experiences of living in this sex, 130–31;
    consistency in, 129; and hermaphrodit-
    ism, 203, 215–16, 275n66; and homo-
    sexuality, 115–16; and intersexuality,
    5; and management/treatment, 126,
    178; and normalization, 164–65; and
    personality, 4; and psychological sex,
    69, 73–75; and psychologization, 57, 73;
    and sex determination, 14–15, 18–44;
    and true sex, 32
sex changes, 7, 16, 105, 114, 127, 136, 172–
    73, 175, 182, 185, 201, 204–6, 277n77;
    and behavior, 116; experiments,
    240n22; and homosexuality, 116, 138;
    and psychological unhealthiness, 172
sex chromosomes: as ambiguous, 148; de-
    termining/testing, 1, 13, 111, 113, 129–
    30, 135, 143, 148–50, 152, 159, 173,

183, 197, 209, 228, 267n52, 275n67; and gender identity, 3, 111, 130, 135, 143, 152, 159, 172, 185, 209; and gender roles, 2, 130, 213, 228; and gonads, 35, 37, 56–57, 68, 114, 116, 118, 129, 180; and hermaphrodites, 267n52; and hormones, 56, 209, 245n30; and intersex studies, 130; sexing of, 270n16; and sexual differentiation, 148; and social learning, 185

sexed body: and hermaphroditism, 29; as scientific construct rather than natural phenomenon, 242n40; as social formation, 228

sex/gender binary, 3–5, 8–11, 14, 20–21, 43, 224, 226, 228–30

sex/gender system, 223–24

sex glands, 27, 43, 53. *See also specific gland(s)*

sex hormones. *See* hormones

Sex Orientation Scale, 203

sex reversals, 34, 66

"Sex-Role Learning in Childhood and Adolescence" (panel), 215

sex roles, 3, 128, 216, 219, 224; and behavior, 6; and culture, 97; learned, 85; and ontogenetic factors, 265n31; and ontogeny, 265n31; and personality, 87–88, 105, 109; and psychology, 68, 97; and sexual orientation, 62–63, 72; and socialization, 216; and social sciences, 85. *See also* gender roles

sex/sexual determination, 4–5, 10, 16, 56, 58–60, 63, 74, 107, 113, 125–26, 147–48, 217, 222, 250n2, 267n53; and sex assignment/reassignment, 14–15, 18–44

sexual ambiguity, 29, 44, 56–57, 66, 105–6, 123, 184

sexual behavior, 7, 35, 58–59, 62, 74, 98, 100, 102, 108, 119, 125, 131, 137, 182, 208, 210, 281n67. *See also* behavior

Sexual Behavior in the Human Male (Kinsey, Pomeroy, and Martin), 137

sexual deviance, 8, 36, 95–96, 102, 137

sexual difference(s), 87, 195–96, 215, 219, 222, 224, 226, 228, 230

sexual differentiation, 26, 148

sexual difficulties, 74

sexual direction. *See* sexual orientation

sexual fantasies, 58, 60, 102, 116, 199

sexual intermediaries, 8

sexual inversion, 8, 63, 103, 251n31, 262n94. *See also* gender inversion

sexuality, 240n20; as deeply personal expression of individual freedom and personhood, 7; and gender, 4; and sex, 4

"Sexuality and Psychoanalysis Revisited" (talk at the Sixth Symposium of the Society of Medical Psychoanalysts), 221

sexual morality, 101. *See also* social mores

sexual neutrality, at birth, 184–85

sexual norms, 7, 33, 87, 137, 159, 239n17. *See also* biological norms; gender norms; social norms

sexual orientation, 131; and behavior, 107; and hermaphroditism, 62–63; and homosexuality, 137; and psychosexuality, 67; and sex roles, 62–63, 72; and sexual preference, 266n45; term, usage, 266n45

sexual politics, 216–18

Sexual Politics (Millett), 217–18

sexual psychology. *See* psychological sex

Shankman, Paul, 219, 285n128

Sharman, Jim, 281n62

sickness, 76

Sigmundson, H. Keith, 212, 283n94

Simon, Theodore, 259–60n77

Sisterhood Is Powerful (Morgan), 218–19

Smith, Andy/Ann, 141–42, 144, 151

Smith, Dr. (Miller colleague), 46

Smith, Freda, 286n141

social causes, 26–27, 228–29

social change, 96, 220

social determination, 85–86, 88

social determinism, 6, 108, 132, 139–40. *See also* biological determinism; environmental determinism

social engineering, 6, 8, 15, 71, 85–86, 89–90, 139–40

socialization, 74, 87, 93, 216, 219–20, 222, 227–28

social learning, 103, 185, 222

social mores, 222. *See also* sexual morality

social norms, 3, 5–6, 16, 86, 212, 214–15, 221; and biological norms, 21, 116, 164, 216; and heterosexuality, 10, 29, 43, 119; and normalization, 142, 144, 153; and true sex, 26, 36, 42–43. *See also* biological norms; gender norms; sexual norms

social ostracism, 174

social relations: and anthropology, 257n46; in clinic, 99–106; and cultural patterns, 99–106; and psychology, 94–96; and social sciences, 92–94

social sciences, 15–17; and behavioral sciences, 85; biological, 8; and cultural patterns, 86–90; and culture, 139, 259n64; and human nature, 85; and ICM, 108; and learned behavior, 10–11; and motherhood, 71; and personality, 15, 93; and psychiatry, 71; and psychology, 5; and sex roles, 85; and social relations, 92–94; and terminology/vocabulary, 3, 94; and transformation of sex, 4

Society for the Scientific Study of Sex, 202, 279n26

Society of Medical Psychoanalysts, 221

Society of Pediatric Urology, 65

sociology, 257n46, 258n52; and anthropology, 3; and psychology, 118; and sex roles, 3

somatic sexuality, 34, 181–83

Spelman, Elizabeth, 288n11

Stanford-Binet test, 48, 116, 259–60n77

Stanford University, 207

Starling, Ernest, 24

Steinach, Eugen, 26, 240n22

stereotypes, 56, 58, 106, 133, 216, 220–23, 227, 229, 286n140

sterilization, 255n25

steroid hormones, 19, 39, 243n4. *See also* cortisone

stilbestrol, 32, 60–61, 73–74, 78–79, 199

Stoller, Robert J., 196–204, 211, 217–22, 277–78n2, 279n29, 284n112, 285n131, 286n139

Stone, Calvin, 140

Stryker, Susan, 253n72, 279n34, 286nn140–41

suffragettes. *See* women's emancipation/liberation

Sulkowitch, Hirsh W., 57

suprarenal glands. *See* adrenal glands

Talbot, Nathan B., 24, 32, 169, 265n24, 272n13

TAT. *See* thematic apperception test (TAT)

TeLinde, Richard Wesley, 72, 147, 270n13

Temple University, Lewis Katz School of Medicine (Philadelphia), 180

Terman, Lewis Madison, 259–60n77

Terman-Miles Attitude-Interest Analysis test, 60

testosterone, 31, 36, 152, 159, 208

Textbook of Pediatrics (Nelson), 176, 180

thematic apperception test (TAT), 60, 95, 100, 116

"Three Essays on the Theory of Sexuality" (Freud), 63

Time (magazine), 205–6, 215

Tinbergen, Nikolaas, 133

tomboyism, 69, 160, 212–13

Toronto General Hospital, Dept. of Medicine, 181

Toward a New Psychology of Women (J. B. Miller), 217

"Traffic in Women, The" (Rubin), 223–24

trans activism, 203, 279n34

transfeminism, 222, 229, 286n141

transgender, 3, 10, 195–96, 223, 229, 281n62, 286n140

"Transsexualism" (Stoller), 221

transsexuality, 195–96, 216–17, 221–22, 224, 229; chromosomal setup of, 130; clinics for, 3; and feminism, 286n140; and gender identity, 200–207, 286n139; and gender stereotypes, 286n140; and hermaphroditism, 203; and hormones, 239n14; and maladjustment, 239n14; sensationalism of, 138; social history of, 10; and stereotypical gender behavior, 220; study of, 85, 148, 267n53; and surgeries, 206. *See also* gender identity

Transsexual Phenomenon, The (Benjamin), 202–3

transvestitism, 8, 138, 201, 203, 223

treatment plans, 6–7, 16, 37, 44, 135–38, 151–56, 170, 192. *See also* case management

true sex: and best sex, 37, 113; and better sex, 14–15, 18–44, 148; biological, 283n100; determining, 15, 36, 129; diagnosing, 53; and gender, understanding of, 44; general confusion in terms of, 36; and hermaphroditism, 27, 113; insisting on, 36; and intersexuality, 34; and nature, push of, 44; and obvious sex, 44; organs as determiner of, 36–37; psychological vs. anatomical, 57; and psychologization, 57; and psychosexuality, 28–29, 60, 74–75, 97; sex characteristics as determiner of, 37; and social functionality and personal happiness, 140. *See also* better sex; biological sex; proper sex

Turner's syndrome, 275–76n67

UCLA Medical School, Dept. of Psychiatry, 196, 199

United Nations Education, Scientific and Cultural Organization (UNESCO), 87

University Children's Hospital (Zurich), 16, 170–77, 231, 233, 272n16

University of California, 65, 196, 282n79

University of Indiana, 260n83

University of Kansas, 208

University of Maryland, Dept. of Psychiatry, 58

University of Maryland Medical School, 69

University of Minnesota Medical School, 207

University of New Zealand, 91

University of Otago (Dunedin), 91

University of Pennsylvania Hospital, 113–15, 117

University of Washington (Seattle), Gender Identity Research and Treatment Clinic, 168, 207

University of Zurich (Burghölzli), 173

UPMC Psychiatric Hospital (Pittsburgh), 92, 100

vaginal dilation, 191–92, 271n48

vaginoplasty, 122, 161, 212

Van Wyk, Judson, 148–49

Velkas, M. C. Frank, 279n38

Vicedo, Marga, 133–34, 239n14

Victorianism, antisexualism and anti-masturbation hysteria of, 100

Vidal, Gore, 281n62

Vidich, Arthur, 93–94

virilism, 27–28, 79

virilization, 1, 18–19, 25, 31–32, 40–41, 69, 73–74, 78–79, 110–11, 121, 145, 152, 156–57, 159–60, 165; de-/reverse, 41, 72; and drugs, 31; and feminization, 41, 74; and hyperadrenocorticism, 266n41; precocity and somatic, 266n41; short-duration studies, 249n91; signs of changes in, 249n91

Washington Post, 42, 249n97

Waskowitz, C. H., 48

Wechsler, David, 99–100, 260n78

Wechsler-Bellevue Intelligence Scale, 60, 99

Weitzman, Lenore J., 219

West Coast Lesbian Conference (1973), 286n141

Western State Psychiatric Institute and Clinic (Pittsburgh), 92, 100

"What Makes a Person Want to Switch Sexes?" (*National Observer*), 207

Whitehorn, John C., 107, 111, 167

Wilkins, Lawson, 4, 18, *20*, 96, *112*, 243n4, 246n51; on adaptation, 33; and adrenalectomies, 28; on adrenal glands, 31–32, 38; as America's first pediatric endocrinologist, 19, 23–24, 30, 97, 169–70, 186; and anti-adrenal drug, 38; as authority figure, 125, 172–73; and Barr body test, 130, 148; on better (vs. true) sex, 43; and biomedicine, 23; and CAH, 2, 30–40, 43–44, 45, 65, 68–73, 78–79, 121, 127, 144–46, 151, 165, 170–73, 272n11; clinical approach, 14–15, 32–33, 40, 43, 68, 75, 113, 129, 168; and clitoridectomies, 35, 152, 155; contemporaneous approach, 65; and cortisone treatments, 37–39, 42, 45, 66, 71–72, 109, 110–11, 115, 152, 156–57, 170–71, 186, 249n97, 264–65n24, 272n12; death of, 69, 177; diagnoses/prognoses, 51–52, 68, 74, 79, 147, 150, 172, 174; focus on genitals, 265n29, 266n51; and gender roles, 15, 136, 170; and gonadal sex, 65; on heredity and disease, 73; and Hinman, 65–66, 72; and homosexuality, 116; on hormonal body, 34; and intersex patients, 2, 35, 169–70; as leading expert on CAH, 2; and learned gender role formulation, 15; on maladjustment, 15, 154; medical authority, 171; and Miller, 46; and Money, 84; and patient care, 22, 33–34; and patients, 30, 68–69, 78–79, 118–19, 142, 149, 157, 161, 188, 263n6; and psychological sex, 75; and research, 169; and scientifically grounded medicine, 22; on sex changes, 277n77; and sex transformation, 43–44; and social expectations, 33–34; and standardized recommendations for diagnosing sex, 68; on stilbestrol, 74; and surgical intervention, 160, 170, 271n36; textbook, 24, 34, 36, 177, 180, 244n21, 247n57,

Wilkins, Lawson (*cont.*)
  272n13, 274n44, 275n61; therapeutic
  achievements, 249n97; and therapeutic intervention, 171; and treatment
  recommendations, 29–30, 33–34; and
  Van Wyk, 148–49. *See also* Pediatric
  Endocrinology Clinic (Johns Hopkins)
women: and behavior, 218; and biological destiny, 245n31; and careers, 219;
  education for, 220; erotic practices of,
  7; and gender, 3, 142, 158–59, 218, 220,
  230, 289nn17–18; and health activism,
  120; institutionalized roles of, 87–88; as
  mothers, 215; and personality, 218; as
  sex objects, 67, 227; and sex roles, 35;
  socially constructed characteristics of, 3;
  social roles of, 136

Women: A Feminist Perspective, 219
Women and the Public Interest (Bernard),
  218
women's emancipation/liberation, 3,
  253n64; and gender, 183, 214–16.
  See also feminism
Wylie, Philip, 70–71, 253n66

Yerkes, Robert, 259–60n77
Young, Hugh Hampton, 19, 28–32, 34, 53,
  58–59, 65, 67, 73–74, 77–79, 119, 152–
  53, 178, 249n100
Young, William C., 168, 207–9

Zondek, Bernhard, 26
Züblin, Walter, 173–74, 274n36
Zuger, Bernard, 184–86, 276n75, 277n77

Ingram Content Group UK Ltd.
Milton Keynes UK
UKHW021909290323
419370UK00006B/246